Pediatric Cancer in Africa

Daniela Cristina Stefan • Mhamed Harif

Pediatric Cancer in Africa

A Case-Based Guide to Diagnosis and Management

Springer

Daniela Cristina Stefan
South African Medical Research Council
Cape Town, South Africa

Mhamed Harif
Université Mohammed VI des
Sciences de la Santé
Cheikh Khalifa Hospital
Casablanca, Morocco

ISBN 978-3-319-17935-3 ISBN 978-3-319-17936-0 (eBook)
DOI 10.1007/978-3-319-17936-0

Library of Congress Control Number: 2016957721

Printed on acid-free paper

This Springer imprint is published by Springer Nature
The registered company is Springer International Publishing AG
The registered company address is: Gewerbestrasse 11, 6330 Cham, Switzerland

Dedicated to my father whom I am very proud of, to my two amazing daughters, I could have not asked for more and my loving husband who is my pillar of support.

Daniela Cristina Stefan

To my friends and colleagues throughout Africa who struggle every day to offer new hope and justice to children with cancer and their parents in this world.

Mhamed Harif

Foreword

This is the first book on children with cancer in Africa and is intended to serve as a practical manual for all who are involved, in a way or other, in treating or taking care of children affected by malignant disease on our continent. It is a tool to help identifying the best feasible approach, in African circumstances, to diagnosing and treating such patients. Cancer in children might not be as common as it is in adults, but the emotional impact on the family and society is tremendous.

When interacting with Cristina Stefan, in her capacity as Vice President of the South African Medical Research Council and member of the Advisory Committee on Cancer of the Minister of Health, I could understand that full dedication, passion and complete commitment to sustained care, combined with team effort, are indispensable for the success in overcoming this disease. Childhood cancer is a curable disease in many parts of the world and this should also be the case in Africa. This book describes real patients as a starting point for discussing the approach to diagnosis and treatment and presents protocols adapted to African specifics. As an important step forward in advancing and sharing local knowledge, the manual also contributes to raising the level of awareness regarding the burden of cancer among our children.

This book was written by two authors living at the extremities of the continent: Cristina Stefan, a South African and Mhamed Harif, a Moroccan. Their collaboration shows that distance and language should not be an obstacle to achieving common objectives. Beyond the scientific discourse, this work enables us to contemplate the vast potential of conjugating African intellects, beyond national boundaries.

Malebona Precious Matsoso
Chairman of the Executive Board of World Health Organization
Director General Department of Health South Africa

Foreword

Cancer is considered in low mid income countries as a taboo subject. It is more so when it comes to child cancer which, in addition, remains unknown to the public.

Pediatric oncology was largely unknown until recently. It was not until the last 30 years that a group of African doctors has attempted to overcome this challenge across the continent. They demonstrated that through commitment, solidarity and data sharing, treatment of pediatric cancer in Africa can become a reality.

Professor Harif was one of these African leaders of change through his vision, perseverance and humility. This publication reflects his commitment to the cause of the African pediatric oncology. Through this reference book, Professor Harif and his co-author demonstrate that, with the development of appropriate and effective protocols, we can actually save the lives of many children with cancer.

Based on my professional experience, I am convinced that the adoption of simple protocols, adapted to local conditions, will help change the perception of cancer and will give hope to thousands of families.

Continuous commitment, education and access to health care will warrant a better future for pediatric oncology in Africa.

Rachid Bekkali
Lalla Salma Foundation
Rabat, Morocco

Introduction

Manuals of pediatric hematology-oncology are written by specialists from high-income countries and usually target an audience with a sub-specialist level of training, often assisted by cutting-edge diagnostic and treatment facilities. However, approximately 80 % of new cases of cancer in children appear in middle- and low-income countries. Almost invariably, general practitioners, general pediatricians or general surgeons without special training in oncology will look after children with malignancies who enter the health care system in these countries. The diagnostic facilities are often limited: the ultrasound machine will be usually available, but the positron emission tomography will not. The treatment options would be limited too. The survival figures in these conditions are somewhere around 20 %, while in high-income countries they are in the range of 80 % for many childhood cancers.

To the authors' knowledge, no manual has been written yet which provides specific guidance in the domain of childhood cancer, applicable to Africa. This happens while almost 50 % of the population of the continent is constituted by children. Although the book is designed primarily for health professionals—doctors, nurses and students—working in African settings, similar conditions would exist in numerous low- and middle-income countries and the diagnostic and therapeutic approaches described here might apply with success elsewhere in the world.

The experience of the authors, similar to that of other pediatric oncologists working in limited resources settings, is that, with efficient use of limited means, with minimal expenditure on treatments and with a sound knowledge of the essential pediatric hematology-oncology, many more children can be cured. There is a need to disseminate the essential components of the discipline, filtered through the experience of specialists from developing countries, with solutions adequate to the specific health care environment in such countries.

Each clinical chapter of this book starts with a case scenario modelled after a real patient, meant to anchor the theory in the reality of practice. The emphasis is, every time, on diagnosis assisted by a minimum of effective investigations and on adapted therapeutic protocols. Alongside the section on clinical pediatric hematology-oncology, the important aspects of cancer registration, good clinical practice, nursing specifics and the constitution and role of parent support groups are presented. To complete the book, chapters on clinical research, research ethics, essentials of health economics and telemedicine have also been included.

The authors are experts in pediatric hematology-oncology with solid practical and research experience in Africa. Professor Mhamed Harif, Chairman of the Franco-African Paediatric Oncology Group (GFAOP), presently Director of the Cheikh Khalifa Hospital in Casablanca, is a prominent Moroccan academic and clinician. He initiated a new pediatric oncology unit in Marrakech. Professor Cristina Stefan previously the Head of Paediatric Haematology-Oncology at Stellenbosch University is now the Vice-President of The South African Medical Research Council. She carried out research and educational activities related to oncology in numerous sub-Saharan African countries. Both have tried to distill their professional experience in this handbook, for the benefit of the numerous African children affected by cancer.

Contents

Contributors

Linda Abramovitz School of Nursing, University of California, San Francisco, CA, USA

Eric Bouffet Hospital for Sick Children, Toronto, Canada

Julia M. Challinor School of Nursing, University of California, San Francisco, CA, USA

Guillermo Chantada Department of Hemato-Oncology, Hospital JP Garrahan, Buenos Aires, Argentina

Kenneth Dollman Childhood Cancer International, Nieuwegein, South Africa

CHOC Childhood Cancer Foundation South Africa, Cape Town, South Africa

Jean M. Fourie SA Medical Research Council, Cape Town, South Africa

Carlos Rodriguez Galindo Department of Pediatric Oncology, Dana-Farber/Boston Children's Cancer and Blood Disorders Center and Harvard Medical School, Boston, MA, USA

Michelle Galloway SA Medical Research Council, Cape Town, South Africa

Norbert Graf Department of Pediatric Oncology and Hematology, Saarland University Hospital, Homburg, Germany

Khalil Haouach Hôpital Arrazi, Centre Hospitalier Universitaire Mohammed VI, Marrakech, Morocco

Laila Hessissen Service d'Hématologie et Oncologie Pédiatrique, Hôpital d'Enfant, Centre Hospitalier Universitaire Ibn Sina, Rabat, Morocco

Jaques van Heerden Pietermaritzburg Metropolitan Hospital Complex Kwa zulu Natal Health South Africa

Jamila El Houdzi Centre d'Oncologie et Hématologie, Centre Hospitalier Universitaire Mohammed VI, Marrakech, Morocco

Ilde-Marie Kellerman Department of Human Nutrition, Tygerberg Hospital, Cape Town, South Africa

Andre Pascale Kengne Non-communicable Diseases Research Unit, South African Medical Research Council, Cape Town, South Africa

Department of Medicine, University of Cape Town, Cape Town, South Africa

Natalie McCall Department of Pediatrics, Yale University, New Haven, CT, USA

Rwanda Human Resources for Health Program, Kigali University Teaching Hospital, Kigali, Rwanda

Monika L. Metzger Department of Oncology, St. Jude Children's Research Hospital, Memphis, TN, USA

Claude Moreira Centre Hospitalier Universitaire Le Dantec, Dakar, Senegal

Dr. Jaume Mora Scientific Director, Department of Pediatric Hemato-Oncology Hospital Sant Joan de Déu. Barcelona

Blaise Nkegoum University Hospital Cameroon

Chane Kay Department of Paediatrics and Child Health, Stellenbosch University and Tygerberg Hospital, Cape Town, South Africa

Mariana Kruger Department of Paediatrics and Child Health, Stellenbosch University and Tygerberg Hospital, Cape Town, South Africa

Jan du Plessis Department of Paediatrics and Child Health, Paediatric Haematology and Oncology, University of the Free State and Universitas Hospital, Bloemfontein, South Africa

Raul R. Ribeiro St Jude Children's Research Hospital, Memphis, TN, USA

Paul Rogers Division of Pediatric Oncology/Hematology/BMT, BC Childrens Hospital & University of BC, Vancouver, BC, Canada

John Sandlund St Jude Children's Research Hospital, Memphis, TN, USA

David Stones Department of Paediatrics and Child Health, Paediatric Haematology and Oncology, University of the Free State and Universitas Hospital, Bloemfontein, South Africa

Fousseini Traoré Hematology/Pediatric Oncology Unit, Centre hospitalier Gabriel Touré, Bamako, Mali

Gordan M. Vujanic Department of Cellular Pathology, Cardiff University School of Medicine, Heath Park, Cardiff, UK

Atteby Jean-Jacques Yao Service de Pédiatrie, CHU de Treichville/Abidjan (Côte d'Ivoire), Abidjan, Côte d'Ivoire

Anel van Zyl Department of Paediatrics and Child Health, Paediatric Haematology and Oncology, Stellenbosch University and Tygerberg Hospital, Cape Town, South Africa

Chapter 1
Epidemiology of Childhood Cancer in Africa

Case Presentation

Ismail, 6-year-old boy, is admitted for a left thigh alveolar rhabdomyosarcoma. His 42-year-old mother has been treated 3 years ago for breast cancer. He reported also that his nephew had a fatal bone tumor.

- Is there a predisposition to the development of cancers in this family?
- How can we confirm this predisposition?
- In this case, what are the precautions to take to avoid the occurrence of cancer in the family or make early diagnosis?

Epidemiology of cancer is crucial to identify possible etiologic factors and development of preventions, early diagnosis or adapted treatment programs. Cancer in children represents however less than 3 % of human cancers. It is the second cause of death among children in developed countries after the death by accident. In Africa, there are no reliable data. The burden of childhood cancer in Africa is probably higher because the proportion of children in the population is higher than in developed countries.

The features of cancer in children are different from adults. This difference is related to mechanisms of carcinogenesis. The incidence and distribution of childhood cancers vary however according to regions reflecting the impact of ethnic/genetic and environmental factors.

D.C. Stefan, M. Harif, *Pediatric Cancer in Africa*,
DOI 10.1007/978-3-319-17936-0_1

Geographical Variations

There is heterogeneity of distribution of childhood cancers in the world (Fig. 1.1). In developing countries, data are primarily hospital based and not population based registries and surveys limited in time. Low access to care, diagnosis, and treatment capacities of hospitals as well as the quality of the health information system are all factors that contribute significantly to the poor quality of census of the cancers in children in Africa.

The incidence rates of childhood cancer range between 96 and 138 per million children per year for boys, and from 70 to 116 per million children for girls. Leukemia, CNS tumors, and non-Hodgkin lymphomas (NHLs) are the most frequent pediatric cancers in high-income countries, representing 60 % of all cases, whereas in low-income countries, NHL are more common than leukemia and brain tumors.

Middle-income countries have an intermediate pattern. However, it is important to note that a large heterogeneity is observed across continents.

According to GLOBOCAN, the estimated incidence of all pediatric cancers (0–14 years) in Africa is 99 and 73/million for boys and girls, respectively.

There is a wide variation in rates, with the highest rates being recorded in Malawi (220/million for boys) and Uganda (140/million among girls) while the lowest incidence rates are observed in Guinea (43 and 29/million among boys and girls, respectively).

Acute Leukemias

Acute Lymphocytic Leukemia is the most frequent cancer in childhood in developed countries with a peak of incidence between 1 and 4 years and a male predominance. Its incidence increases with economic development. Early exposure to infections seems to have a protective effect. The incidence of acute non-Lymphocytic Leukemia or acute myeloid leukemia seems less frequent in black population. Chronic myeloid leukemia is rare in children whilst chronic lymphocytic leukemia is not a disease of childhood.

Lymphomas

NHL is the most frequent tumor of children in African units. This is due to high frequency of Burkitt lymphoma in sub-Saharan area of Africa. In North Africa this tumor is less frequent. Male predominance is reported in most series.

Hodgkin disease seems to occur at an earlier age in African children with also higher frequency of mixed cellularity subtype. Infection with the Epstein-Barr virus is considered as an important contributor to lymphomagenesis. Its genoma is also often found in the tumor tissue.

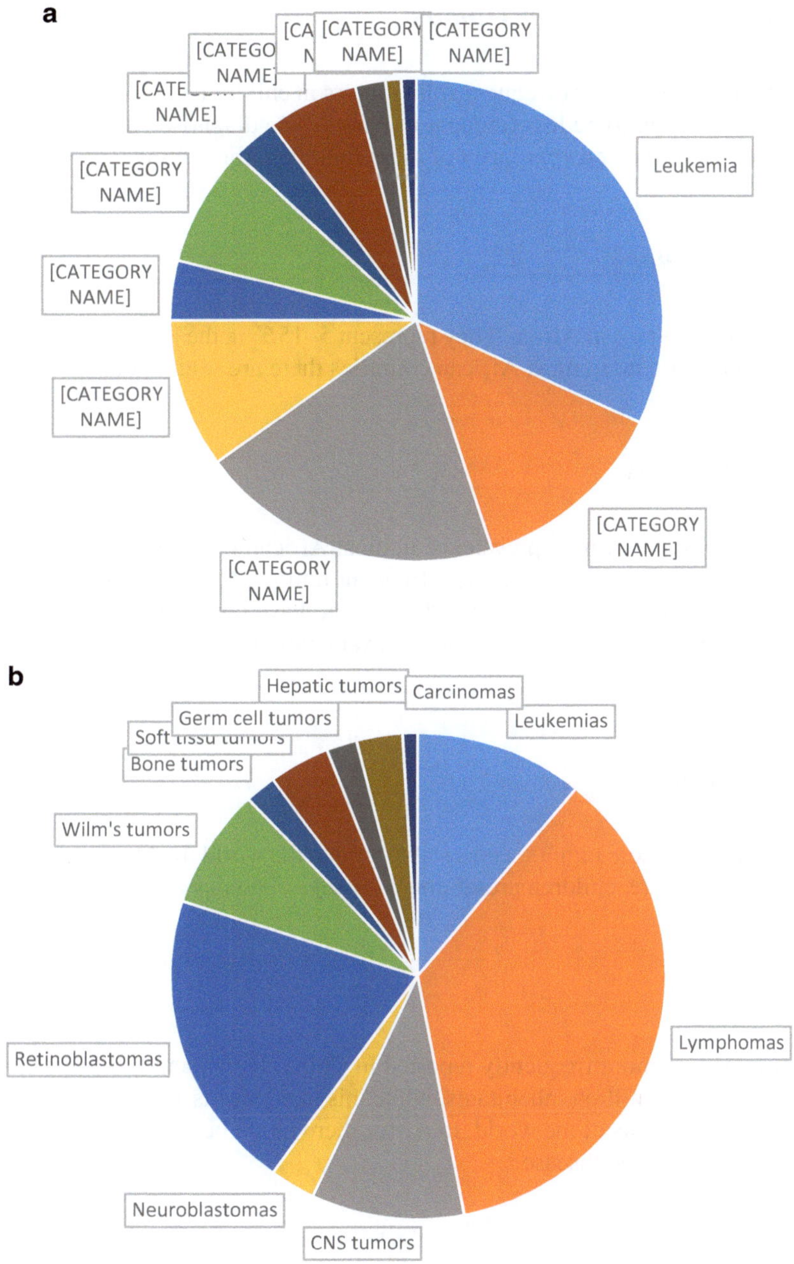

Fig. 1.1 Distribution of childhood cancers in developed (**a**) and limited resources countries (**b**)

Central Nervous System Tumors

These tumors are the most frequent solid tumors in children in developed countries. These tumors seem to be less frequent in Africa. The diagnostic difficulties probably contribute to the apparent rarity of these tumors in this setting.

Neuroblastomas

These tumors are rare in Africa. They represent 5–15 % in the European populations and North American. In most African countries there are seldom diagnosed.

Retinoblastomas

These tumors seem of high prevalence in most African units of pediatric oncology representing the second or third most frequent tumor. Most patients are diagnosed at late stages, present with advanced disease and have consequently a bad prognosis. It is a tumor easy to diagnose and the examination of the eye should be part of each visit to the clinic.

Kidney Tumors

The incidence of these tumors seems stable around the world. In Africa it is also most often diagnosed late, children presenting with huge abdomen and lung metastasis.

Liver Tumors

Liver tumors are more frequently reported in China, Japan, and Fiji Islands, where they exceed 3 per million inhabitants, while this incidence is 1–2 per million inhabitants in other regions of the world. In Africa there might be missed opportunities to diagnose and treat the disease.

Osteosarcoma

Incidence of osteosarcoma is low in Asia (1–2 per million), intermediate (2–3.5 per million inhabitants) in North America and Europe, and high (more than 3.5 per million inhabitants) in the black American population and Brazil. In Africa, this tumor seems rare but the real incidence is not known.

Ewing Sarcoma

This tumor is rare in children in Asia and Africa, not diagnosed or reported.

Mesenchymal tumors

The incidence of these tumors is less than 5 per million in Asia. This incidence is around 8 per million inhabitants in Africa and Europe.

Germ Cell Tumors

The incidence of germ cell tumors is higher in Japan and New Zealand. The peak incidence is bimodal, between 0 and 4 years with a male predominance and between 10 and 14 years with a female predominance.

Thyroïd Carcinomas

These tumors are rare in children. A surge in the number of the tumors occurred in the population of Belarus after the accident of Chernobyl nuclear plant with a high female predominance.

Nasopharyngeal Carcinomas

These tumors are more common in North Africa and Asia (outside Japan) with predominance in adolescents and a male. Epstein-Barr virus is considered as initiating factor in the occurrence of this cancer.

Environmental or Iatrogenic Risk Factors

Identifying environmental or iatrogenic factors is important in order to put in place preventive measures. Their causation is in many cases not demonstrated. Their association to genetic factors significantly potentiates carcinogenesis.

Ionizing Radiation

Radiation is an established risk factor for cancer development. Excessive exposure in utero to X-ray or in childhood increases the risk of developing cancer. Radiation therapy may also be the origin of secondary cancers, especially acute leukemias, cancers of the thyroid, brain tumors, bone tumors, and breast cancers.

Chemotherapy

Secondary cancers are reported following treatment with the alkylating agents, epipodophyllotoxins, nitrosoureas, and anthracyclines. The risk is higher when chemotherapy is associated to radiation therapy. Secondary cancers usually occur 5 years or later after treatment.

Electromagnetic Fields

Exposure to electromagnetic fields from high voltages, electrical appliances, or radio frequency transmission lines has been suspected as carcinogenesis factor. This has not been yet confirmed by controlled studies.

Chemical Exposures

Extended exposure to pesticides increases the risk of leukemia, lymphoma, central nervous system tumors, neuroblastoma, and Wilms tumor. Exposure to solvents increases also the risk of leukemia. Maternal occupational exposure to coal, oil, dyes, or pigments is associated to an increase of the risk of occurrence of hepatoblastoma. Hodgkin disease and CNS tumors are also reported to occur with higher frequency in case of exposure to benzene and hydrocarbons. It was reported that the agricultural child labor in Africa increases the risk of occurrence of Ewing sarcoma which has not been demonstrated.

Parental Smoking

Several studies associated parental smoking with an increased risk of occurrence of non-Hodgkin, lymphoma, central nervous system tumors, neuroblastoma, and hepatoblastoma.

Parental Alcoholism

Maternal alcoholism during pregnancy increases the risk of neuroblastoma. Preconceptual paternal alcoholism also appears to increase the risk of tumors of the central nervous system.

Birth Weight

A high birth weight seems to be a predisposing factor to acute lymphoblastic leukemia and Wilms tumor while low birth weight predisposes to hepatoblastoma.

Breast Feeding

Studies have shown a protective effect of breast-feeding children against cancer and in particular in case of maternal consumption of vegetable protein in the year before pregnancy. The administration of folate and iron during pregnancy seems also to have a protective effect.

Hair Dye

Hair dye used during pregnancy appears to increase the risk of childhood brain tumors.

In Vitro Fertilization

There is an increased risk for children born after in vitro fertilization to develop childhood cancer.

Infection

HIV infection increases the risk of developing chidlhood cancer and the occurrence of B-cell lymphoma and leiomyosarcoma. In this context, Kaposi sarcoma is more common and occurs after HHV8 virus coinfection. The EBV is associated in most cases of Burkitt Lymphoma in sub-Saharan Africa. It is also associated with Hodgkin lymphoma and carcinoma of the nasopharynx in North Africa and Southeast Asia. Hepatitis B and C are associated with hepatocellular carcinoma especially in older children and children not immunized. On the other hand, nursery attendance, chicken pox, poliomyelitis, and rubella appear to have a protective effect due to an increase in immunity.

Genetic Risk Factors

Genetic risk factors are exceptionally encountered in clinical practice but may have a crucial importance in diagnostic or prognosis approaches. The association to malformations can be the initial indicator. A genetic risk factor should also be suspected when there is a family history of cancer in the family, in the bilateral cancers, multifocal and unusual tumor locations or at an unusual age for the specific diagnostic.

Despite their rarity, these situations contribute significantly to understanding of pathophysiological mechanisms of cancer and lead in many cases to preventive measures or to a monitoring program for early diagnosis of cancer. Genetic abnormalities are variable and are currently well documented (Table 1.1). The mechanism of carcinogenesis is however not always clear.

Down Syndrome

Down syndrome occurs in 1 in 1000 births with a higher frequency when the age of the mother is more than 35 years. The risk of leukemia is 10–20 times higher in this population. Acute myeloblastic leukemia (AML) and in particular the type 7 (megacaryoblastic) are often associated with trisomy 21.

These children may develop in 10 % of cases a transient myeloproliferative syndrome (TMS), characterized by an organomegaly, a leukocytosis with circulating blasts and thrombocytopenia. The TMS can evolve to open acute leukemia but in the majority of cases decline spontaneously.

Exact genes involved in the genesis of leukemias in this context are not identified; however the GATA1 gene mutations are found in the majority of cases of AML7 and the TMS. Mutations in JAK2 are also found in the case of ALL.

AMLs observed in this context are usually of good prognosis. These infants have greater susceptibility to toxicity of chemotherapy besides their higher risk of infection. A dose reduction of chemotherapy is recommended.

Li–Fraumeni Syndrome

Li–Fraumeni syndrome is due to a mutation in the anti-oncogene p53, anti-oncogene involved in the control of apoptosis. Transmission of this abnormality is autosomal dominant. In these families there is a high risk of development of soft tissue tumors, cortico-surrenaloma, osteosarcoma, leukemia, brain tumors, or lung and breast cancers at a young age (Table 1.2). The risk of having a cancer before reaching the age of 45 is 41 % in men and 84 % in women and increases exponentially with age. These patients have also higher risk of second tumors. Alterations of p53 activity

Table 1.1 Main genetic syndromes predisposing to cancer in children

Genetic syndrome	Tumor	Transmission	Gene
Ataxia-telangiectasia	Leukemia, lymphoma	Recessive	ATM
Fanconi anemia	Leukemia	Recessive	FANCA
Beckwith–Wiedemann	Wilms tumor, hepatoblastoma, adrenal cortico-surrenaloma, rhabdomyosarcoma	Dominant	CDKN1C, LIT1, IG2, H19, KCNQ1OT1
Bloom Leucémie	Lymphoma	Recessive	BLM
Costello	Neuroblastoma, rhabdomyosarcoma, bladder carcinoma	Dominant	HRAS
Denys–Drash	Wilms tumor	Dominant	WT1
Multiple exostosis	Osteosarcoma	Dominant	ETX1, 2
Gardner	Colorectal polyposis and adenocarcinomas, soft tissue tumors	Dominant	APC
Klinefelter	Mediastinal germ cell tumors, breast cancer	X-linked	XY (+X)
Li–Fraumeni	Soft tissue tumor, osteosarcoma, breast tumor cortico-surrenaloma, leukemias, CNS tumors	Dominant	TP53, CHEK2
Type 1 neurofibromatosis	Neurofibroma, optic pathway glioma, peripheral neurogenic tumors	Dominant	NF1
Type 2 neurofibromatosis	Vestibular Schwannoma, meningioma, ependymoma, astrocytoma	Dominant	NF2
Familial polyposis adenomatosis	Colorectal polyposis/ adenocarcinoma, soft tissue tumors, desmoïd tumors	Dominant	APC
Familial retinoblastoma	Retinoblastoma, sarcoma (osteosarcoma on irradiated field), malignant melanoma	Dominant	RB1
Rothmund-Thomson	Skin tumors, bone tumors	Recessive	RECQL4
Shwachman-Diamond	Leukemia, myelodysplasia	Recessive	SBDS
Sclérosis tubéreuse	Hamartoma, kidney clear cell sarcoma	Dominant	TSC1, 2
Sotos	Leukemia, lymphoma	Dominant	NSD1
Down	Acute leukemia		Trisomy 21
Turcot	Colorectal polyposis, adenocarcinoma, CNS tumors (medulloblastoma, glioma)	Dominant	APC
Von Hippel–Lindau	CNS and retina hemangioblastoma, kidney carcinoma, pheochromocytoma	Dominant	VHL
WAGR	Wilms tumor, Gonadoblastome	Dominant	WT1
Xéroderma pigmentosum	Skin tumors, leukemia	Récessif	XPA, XPC, ERCC, 3, 4, 5

Table 1.2 Clinical criteria in Li–Fraumeni syndrome

Classical form
• Sarcoma occurring before the age of 45 years
• Cancer occurring before the age of 45 in a first degree relative
• Cancer of any type in a first degree relative or second degree before the age of 45 years or sarcoma regardless of age
Variant: Birch criteria
• Childhood Cancer or Sarcoma, CNS tumor or adrenocortical carcinoma before the age of 45 years
• Sarcoma, breast cancer, CNS tumor, adrenocortical carcinoma, or leukemia in a parent of first or second degree regardless of the age
• Cancer of any type in a parent of first or second degree occurring before the age of 60 years
Eeles definition
Two parents of first or second degree developing sarcoma, breast cancer, a brain tumor, an adrenocortical carcinoma or leukemia

are one of the mechanisms of resistance to chemotherapy and radiotherapy. Children with Li–Fraumeni syndrome should be closely followed and monitored using full blood counts and abdominal ultrasound should be part of their regular check-ups.

Ataxia Telangiectasia

This syndrome combines ataxia, skin and scleral telangiectasia, immune humoral deficiency, chromosomal instability, and hypersensitivity to ionizing radiation. These patients have a 5–8 time higher risk of development of malignancy, especially NHL.

The syndrome is an autosomal recessive condition interesting the ATM gene located at the 11q22.3.

Hereditary Retinoblastoma

The hereditary form of retinoblastoma is usually monolateral bilateral or multifocal cancer of retinal cells of the eye. Transmission is autosomal dominant with a high risk of occurrence in the siblings and offspring. According to the model of Knudson, two genetic mutations are required for the occurrence of retinoblastoma. In the hereditary forms, the first mutation occurs at the level of the germ cell and is present then in all body cells, the second mutation occurs at the level of the retinal cells. This hypothesis explains the significant risk of second cancers in patients presenting with hereditary forms. The responsible gene for the disease has been identified as an anti-oncogene located at level 13q 14. The loss of both alleles is required for oncogenesis. Alteration may be a deletion highlighted by cytogenetic but more often it is a point mutation resulting in a transcript of incomplete or absent mRNA of the retinoblastoma gene. This gene is close to the gene of esterase D, measurement of esterase in the red blood cell activity may be used for the identification of patients with deletion.

In 5 % of cases, there is an association with other anomalies and in particular syndromes related to deletion of chromosome 13.

Fanconi Anemia

It is an autosomal recessive condition due to a genetic instability. These gene alterations are related to DNA repair defect. It occurs with an incidence of 1/300,000 but is more frequent among Ashkenazi Jews. These patients have short stature, forearm skeletal anomalies, skin pigmentation and a higher risk of developing leukemia, particularly AML and nephroblastoma, skin or genitourinary cancer. The diagnosis of Fanconi disease is based on the persistence of alterations in chromosome after exposure of the cells of these patients to some antimitotic agents compared to normal cells with normal repair capabilities. This explains also reduced tolerance to chemotherapy and radiotherapy of these patients.

Syndrome of Rhabdoid Predisposition

Called also atypical teratic/rhabdoid tumors, rhabdoid tumors are localized mainly in kidney and are associated in 15 % of the cases with the central nervous system synchronously or as secondary location. They usually occur before the age of 3 years and are particularly aggressive. Gene alterations are found at the level of the 22q11.2 region.

Xeroderma Pigmentosum Syndrome

This syndrome has an incidence of 2.3 per million live births in Europe and seems more common in North Africa. It is autosomal recessive transmitted disease. Alteration of the interested genes induces a reduction in the ability to repair of UV-induced DNA damage. These patients have an increased risk of cancers skin that is proportional to UV exposure. The increase in the risk of basal cell carcinoma development has thus been estimated 10,000 while for malignant melanoma it has been estimated 2000 times compared to normal population. The risk is also higher for other cancers, including the central nervous system.

Table 1.3 Diagnostic criteria for type 1 neurofibromatosis 2 or more criteria are needed for diagnosis

• Six or more hyperpigmented "café au lait" spots of 5 mm, or 1 of more than 15 mm
• Two or more neurofibromas or 1 neurofibroma plexiform
• Inguinal or axillary freckles
• Optic glioma
• Two or more iridien hamartoma (Lisch nodules)
• Bone involvement
• NF1 in a first degree relative

Phacomatosis

It is a group of disorders having in common ectoderm anomalies giving skin, neurological or retinal lesions.

- **Neurofibromatosis Type 1 (NF1)**, called also von Recklinghausen disease, is an autosomal dominant transmitted condition occurring with an incidence of 1/2500 births. The diagnosis is often established in childhood by clinical criteria (Table 1.3).

- Alterations in the gene NF1 (17q11.2) encoding the neurofibromin lead to the formation of skin neurofibromas or neurofibromas plexiform, low grade gliomas of optic nerve or in the central nervous system. Hyperpigmented macules related melanocytes proliferation are found at young age of the childhood and then develop as neurofibromas along the nerve endings in the plexiform type or more deeply at the level of the nerve roots (particularly at the cranio-facial and para-spinales regions). Glioma of the optic way represents nearly 5 % of tumors of the nervous system, but about 50 % of the cases are related to NF1.
- **Neurofibromatosis Type 2 (NF2)** is less frequent than NF1 (1/30,000 or 40,000). Its clinical expression is more discrete. It is frequently associated with a cochlear schwannoma which usually occurs in teenagers or young adults. Other tumors of the nervous system are also associated to NF2.
- **Tuberous sclerosis of Bourneville (STB)** is neuro-cutaneous syndrome transmitted according to autosomal dominant mode. The STB is associated primarily with angiofibromas or skin adenomas, hypo-pigmented maculas, and seizures. Tumors of the central nervous system are the main cause of morbidity and mortality. The STB is linked mutations of one of the anti-oncogene TSC1 located in chromosome 9 or TSC2 in the chromosome 16.
- **Von Hippel–Lindau syndrome (VHL)** is a rare autosomal dominant disorder giving rise to skin lesions and retinal, kidney, or CNS hemangiomas. It is also associated to renal carcinoma and pheochromocytoma. VHL anti-oncogene activity gene is located at chromosome 3p level. Loss of function of this gene leads an upregulation of proteins inducing angiogenesis process which would be at the origin of carcinogenesis.

Nephroblastoma and Anomalies of the WT1 Gene

Near 5 % of cases of nephroblastoma are related to a genetic susceptibility. The WT1 anti-oncogene is located at chromosome 11 level. Mutation or deletion of this gene leads to persistence of an immature mesenchymal tissue. The WT1 gene plays an important role in the maturation and morphogenesis of the urogenitale tractus. According to the model of Knudson secondary somatic mutation induces malignant transformation.

- **Wilms, Aniridia, Genitourinary anomalies, mental Retardation (WAGR) syndrome:** This syndrome is linked to the loss of the short arm of chromosome 11 and in particular the 11p14-p12 region leading to the loss of anti-oncogene WT1 activity. Almost 25 % of patients with WAGR syndrome develop renal disease which may lead to terminal renal failure.
- **Denys–Drash syndrome** is due to a mutation interesting the WT1 gene. It is associated to a sexual ambiguity and nephropathy leading to nephrotic syndrome with a progressive evolution towards a mesangial sclerosis and a terminal renal failure. The recommended treatment in this case is bilateral nephrectomy with kidney transplant.
- **Beckwith–Wiedemann syndrome (BWS)** has an incidence of 1/15,000 live births. This syndrome combines varying degrees a hemi-hypertrophy, genitourinary, cardiac, or musculo-skeletal malformations and a high risk of embryonic tumor and in particular the nephroblastoma and also hepatoblastoma, adrenocortical carcinoma, or neuroblastoma. Nephroblastoma occurs in 5–7 % of patients with BWS. Alteration of the growth regulator gene located at chromosome 11 is found in this syndrome.

Key Points and Practical Recommendations

- Childhood cancer is the second most common cause of mortality in children in developed countries. The burden of childhood cancer is not known in most African countries.
- The distribution of cancers varies according to the regions of the world

NHL is the most frequent tumor type, corresponding to 22.8 % of all cancers diagnosed in children living in Africa, followed by leukemia and kidney tumors for both sexes.

In Africa, HIV infection is an important cause of childhood cancer. Studies have shown an excess of Kaposi sarcoma and Burkitt lymphoma among HIV-infected children. On the other hand, leiomyosarcoma, which is frequently reported among HIV-positive children living in developed countries, is rarely reported in African countries.

- Risk factors are unlike the adult cancer rarely found and can be extrinsic or intrinsic.
- The extrinsic risk factors are mainly irradiation, some viral infections and in particular HIV and cancer chemotherapy.
- Genetic factors should be suspected in case of reported cancer in the family with or without associated malformation.

Epidemiology of childhood cancer in Africa has different features then in developed countries. Preventive measures do not play an essential role in childhood cancer.

Suggested Reading

D'Orazio JA (2010) Inherited cancer syndromes in children and young adults. J Pediatr Hematol Oncol 32:195–228

Howard SC, Metzger ML, Wilimas JA et al (2008) Childhood cancer epidemiology in low-income countries. Cancer 112(3):461–472

Smith MA, Seibel NL, Altekruse SF et al (2010) Outcomes for children and adolescents with cancer: challenges for the twenty-first century. J Clin Oncol 28(15):2625–2634

Stiller CA, Parkin DM (1996) Geographic and ethnic variations in the incidence of childhood cancer. Br Med Bull 52:682–703

Chapter 2
Early Warning Signs and Diagnostic Approach in Childhood Cancer

Case Presentation

Abdu, a 14-month-old boy, presents with fever. He has a poor appetite and has developed peri-orbital bruises in the absence of any trauma. Whenever his mother picks him up, he seems to be in pain.

Weight = 12 kg, height = 78 cm (Fig 2.1)

On examination the child appears unwell, irritable, and in pain. His pulse rate is 160/min, respiratory rate 40/min, and his temperature 38 °C. His blood pressure and oxygen saturation are normal. He is very pale. Left-sided peri-orbital bruising is present, as well as mild proptosis of the left eye. His right upper arm and left knee are tender to touch. His abdomen is distended, but not tender. A left flank mass (8 × 10 cm) is found. It is not ballotable. The liver is palpable 4 cm under the costal margin.

What diagnostic investigations should be requested in this case?

Hematology: Complete blood count, reticulocyte count and peripheral blood smear, clotting profile

Biochemistry: U&E, LDH, ferritin, urine VMA and HVA

Abdominal sonar, followed by a CT or MRI abdomen if available

Biopsy of abdominal mass

Once neuroblastoma has been confirmed: MIBG scan and bone marrow aspirate and biopsy

Diagnostic Delay in Childhood Cancer

The majority of children with cancer in developing countries are diagnosed too late, when advanced disease is already present, and many more die without ever being diagnosed. Various factors contribute to the diagnostic delay (Fig. 2.2).

D.C. Stefan, M. Harif, *Pediatric Cancer in Africa*,
DOI 10.1007/978-3-319-17936-0_2

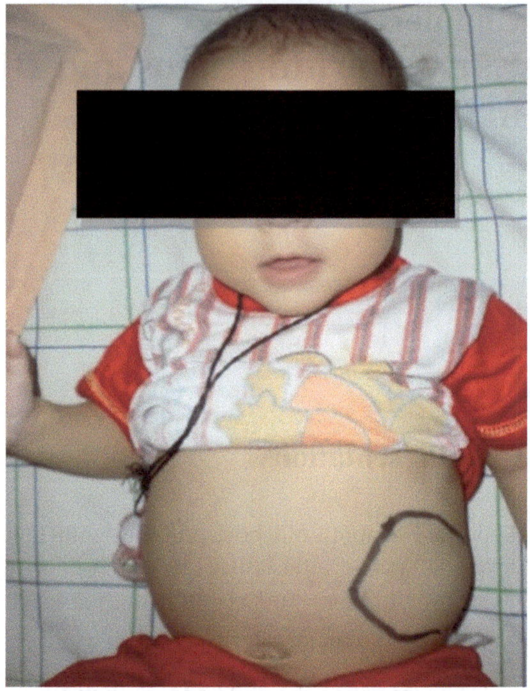

Fig. 2.1

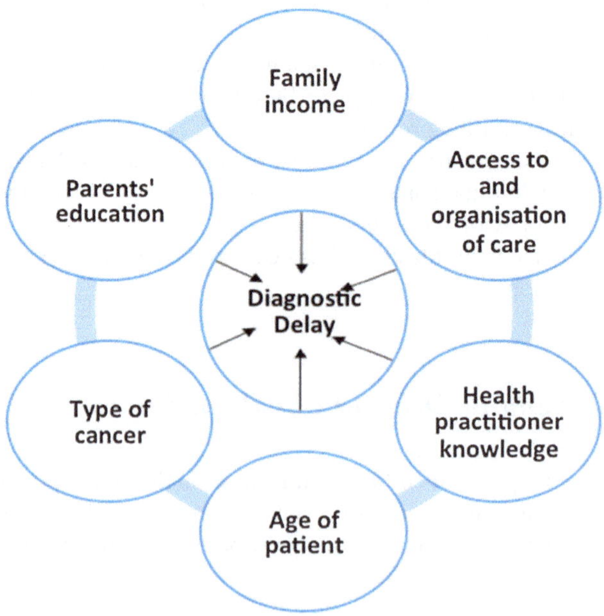

Fig. 2.2 Factors contributing to diagnostic delay and abandonment of treatment

The site of the solid tumor will determine if the presentation is early or late. If it is in the close proximity of a vital structure such as the airway, it may present earlier, as compared to a tumor in the parenchyma or pleura. A high proliferation rate may also ensure that a tumor is noted earlier, e.g., Burkitt lymphoma or acute leukemia. Systemic symptoms, like night sweats or fever may prompt a visit to the doctor and lead to a cancer diagnosis or may be misdiagnosed with common infection.

In young babies it may be difficult to note neurological signs and symptoms early, since the tumor can grow to a significant size due to the pliable skull bones and open fontanelle. Adolescents may not want to discuss their health problems with their parents for various reasons, including cultural reasons or privacy issues.

Parents may not recognize symptoms as possible early warning signs of childhood cancer. In the African setting, because of difficulties in accessing health care and also because of religious and social beliefs, parents often first seek help from traditional healers. Therefore awareness campaigns and education in the community are extremely important, as well as ensuring access to health care and specified referral pathways. However, a South African study showed that the biggest reason for delay in diagnosis in their setting was the failure of health care practitioners to recognize the warning signs. Thus health care practitioners should be adequately trained regarding the suspicion and early diagnosis of childhood cancer. Awareness and outreach campaigns among health care practitioners are important to keep the focus on childhood cancer.

Early Warning Signs of Childhood Cancer

The early warning signs of childhood cancer are present in about 85 % of childhood cancers, although they are not specific for cancer. They are easy to remember and easy to identify on history or clinical examination. Every country should have simple pamphlets or posters of early warning signs to be distributed among health care practitioners and the community (Fig. 2.3). A study performed in South Africa showed that after an awareness campaign using the "Saint Siluan early warning signs of childhood cancer" was started, an increased number of new cancer cases were diagnosed (Fig. 2.4). The Saint Siluan signs have been adopted by SIOP-PODC (International Society of Pediatric Oncology's Committee on Developing Countries) and the International Confederation of Childhood Cancer Parent Organization (ICCCPO).

Another example of a list of warning signs is "CHILD CANCER," an acronym which is also endorsed by international childhood cancer organizations (Table 2.1).

Children with a High Risk of Cancer

High-risk groups should be identified early and follow-up/surveillance programs should be instituted as soon as possible. Conditions with a high risk for cancer include neurocutaneous syndromes (neurofibromatosis, tuberous sclerosis), certain

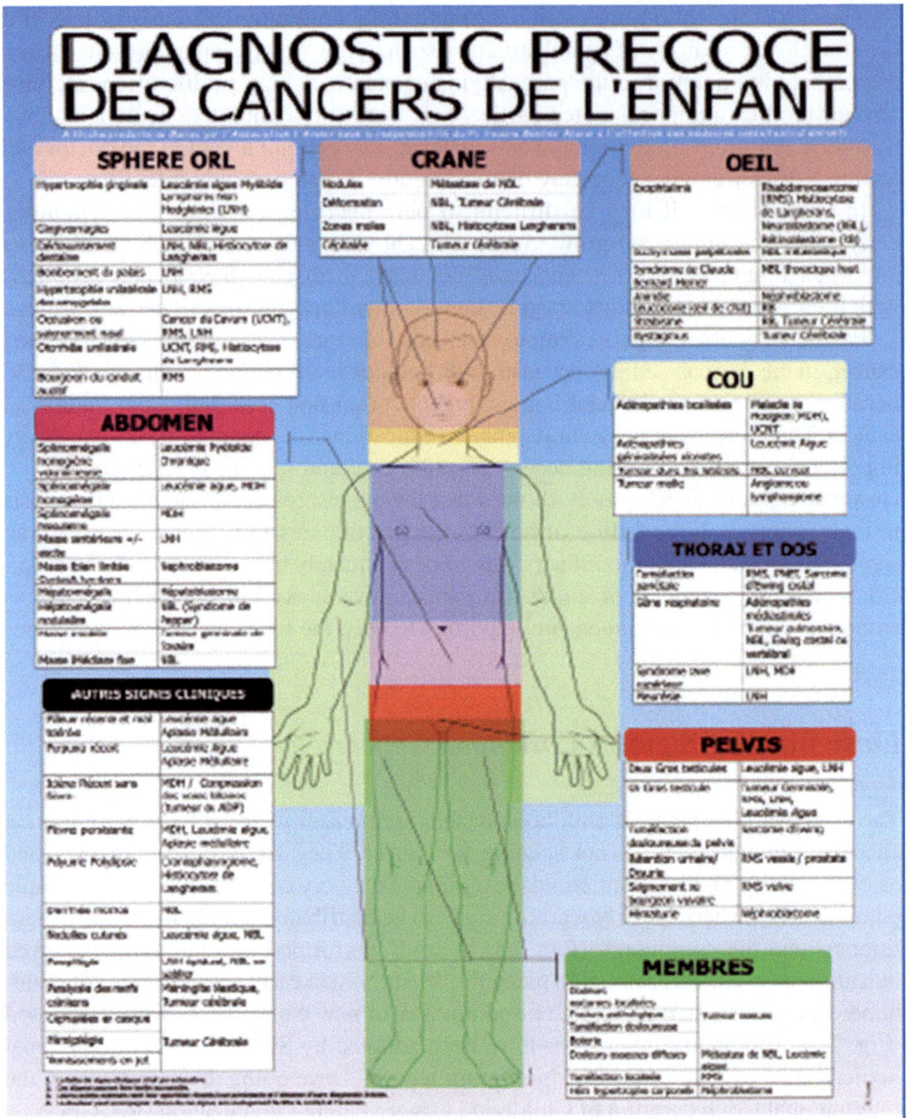

Fig. 2.3 Poster for caregiver's awareness program in Morocco

genetic disorders (Down syndrome, Fanconi anemia, Beckwith–Wiedemann syndrome, etc.), primary and secondary immunodeficiency disorders, history of a previous malignancy, as well as congenital malformations (aniridia, hemi-hypertrophy). Some conditions will require regular clinical follow-up and others intermittent abdominal ultrasound investigations.

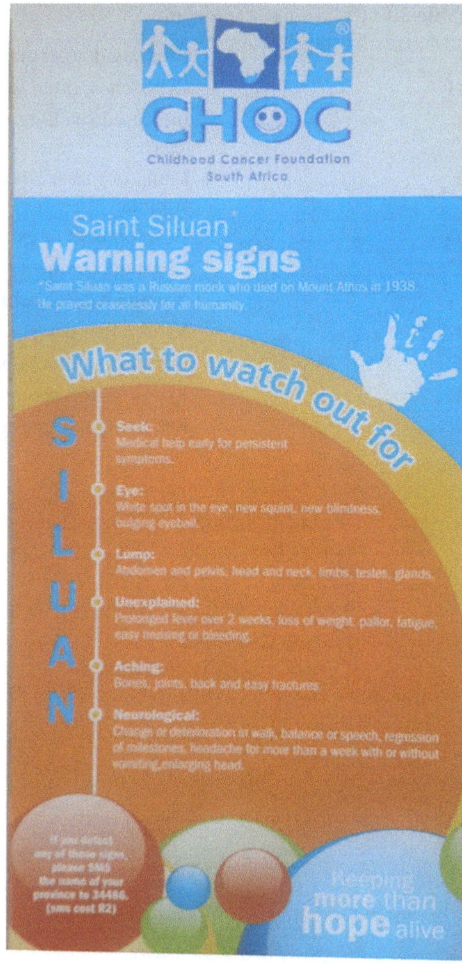
CHOC
Childhood Cancer Foundation
South Africa
Saint Siluan*
Warning signs
*Saint Siluan was a Russian monk who died on Mount Athos in 1938.
He prayed ceaselessly for all humanity.
What to watch out for
S Seek:
Medical help early for persistent symptoms.
I Eye:
White spot in the eye, new squint, new blindness, bulging eyeball.
L Lump:
Abdomen and pelvis, head and neck, limbs, testes, glands.
U Unexplained:
Prolonged fever over 2 weeks, loss of weight, pallor, fatigue, easy bruising or bleeding.
A Aching:
Bones, joints, back and easy fractures.
N Neurological:
Change or deterioration in walk, balance or speech, regression of milestones, headache for more than a week with or without vomiting, enlarging head.
Keeping more than hope alive

Fig. 2.4 St Siluan early warning signs of childhood cancer (South Africa)

Clinical Diagnosis of Childhood Cancers

In Africa, where resources are limited, a thorough history and meticulous examination are essential and often form the backbone of the diagnosis. A histological diagnosis is always required whenever is possible. Besides signs and symptoms, knowledge regarding the age of onset of the different malignancies is also helpful (Fig. 2.5).

Signs and symptoms of childhood cancers can be divided into four main groups (Fig. 2.6). The most frequent signs are related to the tumor mass. Childhood cancer is often rapidly growing and a mass may be palpable or visible. Depending on its site, the mass is more or less noticeable. Complications, symptoms, and signs due to compression/obstruction are frequently present with tumors of the digestive tract, chest, and orbit, while they often appear late with abdominal tumors.

Table 2.1 Child cancer acronym

C	**C**ontinued, unexplained weight loss
H	**H**eadaches, often with early morning vomiting
I	**I**ncreased swelling or persistent pain in the bones, joints, back, or legs
L	**L**ump or mass, especially in the abdomen, neck, chest, pelvis, or armpits
D	**D**evelopment of excessive bruising, bleeding, or rash
C	**C**onstant, frequent, or persistent infections
A	**A** whitish color behind the pupil
N	**N**ausea that persists or vomiting without nausea
C	**C**onstant tiredness or noticeable paleness
E	**E**ye or vision changes that occur suddenly and persist
R	**R**ecurring or persistent fevers of unknown origin

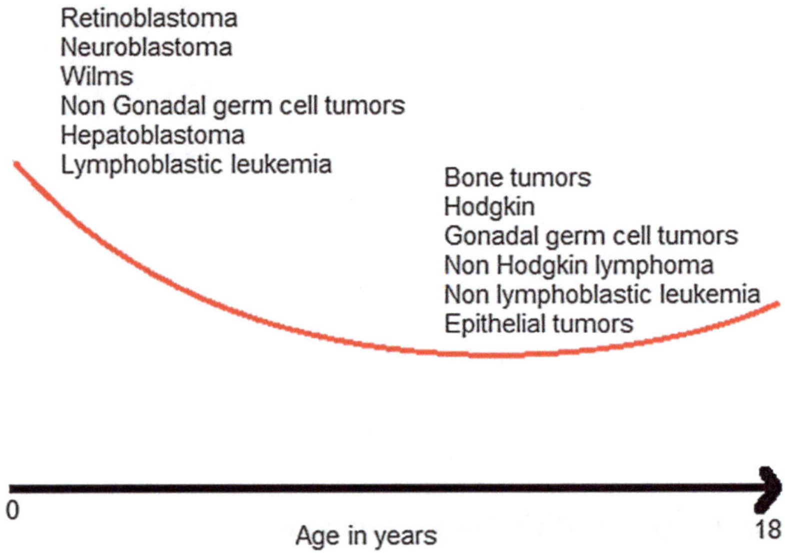

Fig. 2.5 Typical age of onset in different childhood cancers

Symptoms and signs due to metastases may prompt a patient to present, but are most often only found during the diagnostic workup. Bone metastases often present with pain, pathological fractures (less common), or masses. General signs and symptoms and particularly fever, are not specific and do not occur with all cancers in childhood. They become meaningful when they are associated with a mass, lymphadenopathy, or another clinical feature of cancer. Paraneoplastic signs and symptoms occur rarely.

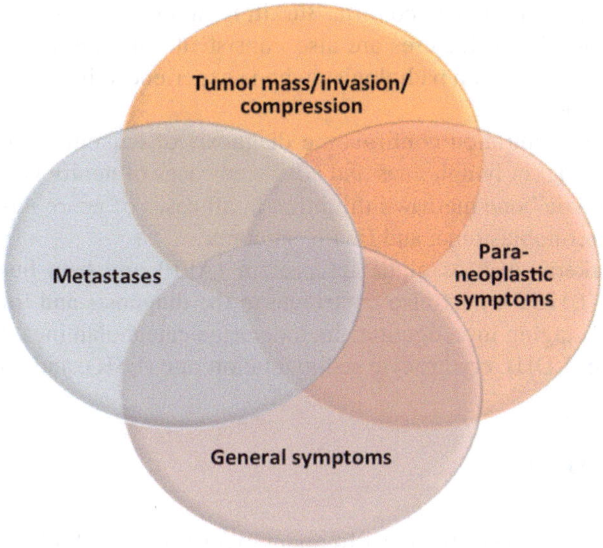

Fig. 2.6 Modes of cancer expression

Diagnostic Procedures

Diagnostic procedures should be adapted to local and national available resources. In Africa, the cost thereof and potential delay should be taken into account. In this setting, clinical signs and symptoms remain the most important factor. A confident diagnosis needs to be made, however, before therapy is initiated. The development of telepathology and/or teleradiology systems may be very helpful.

In the case of life-threatening situations, specific treatment may need to be started while diagnostic procedures are still being performed. In most cases, a fine needle aspiration or biopsy is necessary for diagnostic confirmation. In the case of retinoblastoma, some brain tumors and tumors of the kidney, clinicoradiological diagnosis may be sufficient.

A surgical biopsy is the gold standard for the diagnosis of solid tumors. It must be performed by an experienced surgeon, preferably by the surgeon who will be in charge of tumor excision. When complete resection is possible without performing mutilating surgery, the surgeon should consider this option. The pathologist involved should provide guidance as to the type of biopsy and preservation technique. If a tumor is excised, the margins should be identified as anterior, posterior, etc. Percutaneous biopsy or aspiration is best performed under ultrasound or CT guidance. When good clinical evaluation and communication with the pathologist is in place, most of childhood cancers can reliably be diagnosed by standard HE pathology staining. Good quality of staining is important for accurate diagnosis. Immunohistochemistry and genetic or molecular studies to characterize these tumors are sometimes required.

Fine needle aspiration may confirm Burkitt lymphoma, the most frequent tumor in Africa, when clinical features are also consistent with the diagnosis. It should preferably only be used if a pathologist, who is experienced in cytological interpretation, is available.

Bone marrow aspiration confirms the diagnosis of leukemia and also in some cases of non-Hodgkin lymphomas and advanced cases of neuroblastoma. It should be done to exclude bone marrow infiltration in all cases of neuroblastoma, rhabdomyosarcoma, retinoblastoma, and Ewing sarcoma.

Tumor markers, such as alpha fetoprotein (AFP) and beta human chorionic gonadotropin (BHCG), may also contribute to the diagnosis and follow-up. Other diagnostic and staging investigations include urine catecholamines, ferritin, lactate dehydrogenase (LDH), erythrocyte sedimentation rate (ESR), and bone scan.

Abdominal Mass

Abdominal mass is one of the most frequent expressions of childhood tumors. The age of onset is important. The clinical examination must note the tumor volume, mobility, and consistency. In the neonatal period, the origin is often congenital malformation. Between 1 and 5 years of age, nephroblastoma and neuroblastoma are the most frequently encountered malignancies. Non-Hodgkin lymphoma, especially Burkitt lymphoma, usually presents with several confluent masses associated with pain, vomiting, and constipation. Not infrequently, Burkitt lymphoma presents with acute intussusception or perforation, requiring urgent surgery.

An association with other signs may also help in narrowing down a diagnosis:

- A facial mass with or without an abdominal mass is most often due to Burkitt lymphoma. This tumor is endemic in Africa.
- The presence of macroscopic or microscopic hematuria is usually associated with a renal tumor.
- Aniridia, hemi-hypertrophy or genitourinary abnormalities are associated with nephroblastoma.
- The presence of subcutaneous nodules, peri-orbital bruising, proptosis, or opsomyoclonus point towards neuroblastoma.
- Finally, precocious puberty associated with an abdominal mass is suggestive of gonadal or adrenal tumors.

Abdominal ultrasound is the first step in the diagnostic evaluation. If performed by an experienced radiologist, it is in the majority of cases sufficient to clarify the origin of the tumor and its locoregional impact. Plain abdominal radiography can identify calcifications, which are sometimes seen in teratomas or neuroblastoma and are helpful if an acute abdomen is present. CT scan or MRI, when available, is the investigation of choice and provides detailed anatomical information. Further staging investigations are determined by the type of malignancy, as well as the availability of special investigations. Tuberculosis with or without HIV infection should be considered in most parts of Africa.

Intra-Thoracic Masses

Most intra-thoracic tumors are located either in the mediastinum or the thoracic wall. The most common symptom of mediastinal tumors is dyspnea. In more advanced disease, superior vena cava syndrome may develop. It is a medical emergency and needs to be treated without delay. Mediastinal masses are more frequent in older children and are most often due to T-cell lymphomas and leukemias. These malignancies are often associated with airway compression and/or pleural effusion. Masses in the middle mediastinum are usually hilar lymph node metastases or Hodgkin disease. Neurogenic tumors, particularly neuroblastoma, ganglioneuroma, or neurofibroma, are found in the posterior mediastinum. Sometimes intraspinal extension of the tumor can occur, giving rise to spinal cord compression, which is also a medical emergency.

Careful analysis of the chest X-ray may be very helpful. Ultrasound and CT scan provide details regarding possible pleural or pericardial effusion, the exact site of the tumor and locoregional extension of the tumor. In the event of acute lymphoblastic leukemia, the diagnosis is confirmed by a CBC, peripheral blood smear and bone marrow biopsy. In the case of non-Hodgkin lymphoma, cytology of the pleural fluid may be sufficient for the diagnosis. Otherwise a lymph node biopsy or biopsy of the chest wall mass should be performed. Chest wall tumors are usually due to Ewing sarcoma or soft tissue sarcomas.

Intracranial Masses

Clinical symptoms and signs of brain tumors vary according to the age of the child, the site of the tumor, and its aggressiveness. Diagnostic delay is usually longer for supratentorial tumors. The diagnosis is made by CT or preferably MRI. Initially, an ultrasound may be helpful to identify a mass and hydrocephalus in babies with an open fontanelle.

Headaches are the most common symptom. It is indicative of raised intracranial pressure when they occur early morning, and are associated with vomiting and papilledema. In a young child, behavioral changes or learning problems may be observed. Very often, focal neurological signs (motor deficit, cranial palsy), seizures, ataxia, or a visual field deficit are found.

Lymphadenopathy

Lymphadenopathy is a common finding in children of all ages. Reactive lymphadenopathy needs to be distinguished from sinister lymphadenopathy. The site, size, consistency, mobility, progression in size, and associated signs are of major importance. Nodes are considered to be pathological if their size exceeds 1 cm (cervical and axillary) and 1.5 cm (inguinal). Any supraclavicular lymphadenopathy must be considered to be pathological. Left-sided supraclavicular lymphadenopathy may be related to metastases of an intra-abdominal tumor, particularly neuroblastoma, while the right side can be due to metastases of intra-thoracic tumors. Malignant lymph nodes are usually firm or hard, fast-growing, and can become confluent and fixed.

In the event of suspicious lymph nodes without an obvious etiology, the evaluation should include a CBC, reticulocyte count and peripheral blood smear, chest X-ray, tuberculosis workup and viral tests, particularly HIV. Antibiotic treatment may be given for 1–2 weeks. In the case of cytopenias, circulating blasts or mediastinal lymphadenopathy/mass, a bone marrow biopsy should be performed.

The indications of a lymph node biopsy are: persistent or increasing lymphadenopathy beyond 4–6 weeks, lymph nodes of more than 2.5 cm in the absence of signs of infection or response to antibiotic treatment, supraclavicular involvement and/or an association with fever, night sweats, weight loss or other worrying signs.

The biopsy should be a complete excision of the largest and most accessible lymph node. Lymph node cytology imprints must always be prepared for better characterization.

Soft Tissue Masses

Soft tissue sarcomas may present as a mass literally at any site. Complete resection may be attempted if surgery would not be mutilating or extensive, otherwise a biopsy should be performed.

Bone Pain

Bone pain is a common symptom in children with cancer and is a presenting feature of leukemia. It often reflects metastatic bone involvement in various cancers, such as non-Hodgkin lymphoma, neuroblastoma, osteosarcoma, rhabdomyosarcoma, and some renal tumors. Localized pain may be due to a primary bone tumor, such as osteosarcoma and Ewing sarcoma. Bone pain (and limb or joint swelling) is often attributed to trauma or "growing pains" and not adequately investigated until the tumor is advanced. When bone pain does not respond to analgesia, is not associated with trauma and if swelling is present, an X-ray should be performed and properly interpreted. Lytic lesions, onion skin appearance, Codman triangle, and soft tissue swelling are radiological signs of a bone tumor. A biopsy should be performed as soon as possible.

Summary

Childhood cancer is a relatively rare disease (incidence between 1–10%). The clinical expression is not always specific, which contributes to the difficulties in making a diagnosis. Early diagnosis is crucial, since survival rates are closely correlated to the stage of disease: early stage disease equals excellent patient outcome, while advanced disease usually leads to poor outcomes. Primary care practitioners and parents should be trained to recognize signs and symptoms that may be suggestive of cancer. As soon as cancer is suspected, appropriate basic investigations should be performed without delay, after which patients should be referred as soon as possible to an oncology unit. Children with an increased risk of developing cancer, such as children with Beckwith–Wiedemann or other syndromes, should be identified early and surveillance programs should be instituted for them.

Suggested Reading

Feltbower RG, Lewis IJ, Picton S, Richards M, Glaser AW, Kinsey SE, McKinney PA (2004) Diagnosing childhood cancer in primary care—a realistic expectation? Br J Cancer 90:1882–1884
Haimi M, Perez-Nahum M, Stein N, Ben Arush MW (2011) The role of the doctor and the medical system in the diagnostic delaying pediatric malignancies. Cancer Epidemiol 35:83–89
Okoko AR, Ekouya Bowassa G, Oko AP, Mbika-Cardorelle A, Moyen GM (2012) Epidemiology of palpable abdominal masses in children in Brazzaville. Arch Pediatr 19(8):878–879
Pollock BH, Krischer JP, Vietti TJ (1991) Interval between symptom onset and diagnosis of pediatric solid tumors. J Pediatr 119:725–732
Poyiadjis S, Wainwright L, Naidu G, Mackinnon D, Poole J (2011) The Saint Siluan warning signs of cancer in children: impact of education in rural South Africa. Pediatr Blood Cancer 56(2):314–316
Raab CP, Gartner JC (2009) Diagnosis of childhood cancer. Prim Care Clin Office Pract 36:671–684
Stones DK (2010) Childhood cancer: early warning signs. CME 28(7):314–316
Twist CJ, Link MP (2002) Assessment of lymphadenopathy in children. Pediatr Clin North Am 49:1009–1025

Chapter 3
Cancer Registries and the Value of a Dedicated Pediatric Registry in Africa

Throughout the world, there are approximately 15 million new cancer cases and 9 million cancer deaths estimated for 2015, with 48.2 % and 56.5 % of those being observed in low- and middle-income countries, respectively.

The population in Africa is above one billion. Children represent 41 % of the total population. In some African countries, the population is very young with more than half represented by children below the age of 15 years.

Cancer in childhood is a rare disease. In developed countries, only about 0.5% of all cancer occurs in children younger than 15 years. However, the mortality from childhood cancer occupies the second place following trauma (mostly car accidents).

As a result of the demographic distribution of the world population, 71.4 % of all cancer cases and 83 % of all cancer deaths occurring worldwide are reported among children living in low- and mid-income countries. The African continent is severely affected in terms of new cases as well as increased mortality among children diagnosed with cancer.

Applying the described incidence of 110–140 new cases of cases per million for developed countries, it is expected to report an annual new number between 47,000 and 55.000 children diagnosed with cancer in Africa.

The exact number is not known because of lack of cancer registries, or incomplete registries which do not include data on pediatric oncology cases.

D.C. Stefan, M. Harif, *Pediatric Cancer in Africa*,
DOI 10.1007/978-3-319-17936-0_3

So, What Is a Cancer Registry?

The cancer registry is a critical component of any cancer control program. The data of a cancer registry can be used in several areas including etiology research, primary and secondary prevention, and healthcare services planning.

The cancer registry collects, stores, analyzes, and interprets data on cancer cases.

A pediatric cancer registry refers to data collected on newly diagnosed children in the age group 0–15 years (some of the registries might include data until the age 18 years and some others until 21 years).

Types of Registries

There are two different types of cancer registries: the hospital-based cancer registry, and the population-based cancer registry.

1. The **hospital-based cancer registry** is a register of data collected on all patients treated for cancer in a hospital or in a set of hospitals (central hospital-based cancer registry). The main objectives of a hospital-based cancer registry are to evaluate and improve the quality of patient care, to contribute to professional education, to provide information for hospital administration for planning purposes, and to serve as a basis for clinical research. Furthermore, hospital-based cancer registries can be responsible for controlling the follow-up of patients treated at a specific hospital. Hospital-based cancer registries cannot be used to calculate the incidence of cancer.

   By its very nature, a central registry of hospital-based registries cannot be complete. Nevertheless, it is the most efficient and sustainable way of obtaining data, which can be used in statistical research, as it does not require a substantial expenditure. A minimum of data collected in a hospital-based registry would be: the demographic information (name, age, sex, and address), the type, localization and stage of the tumor, the histological type, the treatment and outcome, as well as the results of annual follow-ups. Should the patient die, the date and cause of the death should be recorded.

   The cost of such a registry is limited to the salary of a data manager who works part time and who collects all the forms from the referring centers, private doctors, and laboratories.
2. **Population-based cancer registries** are registries where information is collected on all cancer cases occurring in a defined population residing within a specified geographic area. Their main objective is the determination of incidence rates (by sex, age, primary site, stage of disease, etc.). Moreover, the data can also be used to conduct epidemiological studies to evaluate the actions of the cancer control program, as well as to assist in the planning of health services for the prevention, diagnosis, and treatment. If mortality data are also collected (which is not done in all cancer registries), a population-based cancer registry can also be used to calculate survival rates (and to estimate prevalence rates).

To compile accurate data, cases for such a registry should be actively sought. Registrars should contact departments of pathology, departments of radiology where radiotherapy is done, other hospital departments (such as surgery), chemical pathology or hematology laboratories, outpatient clinics as well as private clinics and laboratories. They should also study the death certificates and, by all the means described above, identify cases of cancer whose data must then be extracted from the records and entered in the registry.

In most African countries children with cancer are treated in specialized centers, which are at the same time the referring units. Sometimes a hospital-based registry might also represent a population-based registry if the treating hospital is the only one in the country where children with cancer are diagnosed and treated.

What Is the Value of a Cancer Registry?

The value of a cancer registry is entirely dependent on the quality of the data collected. To achieve its objectives, the population-based cancer registry should ensure:

- The inclusion of all new cancer cases in a population (coverage)
- The correct coding and classification of tumors (validity)
- If survival data are also included in the registry, monitoring and follow-up of patients
- Access to estimates of the population at risk (i.e., census data), preferably stratified by gender and age

The main aspects of data quality of a cancer registry are comparability, coverage, and validity. The coverage can be defined as the proportion of incident cases in a population that is included in the registry. Ideally, this number should be as close to 100 % as possible, so that the comparison of changes over time in the population covered by the registry as well as the comparison between registries reflects true differences only in cancer risk. However, full coverage is not achievable in most circumstances for the following reasons:

- The patient does not seek or have access to healthcare and the case is never diagnosed.
- The registry is deficient in their pursuit of cases.
- Under diagnosis of cancer by the health system leading to selection bias (certain cancers tend to be diagnosed more often).

Validity of a registry is measured by the following:

1. The percentage of cases with histological confirmation of the diagnosis (recommended value: >70 %).
2. The percentage of cases reported by death certificate only (recommended: <20 %).
3. Percentage of cases reported as unknown primary site (C80.9) or other and unspecified (C26, C39, C48, and C76) (recommended: <20 %).
4. Percentage of cases with unknown age (recommended: <20 %).

In Africa, the percentage of cases with histological confirmation is unfortunately much reduced as not all cases will have had a biopsy. Very seldom cases reported by death certificate are included in a registry, while the percentage of cases with unknown primary site and unknown age is very high.

International and African Organization of Support of Cancer Registration

1. The International Agency for Research on Cancer (IARC).
2. African Cancer Registry Network (AFCRN).

1. *The International Agency for Research on Cancer* is a unit of the World Health Organization based in Lyon, France and has a division, dedicated to surveillance and cancer registration support worldwide.

   A key objective of the Section of Cancer Surveillance (CSU) is to measure the global burden of cancer and to make available to the public worldwide statistics on global cancer incidence and mortality. On the IARC website, there are many useful tools for cancer registration including the monograph "Cancer Registration: Principles and Methods" as well as the free cancer registration software, CanReg 5 (http://www-dep.iarc.fr/CIN_resources.htm), which is available in many languages.

   GLOBOCAN is a project aiming to provide up-to-date estimates of the incidence, mortality, prevalence, and disability-adjusted life years (DALYs) from major type of cancers, at national level, for 184 countries of the world (including Africa). A specific methodology is utilized to estimate the country-specific burden of cancer, gathering data from population-based cancer registries (national or local), mortality statistics from the WHO, and national population estimates obtained from the United Nations' population division.

   Despite a real value of estimating the total number of cancers in the world, GLOBOCAN cannot replace useful data obtained by local registries.
2. *African support organization of cancer registration in Africa*—the **AFCRN** was formed in 2012, and succeeded and expanded the activities of the East African Cancer Registry Network (EACRN) formed a year earlier.

AFCRN aims improve the effectiveness of cancer surveillance in sub-Saharan Africa by providing expert evaluation of current problems and technical support to remedy identified barriers, with long-term goals of strengthening health systems and creating research platforms for the identification of problems, priorities, and targets for intervention.

Since 2012, the IARC, in the framework of its Global Initiative for Cancer Registry Development in Low- and Middle-Income Countries (GICR), has partnered with AFCRN to provide a network Regional Hub for cancer registration in Sub-Saharan Africa.

Classification of Childhood Cancer

Since childhood cancer differs significantly from that of adult cancer, it is therefore more appropriate to classify childhood cancers according to their histology, rather than the site where the tumor occurs. The first edition of the International Classification of Childhood Cancer (ICCC) classifies childhood tumors into 12 major diagnostic groups: leukemia, lymphomas, central nervous system (CNS) tumors, sympathetic nervous system tumors, retinoblastoma, renal tumors, liver tumors, bone tumors, soft tissue sarcomas, germ cell tumors, epithelial tumors, and other unspecified malignant cancers.

In 1988, IARC published the first volume of the series "International Incidence of Childhood Cancer", describing the incidence observed in the 1970s; 10 years later the 2nd volume was published, and expanded with the inclusion of 15 additional cancer registries. Today IARC is busy with publishing the 5th edition.

The incidence rates of childhood cancer range between 96 and 138 per million children per year for boys, and from 70 to 116 per million children for girls. Leukemia, CNS tumors, and non-Hodgkin lymphomas (NHL) are the most frequent pediatric cancers in high-income countries, representing 60 % of all cases, whereas in low-income countries, NHL are more common than leukemia and brain tumors.

Middle-income countries have an intermediate pattern. However, it is important to note that a large heterogeneity is observed across continents.

According to GLOBOCAN, the estimated incidence of all pediatric cancers (0–14 years) in Africa is 99 and 73/million for boys and girls, respectively.

There is a wide variation in rates, with the highest rates being recorded in Malawi (220/million for boys) and Uganda (140/million among girls) while the lowest incidence rates are observed in Guinea (43 and 29/million among boys and girls, respectively).

NHL is the most frequent tumor type, corresponding to 22.8 % of all cancers diagnosed in children living in Africa, followed by leukemia and kidney tumors for both sexes.

In Africa, HIV infection is an important cause of childhood cancer. Studies have shown an excess of Kaposi sarcoma and Burkitt lymphoma among HIV-infected children. On the other hand, leiomyosarcoma, which is frequently reported among HIV-positive children living in developed countries, is rarely reported in African countries. Of interest is that cervical cancer is the 7th most common cancer diagnosed in children younger than 14 years old. This is probably a reflection of the widespread infection with virulent forms of human papilloma virus as well as the underlying susceptibility caused by HIV.

A recent study looking at the patterns of distribution of childhood cancers in Africa, showed a different distribution between different African countries with a prevalence ranging from 1.4 % to 10 %.

In the same local study it was shown that in Southern Africa, Kaposi sarcoma was the most common malignancy in children in Mozambique (15.8 % of all cases) and the second most common in Zambia (15.6 %) and in Malawi (12.4 %).

In Eastern Africa, Uganda recorded Kaposi sarcoma as the most common tumor in children (22.0 %) while two Kenyan centers reported mainly Burkitt lymphoma (25.1 % and 37.1 %, respectively).

In Western Africa, NHL was the most common in Ghana (53.6 %), the Ivory Coast (73.6 %), and in Mali (32.7 %).

Nephroblastoma remains one of the most common solid tumors in Africa, exceeding 10 % of the total number of pediatric cancers in many countries (Rwanda 26.0 %, Senegal 22 %, Ivory Coast 14.5 %, Mali 17.6 %, Congo 15.5 %, etc.).

The conclusions of the study showed that unlike developed countries, lymphomas, nephroblastoma, Kaposi sarcoma, and retinoblastoma were the most common pediatric tumors in Africa.

GLOBOCAN estimations, despite bringing significant contribution to the registration map, cannot replace the data from local hospital- and population-based registries.

Mortality rate calculation remains difficult in Africa as many patients are lost to follow-up.

Take Home Messages

- A dedicated childhood cancer registry will furnish data on incidence, survival, mortality, and on the epidemiology of newly diagnosed children with cancer.
- A dedicated childhood cancer registry can start as a hospital-based registry and later be developed as a population-based registry.
- The information collected includes demographic parameters (date of birth, gender, age at diagnosis, date of diagnosis, ethnic group) as well as information relating to the pathology (specific cancer), diagnosis, stage, treatment, and outcome (several registry forms are presented below).
- The cost of such a registry should not be prohibitive.
- If a dedicated pediatric registry is not possible, all efforts should be directed to the inclusion of pediatric cases in the general hospital-based or ideally population-based registry (Fig. 3.1).

Suggested Reading

Bray F, Parkin DM (2009) Evaluation of data quality in the cancer registry: principles and methods. Part I: comparability, validity and timeliness. Eur J Cancer 45(5):747–755

Curado MP et al (2007) Cancer incidence in five continents, vol IX. ARC Scientific, Lyon

Kramarova E, Stiller CA (1996) The international classification of childhood cancer. Int J Cancer 68(6):759–765

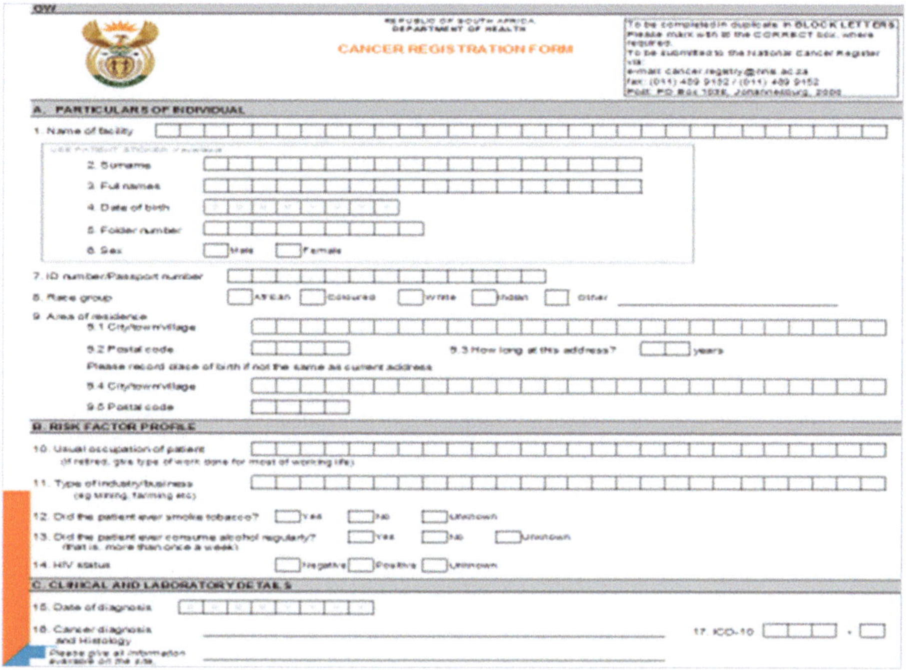

REPUBLIC OF SOUTH AFRICA
DEPARTMENT OF HEALTH

CANCER REGISTRATION FORM

To be completed in duplicate in BLOCK LETTERS
Please mark with ☒ the CORRECT box, where required.
To be submitted to the National Cancer Register via:
e-mail: cancer.registry@nhls.ac.za
fax: (011) 489 9152 / (011) 489 9152
Post: PO Box 1038, Johannesburg, 2000

A. PARTICULARS OF INDIVIDUAL

1. Name of facility
2. Surname
3. Full names
4. Date of birth
5. Folder number
6. Sex ☐ Male ☐ Female
7. ID number/Passport number
8. Race group ☐ African ☐ Coloured ☐ White ☐ Indian ☐ Other
9. Area of residence
9.1 City/town/village
9.2 Postal code 9.3 How long at this address? ☐ years
Please record place of birth if not the same as current address
9.4 City/town/village
9.5 Postal code

B. RISK FACTOR PROFILE

10. Usual occupation of patient (if retired, give type of work done for most of working life)
11. Type of industry/business (eg mining, farming etc)
12. Did the patient ever smoke tobacco? ☐ Yes ☐ No ☐ Unknown
13. Did the patient ever consume alcohol regularly? (that is, more than once a week) ☐ Yes ☐ No ☐ Unknown
14. HIV status ☐ Negative ☐ Positive ☐ Unknown

C. CLINICAL AND LABORATORY DETAILS

15. Date of diagnosis
16. Cancer diagnosis and Histology 17. ICD-10
Please give all information available on the site.

Fig. 3.1 Cancer registration form

Parkin DM (2006) The evolution of the population-based cancer registry. Nat Rev Cancer 6(8):603–612

Parkin DM (2008) The role of cancer registries in cancer control. Int J Clin Oncol 13(2):102–111

Parkin DM, Bray F (2009) Evaluation of data quality in the cancer registry: principles and methods Part II. Completeness. Eur J Cancer 45(5):756–764

Parkin DM et al (1998) International incidence of childhood cancer, vol 2. IARC Scientific, Lyon

Stefan DC, Galindo CR (2014) Pediatric hematology oncology in countries with limited resources—a practical guide. Springer, New York

Stefan DC, Stones DK (2013) Children with cancer and HIV infection: what is different about them? J Pediatr Hematol Oncol 35(8):590–596

Chapter 4
Organization of Care for Children with Cancer in Africa

The establishment of a pediatric oncology unit must fulfill the needs of the community and obey the rules of good practice for appropriate diagnostic and therapeutic support.

The complexity and the risks associated with a pediatric oncology unit require suitable facility, specialized skills, and multidisciplinary team capacity. The unit should implement a program of continuous evaluation of its practice and be open to its medical environment as well as parents' or volunteers' associations. Implementation of a pediatric oncology unit should at best be integrated within the framework of a national or regional cancer plan.

Prerequisite to Put in Place Pediatric Oncology Unit

Before putting in place a unit, it is necessary to ensure that this activity will be large enough to allow the team to acquire appropriate experience. To do this, 50 new cancer cases per year appear to be a minimum to develop sufficient expertise and form a reliable tertiary care facility for children with cancer. Therefore, it is necessary to have an estimation of epidemiology of childhood cancer in the serving area. There must also be a commitment from the health authorities, and if possible, non governmental organizations (NGOs) to support this activity through the provision of minimal required resources.

D.C. Stefan, M. Harif, *Pediatric Cancer in Africa*,
DOI 10.1007/978-3-319-17936-0_4

Human Resources

Human resources must be adapted to the expected activity. The health care team must include full-time doctors and nurses trained in pediatric oncology. The team should be able to meet the demand for urgent situations as well as planned activity.

Physicians should be trained in clinical oncology in children, in prescription and monitoring of chemotherapy and in supportive care. Nurses must also be trained in pediatric oncology, in the preparation and administration of chemotherapy and supportive care. The training should address theoretical and practical issues.

It is important to have in the team a social worker, psychologist, physiotherapist, and nutritionist.

Required Hospital Environment

The pediatric oncology unit can be in a children's hospital (preferably), in an oncology or a hematology centre. In cases where the pediatric oncology unit is outside a children's hospital, it is important to ensure easy access to intensive care unit, radiology, and laboratory. The best location for a pedaitric oncology unit is in a university hospital in order to contribute to the training of young doctors and nurses in that specialty. The unit should be organized in subunits including inpatient unit, a day care unit, and an outpatient clinic.

The inpatient ward should have at least 8–10 beds and be sufficiently large to avoid the crowding of patients and parents. It should be separated from units for patients with other conditions that may constitute a risk of infection for children undergoing chemotherapy. The hospital should strive on offering the possibility of hosting one of the parents if the child or his parents wish so. In Africa, special attention should be given to hygiene requirements (Fig. 4.1).

Day care unit should be put in place because in the majority of cases, initial evaluation, treatment with chemotherapy or supportive care does not require inpatient admission (Fig. 4.2). This reduces the risks associated with hospitalization and also costs and also helps to maintain the child in his family environment.

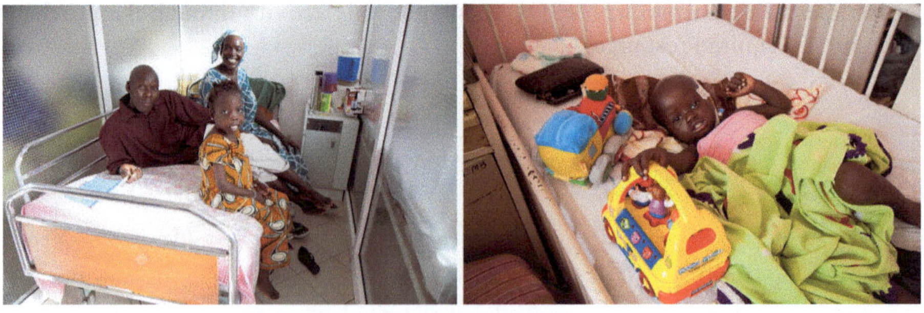

Fig. 4.1 Inpatient facility in sub-Saharan Africa

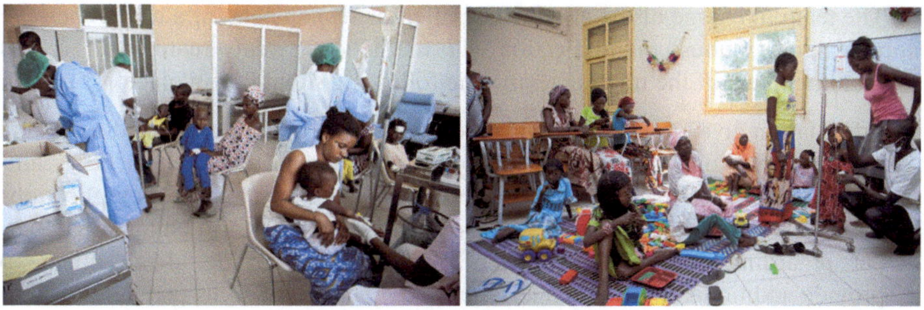

Fig. 4.2 Day care clinic and playroom in sub-Saharan unit

It is also important to have *an intensive care unit* for children within the department or within the hospital where children can be admitted.

The hospital should have resources for diagnosis and prognosis needed for patient's evaluation. These resources must be adapted to specific needs of cancers in children.

Clinical laboratory is of critical importance for appropriate care.

- The hematology laboratory should routinely perform CBC with differential and hemostasis tests and also cytological studies of blood and bone marrow smears. Cytological analysis of masses or lymph nodes fine needle aspiration is also important for diagnostic approach.
- Biochemistry, bacteriology/virology, and parasitology evaluation should be available.
- Radiology department adequately equipped for Xrays, ultrasound, CT scan and ideally other more sophisticated radiological investigations (such as MRI).
- A pathology laboratory adequtely equipped for basic routine investigations (complete blood count, electrolytes analysis, liver function tests, renal function tests, etc).

Other specialized tests will add value to the diagnostic and later to the follow up of the patient.

Additional services must be available to ensure proper care and include:

- Pediatric surgery.
- Pediatric intensive care.
- Radiotherapy adapted for children.
- Blood bank facility.

Functional Organization of Cancer Care

Care for children with cancer is complex and requires a multidisciplinary team. Treatment protocols used are specialized and designed for children. Many protocols are specific for different age groups and also adapted according to the existing resources.

The team in charge of the care of the patient is responsible for a comprehensive approach, continuous communication with the patient/parents/guardian as well as with all members of the treating team. The following should be in place:

- Information given to child and his parents or guardian regarding the disease and its treatment at diagnosis and during follow-up. This information must be streamlined and given so that the diagnosis, prognosis, treatment, and its complications are well understood. Special effort should be given to inform children and parents regarding preventive measures of hygiene. The team should be available to provide additional information as requested by the child or his parents or guardian at all times. This information should be preferably be given by the doctor who is in charge of the patient and who coordinates the care and complemented by a nurse, a social worker, and other resources.
- Treatment of patients according to validated national or international protocols and adapted to the context of care. These protocols must be understood and should be adapted according to the specific needs of each case.
- Providing psychological and social support at different phases of care.
- Holding regular multidisciplinary meetings where documented observations should be discussed. These meetings are of crucial importance for decision-making adapted to each case, to coordinate decision-making as well as teaching opportunity of pediatric oncology for young physicians (Fig. 4.3).
- Preventing and treating immediate complications related to the disease and therapies and in particular the treatment of pain, tumor lysis syndrome, and nutritional support.

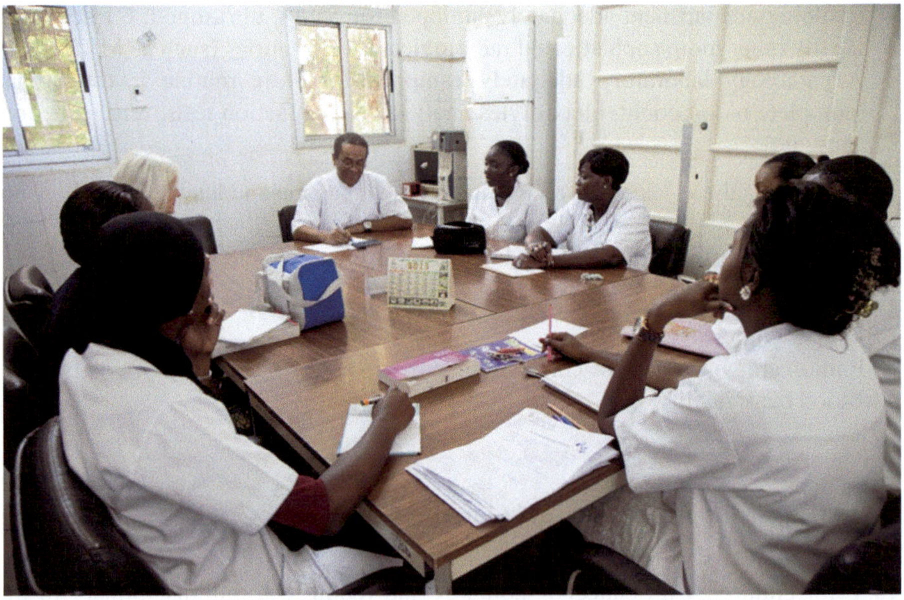

Fig. 4.3 Multidisciplinary team in Dakar

- Preventing and treating long-term complications related to the disease and therapies and especially neurocognitive functions, growth, fertility, cardiac, respiratory, and kidney function. Methods of administration and cumulative doses of radiotherapy and medications must always be assessed in terms of risk–benefit.
- Adapting care so as to reduce the length of hospital stay and trying as much as possible to maintain a social life of the child and in particular his/her schooling.
- Develop a research program in compliance with the principles of ethics.

Integration to Regional, National, or International Programs

The unit must participate in the cancer awareness programs for caregivers and for general population in order to improve early diagnosis. The team should also work on developing a network of care and satellite units in order to provide as much as possible care near the dwelling place of the family.

The unit must also develop professional relationships with other similar units and collaborative work to improve the quality of care and actively participate in continuing education.

Parent Associations

Associations of parents have a major impact in improving support for children with cancer. They contribute significantly to the awareness of childhood cancer in the community. They can provide assistance to improve access to care for children. The parents and parents' associations raise funds to build lodges for parents and children in the vecinity of the hospital. In this way the family can remain for longer period of time close to the unit in order for the child to complete his/her treatment. These various actions have a significant impact in adherence to treatment reducing the number of children lost to follow up and in improving the quality of life of children and their parents.

Health Care Team and Burnout

Doctors and nurses treating daily children diagnosed with cancer , offering emotional support to the patients and their families could found themselves affected by the intensity of the process, by the multitude of various others factors as well as sometimes the unexpected evolution of the disease. The long number of hours working without any breaks or so much needed psychological support, the continuous confrontation with unplanned complications, the very fine line between death and life will add to the major stress which the medical team experiences constantly in their fight against cancer and in their efforts of saving lives of their patients. The sense of emotional vacuum, physical, and mental exhaustion is the first phase of an exhaustion syndrome or "burnout" syndrome. A feeling of powerlessness to provide care settles with an impact on personal life followed eventually by a depression or a loss of the ability to concentrate. If appropriate measures are not taken a state of indifference to the suffering of the patients, a lack of involvement and irritability will eventually settle. The relation to the patients or parents may be dehumanized. At this stage, the absenteeism becomes frequent with a more or less well-expressed will to move to another ward. The main causes are related to cancer pathology in children and the needs of parents considering these caregivers as the last resort. Working environment plays a major role in the genesis of this syndrome. The gap between resources and needs, interpersonal conflicts, and rigid management can significantly contribute. Finally, the personality of the caregiver may predispose to this pathology in particular the difficulties of expression and participation, but also the lack of sharing moments of work fulfillment with the team.

The team and in particular the leaders of the team should strive to create a pleasant, rewarding working environment, in which caregivers have the opportunity to express their opinions and feelings. The leaders should also be able to identify risk situations and strive to help the vulnerable person by all means including temporary change of activity, permissions of temporary leave, and if necessary support of a psychologist. Relaxation techniques and stress management can also be helpful.

Practical Recommendations in Limited Resource Settings

- Ideally a new pediatric oncology unit should be placed within a tertiary hospital and in the vecinity of a medical university. It should serve the needs of the community and should be the referral centre for a larger area.
- A unit with a minimum of 30–50 new patients per year is required in order to develop the expertise desired.
- The location of the unit must take into account the needs of the multi-disciplinarity team treating the children with cancer. It is best located in a university hospital.
- Primary and continuous education program should be included in daily activities.
- The activity must ensure conventional hospitalization with an intensive care unit, a unit of day care and consultation rooms.
- Multidisciplinary coordination of the meetings and good, reliable and constant information for the children and their parents are necessary.
- A research and collaborative work activity must be strongly be considered.
- Parents associations play an important role helping the family with housing, emotional and financial support. They contribute to advocacy and increase in the awareness of childhood cancer in the society offering support to the children and their families as well as supporting also the medical team.

- In limited resource setting, international support and collaboration may have a great impact on the development of a pediatric cancer unit and improve the survival of the patients.
- A positive working atmosphere must be ensured in order to avoid burnout syndrome.

Suggested Selective Reading

American Academy of Pediatrics Guidelines for pediatric cancer centers (2004) Pediatrics 113:1833–1835

Murphy Positive SB (2010) Benefits of cooperative group membership: being part of a networked rapid learning. Syst Pediatr Blood Cancer 55:601–602

Spinetta JJ, Jankovic M, Ben Arush MW, Eden T et al (2000) Guidelines for the recognition, prevention, and remediation of burnout in health care professionals participating in the care of children with cancer: report of the SIOP Working Committee on psychosocial issues in pediatric oncology medical and pediatric oncology. Med Pediatr Oncol 35(2):122–215

Standards for pediatric cancer centers (2014) Pediatrics 134:410–414

Chapter 5
Hematological and Oncological Emergencies

Definition

Oncological emergencies are defined as acute and potentially life-threatening events that are directly or indirectly related to the underlying malignancy or occur as sequelae of its treatment. These events may rapidly result in permanent morbidity or the death of a patient if not anticipated, quickly recognized, and effectively treated.

Respiratory Emergencies

Case Presentation 1

A 9-year-old girl, previously well, presented with a 1-month history of shortness of breath which was attributed to a respiratory infection and asthma. The symptoms worsened, she developed chest pain on the left side, and subsequently she was admitted to hospital.

Findings on Examination

The patient did not look acutely ill, but complained of chest pain.

D.C. Stefan, M. Harif, *Pediatric Cancer in Africa*,
DOI 10.1007/978-3-319-17936-0_5

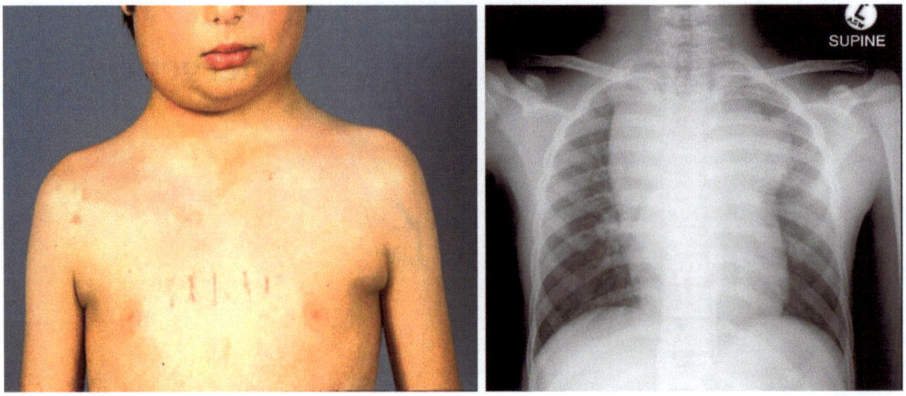

Fig. 5.1 Swollen neck and left side of chest, cervical and submandibular lymphadenopathy and mediastinal lymphadenopathy on chest X-ray

Apart from a respiratory rate of 35/min and a pulse rate of 100/min, her observations were normal. Normal anthropometry was noted. Pallor and mild periorbital edema was present. Her neck and left side of the chest appeared swollen (Fig. 5.1); no skin changes were noted. She had significant cervical and submandibular lymphadenopathy, more prominent on the right side, as well as axillary lymphadenopathy. On examination of the chest, decreased air entry was found on the left side with no adventitious sounds or dullness. Hepatosplenomegaly was present, but the rest of the examination was unremarkable. The chest X-ray showed a mediastinal mass (Fig. 5.1).

Which oncological emergency is most likely present?

This is most likely superior vena cava syndrome (SVCS), due to obstructive lymphadenopathy caused most often by acute (T lymphoblastic) leukemia/lymphoma.

Briefly describe the immediate investigations and management.

Provide supportive oxygen as needed; monitor patient closely.

Monitor intake and urine output.

Full blood and differential count, reticulocyte count and peripheral smear.

Biochemistry (electrolytes, renal function, calcium, magnesium, phosphate, uric acid, lactate dehydrogenase, and other liver enzymes).

Bone marrow aspiration and biopsy.

Choose the diagnostic modality that would confirm a diagnosis in the fastest way: fine needle aspiration for cytology and flow cytometry (if available) or lymph node biopsy and bone marrow biopsy.

Start hyperhydration and allopurinol to prevent/treat tumor lysis syndrome (TLS).

Table 5.1 Common mediastinal tumors in children

Anterior mediastinum
• Non-Hodgkin lymphoma
• Hodgkin disease
• Teratoma
• TB/Kaposi sarcoma
Middle mediastinum
• Lymphoma
• TB/Kaposi sarcoma
Posterior mediastinum
• Neuroblastoma

Superior Vena Cava Syndrome

SVCS or superior mediastinal syndrome (SMS) is a clinical phenomenon that develops when a mass lesion compresses and obstructs the great vessels and heart, especially the right ventricular outflow tract and therefore causes obstruction of the blood flow in the SVC. The collateral veins of the thorax, neck, and head become congested and cause the classical symptoms (see below). The term 'superior mediastinal syndrome' is used when the respiratory symptoms and compromise predominate the clinical picture.

In children, the most likely cause of SVCS is malignant tumors (Table 5.1). The so-called "terrible Ts"—T-cell lymphoblastic lymphoma, T-cell acute lymphoblastic leukemia, malignant teratoma, thyroid cancer, and thymoma—may all cause this syndrome. Other malignancies associated with SVCS include Kaposi sarcoma, Ewing sarcoma, rhabdomyosarcoma, and peripheral neuroectodermal tumor (PNET). In areas endemic for TB, one should always consider TB adenitis, which can also present with a similar clinical picture.

Clinical Presentation

The most common complaints are cough, facial swelling, dyspnea, and orthopnea. Low grade fever and weight loss may or may not be present. Other symptoms include headache, dizziness, visual disturbances, hoarseness, dysphagia, and fatigue. Symptoms worsen in the supine position and patients usually prefer to sit upright. Classical signs include plethora and edema of the head, neck and upper limbs, marked venous distension, laryngeal edema, stridor, wheezing, and anxiety. Significant lymphadenopathy is very often present and may give rise to swelling of the neck, as well as the suprasternal notch. On auscultation of the chest, reduced or absent air entry may be noted.

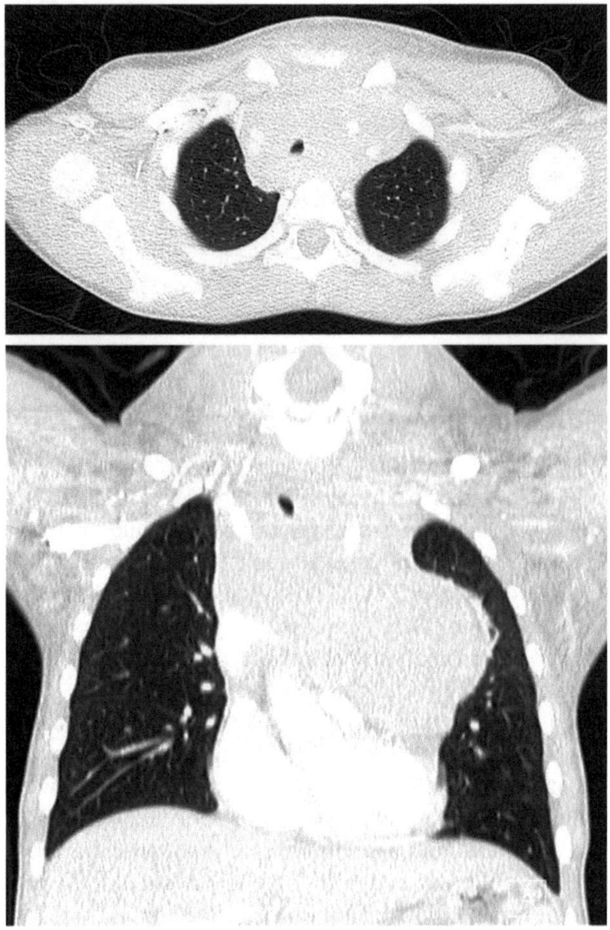

Fig. 5.2 CT chest showing a mediastinal mass and tracheal occlusion by the mass

Diagnosis

The diagnosis of SVCS is usually made clinically. In the majority of the cases, a chest X-ray shows a mediastinal mass or widening of the mediastinum. A pleural or pericardial effusion may be present. Rarely, the chest X-ray may be normal. Computed tomography (CT), if available and if the patient is able to tolerate a supine position, should be used to obtain detailed anatomical information, as well as to evaluate tracheal compression prior to decisions regarding sedation/anesthesia (Fig. 5.2).

Great caution has to be taken when transporting the patient to the radiology department. Ensure that he/she remains in the upright position. Positioning patients in a supine position for CT scan can be extremely risky and even fatal.

A diagnosis should be confirmed by using the least invasive and fastest method. If significant lymphadenopathy is present, a fine needle aspiration (FNA) may be performed if the local pathologist is experienced in the interpretation thereof. Flow cytometry should also be performed on the same specimen. This is usually adequate to confirm the diagnosis of T cell lymphoblastic lymphoma. Examination of the pleural fluid (chemistry, cytology, and flow cytometry) may also be performed. A bone marrow aspiration and biopsy should follow to make the distinction between T cell lymphoma and leukemia on the grounds of the blast percentage. If FNA cannot be performed, an urgent biopsy of the most accessible lymph node should be performed. If no superficial lymphadenopathy is present, a thoracic surgeon should perform a biopsy of the mediastinal mass.

Management

Patients with SVCS have a high risk of airway compromise and often present with life-threatening respiratory distress and stridor, necessitating admission to an intensive care unit. In some instances immediate emergency treatment may need to be given before a definitive diagnosis has been made.

The main aim is always to secure the airway of the patient. Oxygen should be provided via a face mask or rebreather mask and intravenous access should be obtained. A helpful measure to alleviate the respiratory distress is strict bed rest with the patient sitting in a left lateral decubitus position (this helps to "lift" the mass off the airways and right ventricular outflow tract). Inability to tolerate the supine position is an ominous sign and such patients should definitely be admitted to an intensive care unit.

Treatment

Considering that T cell lymphoblastic lymphoma/leukemia is the commonest cause for a mediastinal mass in a child, treatment should be directed against T lymphoblastic lymphoma/leukemia without waiting for a tissue biopsy if the patient's airway is compromised.

Empiric chemotherapy (cyclophosphamide, anthracyclines, vincristine, and prednisone as specified in the CHOP, BFM, or COG protocol) may be initiated. An alternative combination may be used, depending on the most probable diagnosis. The use of intravenous steroids (methylprednisolone 50 mg/m^2/day in 4 divided doses) may contribute to the reduction of the tumor size and rapidly decrease the severity of the clinical symptoms and signs.

Alternatively, radiotherapy (daily dose of 200–400 cGy) may be commenced. As most lymphomas are radiosensitive, improvement is usually seen within 18 hours. Radiation-induced edema might occur and can result in temporary worsening of symptoms and signs. Note that chemo- or radiotherapy could result in distortion of the histology, thus making it difficult to establish a definitive histological diagnosis.

Anticipate TLS in these patients and start hyperhydration and allopurinol as soon as possible. Monitor intake and urine output closely and repeat biochemistry at least twice a day if possible.

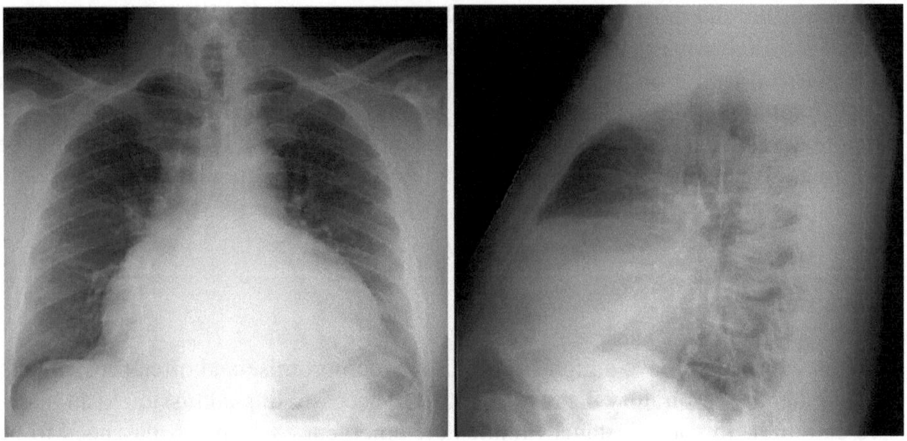

Fig. 5.3 Chest X-ray showing cardiomegaly with a globular heart shape

In critical airway compromise, AVOID sedation for procedures unless an anesthesiologist is present and prepared for a very difficult intubation and involve a pulmonologist/intensivist, if available.

Case Presentation 2

A 9-year-old boy presented with anxiety, restlessness, and a sharp pain in his neck, chest, and shoulder. The chest pain worsened with deep breathing or coughing and he was short of breath. He reported that his discomfort was relieved by sitting upright or leaning forward.

Findings on Examination

The boy appeared pale and gray and was tachypnoeic (rate 40/min). His heart rate was 140/min, his peripheral pulses were weak, and pulsus paradoxus was noted. Distended neck veins were present. The apex was found in the 6th intercostal space lateral to the midline. His heart sounds were very soft and a pericardial rub was heard. The chest X-ray is shown in Fig. 5.3.

Pericardial Effusion/Cardiac Tamponade

Pericardial effusion is an important oncological emergency in children. It is seen with a variety of tumors including lymphomas and metastatic solid tumors. It is often asymptomatic and incidentally observed on a chest X-ray performed to evaluate the lungs or diagnosed as an incidental finding at autopsy.

Inflammation of the pericardium or obstruction of lymphatic drainage from the pericardium of any etiology causes an increase in fluid volume, referred to as a pericardial effusion.

Malignant involvement of the pericardium may be primary (less common) or secondary (spreading from a nearby or distant focus of malignancy). Secondary neoplasms can involve the pericardium by contiguous extension from a mediastinal mass, nodular tumor deposits from hematogenous or lymphatic spread, and diffuse pericardial thickening from tumor infiltration (with and without effusion). In diffuse pericardial thickening the heart may be encased by constrictive pericarditis.

Cardiac Tamponade

Cardiac tamponade is the inability of the ventricle to maintain cardiac output because of extrinsic pressure caused by a mediastinal or an intrinsic mass. It is the most serious consequence of a pericardial effusion, when the accumulation of fluid compresses the heart chambers and results in a reduction of venous return and decrease in cardiac output.

In pediatric patients, cardiac tamponade results from a malignant or reactive pericardial effusion. It is not a common condition and to date only 9 cases have been reported as result of acute myeloid leukemia (3 patients) and one each of acute lymphoblastic leukemia, Hodgkin lymphoma, B-cell lymphoma, medulloblastoma, desmoplastic small round cell tumor, and rhabdomyosarcoma.

Clinical Presentation

Symptoms are similar to those of heart failure and include shortness of breath as the main symptom, cough, palpitations, and chest pain improved by sitting, as well as nonspecific abdominal pain.

On examination, the main findings are jugular venous distension, pulsus paradoxus, soft heart sounds, pericardial rub, and signs of low cardiac output, namely tachycardia with hypotension and poor peripheral perfusion.

Diagnosis

A chest X-ray shows cardiomegaly and an ECG demonstrates low voltage QRS complexes and flattened or inverted T waves. Echocardiography is the best investigation, showing pericardial effusion and atrial or ventricular collapse with hemodynamic compromise.

Treatment

The treatment of choice is percutaneous catheter drainage under electrocardiographic or fluoroscopic guidance. While that is being arranged, an emergency pericardial tap to relieve symptoms can be performed in the ward at the bedside. This has to be done slowly to drain just enough fluid to avoid circulatory collapse. Fluid should be sent for cytology. Once the underlying malignancy is treated, the pericardial effusion will resolve.

Case Presentation 3

An 8-year-old boy, previously treated for T lymphoblastic lymphoma, presented with a 1-month history of shortness of breath and right-sided chest pain.

Findings on Examination

The patient appeared acutely ill. He was tachypnoeic with a respiratory rate of 40/min and tachycardic (pulse rate 110/min). The oxygen saturation in room air was 85 %. There was decreased expansion of the right hemithorax and the trachea was displaced to the left. Stony dullness of the right hemithorax was found, as well as no air entry. The chest X-ray is shown in Fig. 5.4.

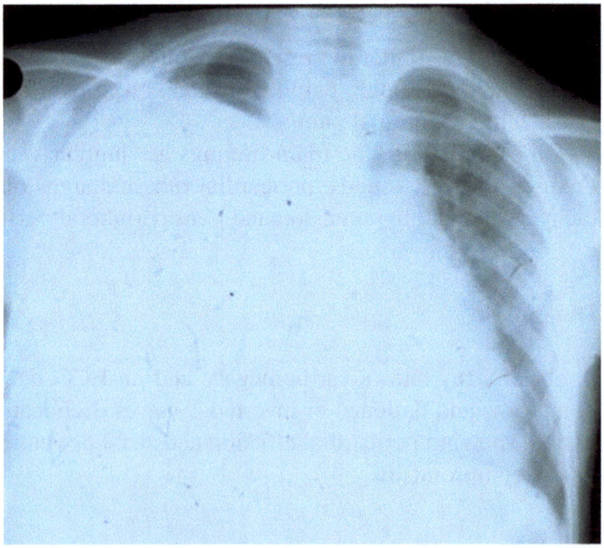

Fig. 5.4 Dense, homogenous opacification of right hemithorax with the mediastinum displaced to the left

Malignant Pleural Effusion

Pleural effusions are often seen in children. Pulmonary tuberculosis frequently presents with a pleural effusion and pneumonia is often complicated by the development thereof. It is also often seen in lymphoma, especially non-Hodgkin lymphoma. Pleuropulmonary blastoma, metastatic sarcoma, and nephroblastoma, as well as Kaposi sarcoma, are other examples of malignancies that can cause effusions. Nonmalignant causes include SVCS, cardiac tamponade, chylothorax, empyema, congestive cardiac failure, and hypoalbuminemia among others. Several antineoplastic agents such as methotrexate, procarbazine, cyclophosphamide, and bleomycin have been reported to cause pleural effusion. Although pleural effusion is not life-threatening, sizeable and rapid accumulation of fluid can compress lung parenchyma leading to respiratory insufficiency.

Clinical Presentation

Symptoms are related more to the rate of pleural fluid accumulation rather than to the total volume of fluid. The most common symptoms are dyspnea, orthopnea, cough, and pleuritic chest pain. The presence of fever suggests atelectasis and/or infection.

Diagnosis

A chest X-ray (anteroposterior and lateral), including a lateral decubitus chest film, is useful in confirming the presence of a pleural effusion. Ultrasonography, and CT where available, is useful in differentiating fluid from a solid mass, especially if a pleural tap and/or biopsy is planned.

Treatment

A diagnostic and therapeutic thoracocentesis (pleural tap) is indicated in patients presenting with respiratory distress. Initially drainage can be performed manually using a large bore needle, attached to a three-way stopcock, and a large volume syringe. This is followed by insertion of tube for more complete drainage. Chemotherapy is initiated once a definitive diagnosis is made.

Case Presentation 4

A 10-year-old girl, previously treated for nephroblastoma, presents with shortness of breath for 3 weeks. She also developed noisy breathing for the past few days.

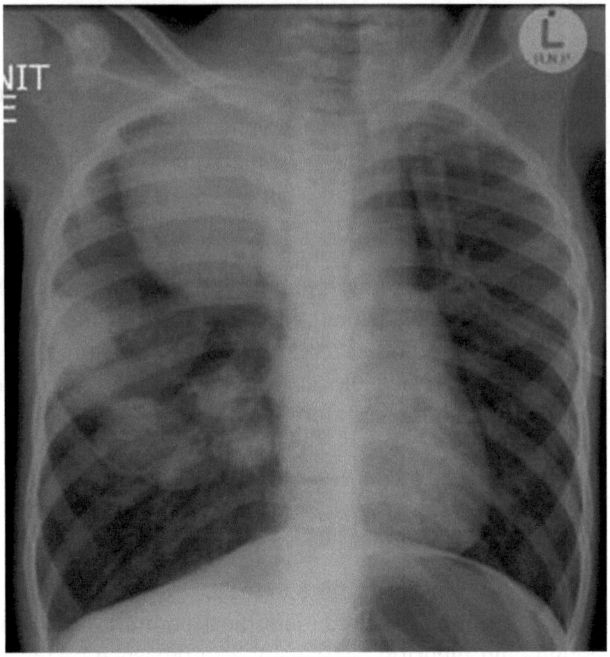

Fig. 5.5 Several round areas of opacification in the right lung with displacement of the trachea and mediastinum

Findings on Examination

On physical examination the patient was apyrexial, but acutely ill and short of breath (respiratory rate of 42/min) with a pulse rate of 133/min and oxygen saturation of 87 % in room air. The trachea was displaced to the left and there was reduced air entry and stony dullness in the right upper zone. Signs of hyperinflation were also noted. The chest X-ray is shown in Fig. 5.5.

Central Airway Compression Syndrome

Airway obstruction is divided into proximal or large airway obstruction (upper airway) or distal (lower) airway obstruction. Mediastinal tumors are a common cause of upper and lower airway obstruction in children with cancer; often also causing SVCS. Kaposi sarcoma is becoming an increasingly common cause of lower airways obstruction.

Clinical Presentation

The clinical manifestations, investigations, and management are similar to that discussed under SVCS.

Treatment

Supportive care (oxygen, positioning, intravenous fluid, monitoring, etc.) should be provided while the diagnosis is being confirmed in the least invasive and fastest way. As in SVCS, treatment may need to be initiated without histological/cytological confirmation of a diagnosis.

Neurological Emergency

Case Presentation

An 8-year-old girl, previously well, presented with a 4-week history of backache and weakness of her legs that led to a fall at school.

Findings on Examination

The girl did not appear acutely or chronically ill. Her observations were normal. She was unable to move her legs (power 1/5) and had increased tone and reflexes in both legs with a Babinski plantar response. A sensory level could be elicited at the level of ±T10. The rest of the examination was unremarkable. An urgent MRI was requested and the images can be seen in Fig. 5.6.

Spinal Cord Compression

Compression of the spinal cord is a medical emergency, because early diagnosis and intervention are critical to preserve and potentially restore neurological function. Tumor compression and associated vasogenic edema of the cord within the rigid space of the spinal canal result in injury of the spinal cord neurons. A variety of solid tumors and about 0.4 % of patients with leukemia can present with spinal cord compression (SCC). In children, the thoracic vertebral segment is most often affected, but it can occur at any site. Tumor invasion of vertebral bodies resulting in collapse can also compromise the spinal cord.

Clinical Presentation

Compression of the spinal cord may present with a long history of nonspecific complaints, i.e. pain and constipation. The most common symptom, however, is back pain, occurring in 80 % of children with SCC. It may occur at any level of the spine

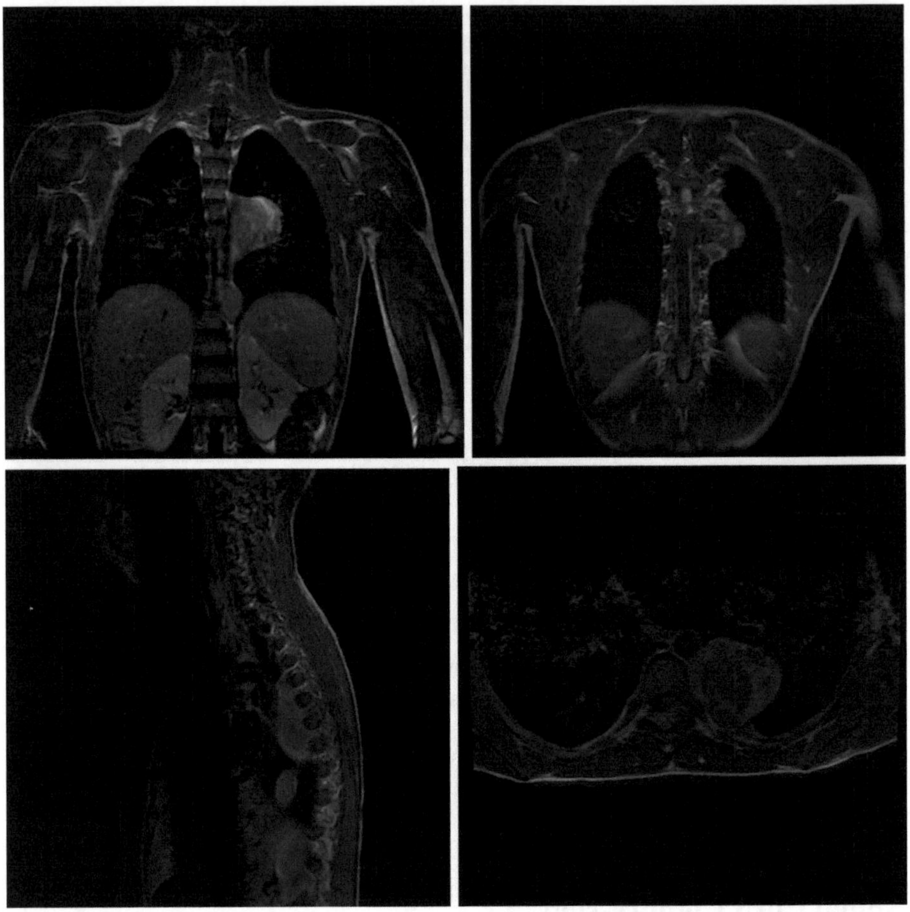

Fig. 5.6 Solid paraspinal mass with intradural extension at T10

and may worsen with movement, straight-leg raising, neck flexion, or the Valsalva maneuver. Partial or complete weakness of an extremity is a worrying complaint. Incontinence develops late due to a neurogenic bladder. Other common signs include tingling, paresthesia, numbness, and radicular pain. Power is usually symmetrically reduced, but asymmetry is also possible, even rarely monoplegia. Sensory deficits are difficult to elicit in younger children, but a sensory level is indicative of a spinal cord lesion. Deep tendon reflexes are increased, an extensor plantar response is seen, and clonus or other signs of an upper motor neuron lesion may be noted.

Diagnosis and Treatment

Patients should be evaluated promptly, since this is a medical emergency. Early consultation with a neurosurgeon, radiation oncologist, and neurologist should be obtained. An urgent MRI should be performed whenever possible, because X-rays and CT scans are not sensitive enough to identify the SCC.

To reduce spinal cord edema, intravenous high dose corticosteroids (dexamethasone 1–2 mg/kg) should be given as soon as the diagnosis is considered, followed by lower doses (0.25–0.5 mg/kg every 6 h) when the diagnosis has been established. Chemotherapy and radiotherapy may be considered in patients with newly diagnosed cancers that are known to be chemo/radiosensitive. Decompression surgery is indicated for patients where the diagnosis is unknown or if chemotherapy or radiotherapy is not readily available.

Hematological Emergency

Case Presentation

A 2-year 6-month-old boy presented with shortness of breath and coughing. On physical examination he was acutely ill; his respiratory rate was 35/min and temperature 37.8 °C. Pallor, petechiae, and echymoses were noted on his skin. He also had generalized lymphadenopathy, hepatomegaly of 4 cm, and splenomegaly of 9 cm.

His full blood count result was as follows:

White cell count	Hemoglobin	Platelets	Neutrophils	Blasts
419×10^9/L	7.3 g/dL	29×10^9/L	4.19×10^9/L	80 %

Leukostasis and Hyperleukocytosis

Hyperleukocytosis is present when the peripheral white cell count (WCC) exceeds 50 or 100 x 10^9/L and is a result of blast formation in patients with leukemia. When white blood cell plugs develops in the microvasculature, it is called leukostasis or symptomatic hyperleukocytosis.

Clinical Presentation

Patients may be asymptomatic or present with symptoms related to the involvement of the central nervous system and/or lungs. Symptoms and signs may include headache, seizures, altered mental status, weakness, papilledema, shortness of breath, hypoxemia, and right heart failure.

Treatment

Symptomatic hyperleukocytosis is a medical emergency. Urgent measures need to be taken to stabilize the patient and to decrease the WCC. Induction chemotherapy can achieve rapid cytoreduction, but there is a significant risk that TLS may develop, thus preventative measures for TLS must be instituted.

Metabolic Emergencies

Case Presentation 1

A 1-year 9-month-old girl presented with a 2-week history of fever, thought to be due to an upper respiratory infection, as well as abdominal distention. She did not respond to two courses of oral antibiotics prescribed by the GP.

Findings on Examination

The patient was acutely ill and pallor, petechiae, and generalized lymphadenopathy were noted. Her abdominal examination revealed hepatomegaly of 4 cm and splenomegaly of 3 cm. Her blood results were as follows:

Full Blood count

White cell count	Hemoglobin	Platelets	Neutrophils	Blasts
130×10^9/L	8.5 g/dL	76×10^9/L	11.8×10^9/L	85 %

Biochemistry

Sodium 142 mmol/L (135–147)	Potassium **5.8** mmol/L **H** (3.4–4.7)	Urea **17.6** mmol/L **H** (1.1–5.0)	Creatinine **267** µmol/L **H** (15–31)
Corrected calcium **1.98** mmol/L **L** (2.12–2.59)	Phosphate **2.74** mmol/L **H** (1.10–1.95)	Magnesium 0.90 mmol/L (0.70–0.95)	Uric acid **>0.89** mmol/L **H** (0.12–0.32)

Tumor Lysis Syndrome

This is an oncological emergency which is caused by massive tumor cell breakdown with the release of large amounts of potassium, phosphate, and nucleic acids into the systemic circulation. It occurs most commonly in children with acute leukemia or lymphoma after initiation of treatment, but can occur in any bulky tumor or even spontaneously before treatment is started.

The breakdown of tumor cells causes the release of potassium, phosphate, and DNA, which is metabolized into uric acid. The hyperuricemia can lead to renal injury with oliguria, fluid overload, pulmonary edema, hypoxia, cerebral edema, and death. The resultant hyperphosphatemia, hyperkalemia, and hypocalcemia can lead to further renal injury, dysrhythmias, and cardiac arrest. The diagnosis is usually made after demonstration of hyperuricemia, hyperkalemia, hyperphosphatemia, and hypocalcemia.

Symptoms and Signs

Clinical signs are caused by the associated metabolic abnormalities and include nausea, vomiting, diarrhea, anorexia, lethargy, hematuria, heart failure, cardiac dysrhythmias, seizures, muscle cramps, tetany, syncope, and sudden death.

Management

Prevention is the best strategy and is achieved by giving hyperhydration and allopurinol to patients who are at risk of developing TLS.

Hyperhydration

Rapid volume expansion (2–3 L/m^2 daily) to achieve normal blood pressure and urine output is indicated, since precipitation of uric acid, xanthine, and phosphate causes renal injury in TLS. Fluid intake and output should be monitored closely; urethral catheterization may be helpful in some patients. The urine output should be kept above 100 mL/m^2/h. Mannitol and furosemide may be considered only once the patient has achieved adequate intravascular volume in order to maintain adequate urine output.

Hyperuricemia

Rasburicase (0.2 mg/kg single dose) should be used, when available, for patients with hyperuricemia. If not available, allopurinol should be used. Urine alkalinization has been used in the past, because uric acid is more soluble in alkaline conditions, but this approach has fallen out of favor and is not advised in patients with TLS.

Hyperkalemia

Hyperkalemia can develop rapidly and lead to dysrhythmia and sudden death. Patients with or at risk of TLS should be monitored closely with continuous cardiac monitoring and frequent electrolyte measurements (6–12 hourly if possible). Potassium-free intravenous fluids should be used. Potassium exchange resins should be used for patients with serum potassium levels ≥6 mEq/L or for symptomatic hyperkalemia. Kayexalate (polystyrene sulfate) at a dosage of 0.25–0.5 g/kg every 6 hours orally or rectally may be used.

Cardioprotective agents should be used for patients with ECG abnormalities or potassium levels>6.5 mEq/L: sodiumbicarbonate ($NaHCO_3$) at 0.5 mEq/kg over 10–15 minutes, followed by 10 % calcium gluconate solution at 0.5 mL/kg over 5–10 minutes. These measures help to move the potassium into the intracellular space, but the effect is only temporary and should only be used until the potassium levels are reduced by Kayexalate and forced diuresis with hyperhydration and furosemide or dialysis. Other potassium-shifting agents may also be indicated, e.g. glucose, insulin, furosemide, and salbutamol.

Hyperphosphatemia and Hypocalcemia

Oral aluminum hydroxide or calcium carbonate (Titralac) taken together with meals can control hyperphosphatemia. Patients with asymptomatic hypocalcemia can be managed with oral calcium carbonate, but symptomatic patients should receive 10 % calcium gluconate 0.5 mL/kg over 5–10 min intravenously. Hypocalcemia cases unrelated to TLS should receive calcium supplementation and vitamin D.

Case Presentation 2

A 12-year-old girl presented with progressive neck swelling. Bilateral cervical lymphadenopathy was found. The rest of the examination was unremarkable. Histology confirmed the diagnosis of Hodgkin lymphoma and on her blood results her serum calcium levels were 5.15 mmol/L (normal values: 2.05–2.56 mmol/L).

Hypercalcemia

Hypercalcemia is the most common life-threatening metabolic complication of malignancy in adults, but rarely occurs in children with cancer. It may be potentially fatal. It has been reported in leukemias, lymphomas, and solid tumors such as rhabdomyosarcoma, neuroblastoma, and Wilms tumor. It can be present at the initial diagnosis of the cancer as for example in acute lymphoblastic leukemia, or it can occur during treatment of relapsed disease. Some patients might have several episodes of hypercalcemia.

Mild hypercalcemia is defined as a total serum calcium of <12 mg/dL, moderate hypercalcemia is 12.0–13.5, and severe hypercalcemia is >13.5 mg/dL.

The mechanism is related to increased local release of skeletal calcium caused by direct erosion of the bone, as well as the release of local and systemic endocrine factors. These interfere with bone metabolism, renal calcium clearance, and intestinal absorption of calcium.

Clinical Presentation

Symptoms of hypercalcemia are dependent on both the serum level of calcium and the rate of the rise. With mild hypercalcemia, patients are usually asymptomatic. When moderate hypercalcemia is present, weakness, anorexia, constipation, polyuria, and polydipsia due to intravascular volume contraction usually develop. Severe hypercalcemia can manifest as a life-threatening metabolic emergency with cardiac and central nervous system effects including encephalopathy, seizure, and coma.

Signs

There are usually no specific physical signs. The patient may appear drowsy and confused and may have signs of dehydration.

Diagnosis

The diagnosis is made on the basis of a raised serum calcium.

Treatment

There are two components to the treatment: correction of dehydration and establishing good urine flow, as well as specific therapy to reduce calcium levels.

Moderate Hypercalcemia

Use intravenous hydration with normal saline (3000 mL/m^2/day) and encourage a high oral fluid intake to promote calcium excretion. Intravenous furosemide (1–2 mg/kg 6–8 hourly) blocks the reabsorption of calcium in the ascending limb of Henle. Regular electrolyte monitoring should be performed.

Severe Hypercalcemia

Intravenous hyperhydration (6000 mL/m^2 per day) should be given. Use furosemide as described above. Calcitonin and a bisphosphonate have been used in refractory cases. Experience with the use of bisphosphonates such as pamidronate and zoledronate in children is limited, so these are not generally recommended. Dialysis (either peritoneal or hemodialysis) is used in patients who are not responding to initial therapy.

Gastroenterological Emergency

Case Presentation 1

A 12-year-old boy diagnosed with acute myeloid leukemia (AML), presented with pain in his mouth, throat, and stomach about 7–10 days after the start of an intensive phase of his chemotherapy. He refused to eat or drink and also had loose stools. On physical examination he was drooling; redness, swelling, and sores were seen in his mouth.

Mucositis

Oral mucositis is the most frequent and severe complication of chemotherapy and radiotherapy occurring in approximately 65 % of children with cancer. Very often the whole gastrointestinal tract, including the esophagus, is affected. It is a painful and distressing experience affecting the quality of life and often leading to hospitalization for hydration or pain control. Food consumption is limited due to pain and inability to chew; the intestinal absorptive surface is reduced, thus increasing the risk of malnutrition. Mucositis in an immunocompromised individual facilitates the entry of microorganisms into the submucosa, which can cause systemic infection. In addition, oral mucositis has become a dose limiting toxicity, leading to a delay in the administration of chemotherapy. Several chemotherapy drugs such as high dose methotrexate at 1 g/m^2 or higher, procarbazine, daunorubicin, doxorubicin, cytarabine, etoposide, and 5-fluorouracil are well known for causing mucositis. Common

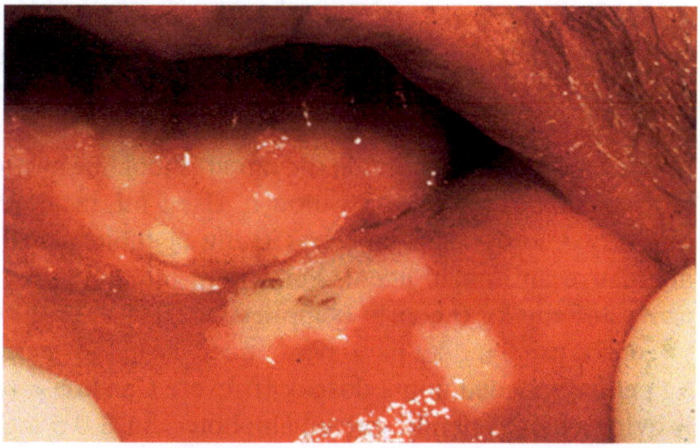

Fig. 5.7 Mucositis

organisms are Candida species and herpes simplex virus (HSV). These organisms are often present simultaneously (Fig. 5.7).

Clinical Presentation

Symptoms occur about 7–10 days after the start of chemotherapy and lasts 5–7 days after the treatment ends: pain in the mouth, throat, or stomach, redness, swelling, or sores in the mouth, throat, or rectum, drooling, refusal to eat or drink, and diarrhea.

Prevention and Treatment

Although there are several potentially useful therapies that have been suggested to be of benefit to patients suffering from mucositis, the evidence for efficacy for the majority of these therapies is not rigorous enough to support a definitive recommendation. However, the use of oral hygiene measures and good oral health status at the onset of therapy are critical in reducing the risk of severe mucositis and its subsequent complications.

Some commonly used preventive measures include good oral hygiene and the use of 0.1 % chlorhexidine gluconate mouth wash. Patients with dental caries should preferably be referred to the dentist before chemotherapy is started.

Treatment

Good oral and dental hygiene is important: the mouth and teeth should be cleaned gently and frequently using a soft bristle tooth brush. The mouth should be rinsed often with nonalcoholic rinses, antibacterial rinses, saline, or plain sterile water. An oral hospital mouth wash as prepared by the local pharmacist may be used. Use pain medication, but avoid the use of antipyretics to avoid masking a fever. Do not use aspirin due to an increased risk of bleeding. Treat infection with intravenous antibiotics. If Candida is suspected, various treatment options are available. Firstly, nystatin oral suspension 1–2 mL 6 hourly (swish and swallow) may be prescribed; in infants and young children the mouth should be swabbed with the suspension and they should be allowed to swallow it. Use 5 mL in adolescents to swish and swallow 6 hourly. Clotrimazole troche 250 mg (1 tablet) sublingually 5 times daily is an alternative antifungal agent. For severe infection, use oral or intravenous fluconazole 3–6 mg/kg 6 hourly (supplied as 50, 100 or 200 mg tablets). For refractory infection, use 5 mg/kg per day, rounded up to the nearest 50 mg (maximum 10 mg/kg per day divided into 2 doses). If severe Candida esophagitis is present and there is evidence of systemic spread, amphotericin B 0.5 mg/kg per day IV may be used for a minimum of 7 days. In cases of herpes simplex mucositis or esophagitis, acyclovir should be prescribed. Topical agents may be used, if available.

Maintain good nutritional intake, encourage plenty of oral fluids, offer soft pureed food, and serve food cold or at room temperature.

Case Presentation 2

An 8-year-old boy, known with relapsed ALL and on second line chemotherapy, presented with watery and bloody diarrhea, fever, nausea, vomiting, and abdominal pain localized to the right lower quadrant about 12 days after an intensive chemotherapy cycle.

Findings on Examination

The patient was febrile and looked acutely ill. Abdominal distension was present, as well as tenderness in the right lower quadrant and absence of bowel sounds. The abdominal X-ray showed an abnormal gas pattern, free air under the diaphragm and no air in the rectum (Fig. 5.8).

Typhlitis

Typhlitis (from the Greek word typhlon, or cecum), also known as neutropenic enterocolitis, is clinically defined by the triad of neutropenia, abdominal pain, and fever. It occurs most commonly in individuals with hematological malignancies such as leukemia and myelodysplastic syndrome, who are neutropenic and have

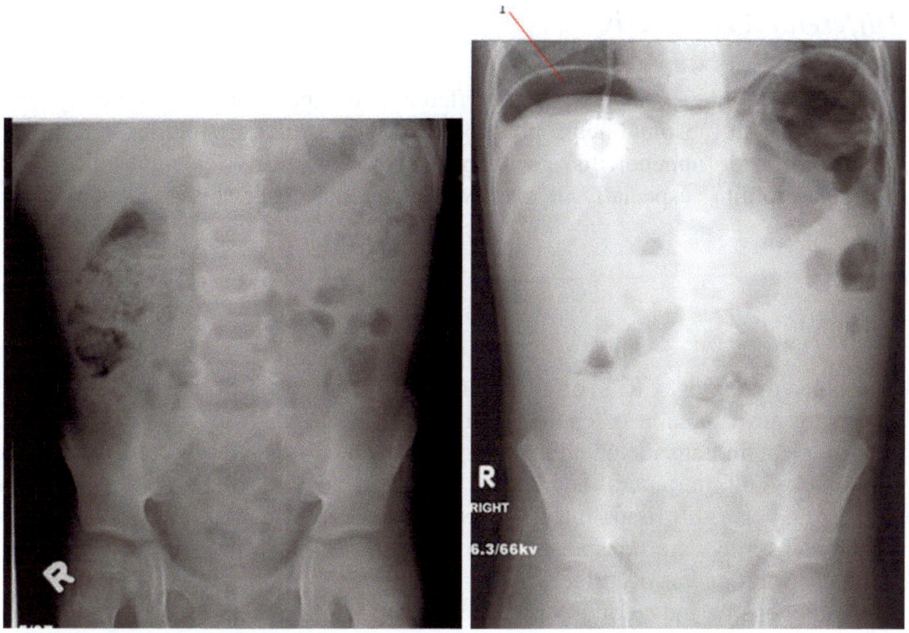

Fig. 5.8 Abnormal gas pattern; free air under the diaphragm; no air in the rectum

breakdown of gut mucosal integrity as a result of cytotoxic drugs. There is inflammation and/or necrosis of the bowel wall. The cecum is almost always affected and the process often extends into the ascending colon and terminal ileum. The bowel wall is infiltrated by various bacteria (gram negative and positive), anaerobes, and/or fungal organisms, e.g., Clostridium and Candida species. Bacteremia or fungemia commonly occur.

Clinical Presentation

Typical symptoms include the following: watery or bloody diarrhea, fever, nausea, vomiting, and abdominal pain which may be localized to the right lower quadrant. Shock could be present secondary to septicemia or colonic perforation. The symptoms often appear 10–14 days after cytotoxic drugs were administered, at a time when neutropenia is most profound and the patient is febrile. The clinical signs are abdominal distension, absence of bowel sounds, tympany, and tenderness, which is usually most prominent in the right lower quadrant. Occasionally there is a palpable mass. Diffuse abdominal pain and rebound tenderness suggests perforation and peritonitis.

Differential Diagnosis

Typhlitis should be considered in the differential diagnosis of any profoundly neutropenic patient (absolute neutrophil count <500 cells/μL). Conditions that mimic typhlitis include appendicitis, pseudomembranous colitis, ischemic colitis, and amoebic typhlitis, especially in areas where amoebic liver abscess is commonly diagnosed.

Diagnosis

Computed tomography (CT) or ultrasonography can be used. Some studies promote CT as the investigation of choice, while others state that ultrasound is superior. Radiological findings include fluid-filled dilated and distended cecum, diffuse cecal wall thickening, intramural edema, air or hemorrhage, localized perforation with free air and/or a soft tissue mass suggesting abscess formation. Findings on plain abdominal X-rays are nonspecific and often not useful in investigating typhlitis, unless perforation has occurred.

Barium enema and colonoscopy in a necrotic bowel in the presence of neutropenia and thrombocytopenia are relatively contraindicated, as they carry a high risk of perforation. Other investigations include blood and stool cultures and, if available, assays for Clostridium difficile toxin.

Treatment

In patients with uncomplicated typhlitis (i.e. no peritonitis, perforation, or severe bleeding), nonsurgical management is advised: bowel rest, nasogastric suction, intravenous fluids, and parenteral nutritional support. Supportive blood product transfusions are often required. Broad-spectrum antibiotics should be prescribed, with cover for Clostridium difficile, if pseudomembranous colitis has not been excluded. Consider adding an antifungal agent, i.e. amphotericin B, if fever persists for more than 72 hours despite broad spectrum antibiotics. Avoid anticholinergic, antidiarrheal, and opioid agents as they may aggravate ileus. Use of granulocyte colony-stimulating factor (G-CSF) should be considered. Delay further chemotherapy until the patient has recovered.

In patients with complicated typhlitis, surgical management is often indicated, e.g. a two-stage hemicolectomy with complete removal of all necrotic tissue.

Patients who develop typhlitis during chemotherapy are prone to this complication during subsequent treatments. Allow sufficient time for complete recovery before the next cycle of chemotherapy is started. Bowel decontamination before chemotherapy is resumed may be helpful.

Other Emergencies

Case Presentation 1

A 10-year-old boy, known with an embryonal rhabdomyosarcoma of the lower limb, presented with urgency, frequency, dysuria, and abdominal discomfort 3 days after receiving chemotherapy, including cyclophosphamide. He also complained that he was unable to empty his bladder.

Hemorrhagic Cystitis

Hemorrhagic cystitis, though uncommon, has a high mortality rate if not treated. It is mainly caused by chemotherapeutic agents like cyclophosphamide or ifosfamide (the urotoxin acrolein is a breakdown product of both drugs), as well as local regional radiotherapy.

Treatment

Hydration

There are no standard fluid instructions for the administration of cyclophosphamide or ifosfamide. Several protocols have different instructions, thus follow the specific protocol instructions. In general, before starting cyclophosphamide or ifosfamide, encourage ample fluid intake for 12–24 hours. If a high dose ($\geq$1 g/m^2) is going to be administered, prescribe 125 mL/m^2 per hour (twice maintenance fluid) of 0.45 % normal saline with 10 mEq KCL/L. The urine output should be >100 mL/m^2 per hour. Administer cyclophosphamide and ifosfamide as per protocol. For at least 18 hours following chemotherapy, continue intravenous fluid administration at 90 mL/m^2 per hour with 0.45 % normal saline with 10 mEq KCL/L or its oral equivalent. Maintain the urine output at 65 mL/m^2 for at least 18 hours. A period of oliguria may occur 8–12 hours after chemotherapy, which may require furosemide 1 mg/kg. The patient should urinate every 2 hours for 18 hours after receiving cyclophosphamide or ifosfamide.

Mesna (sodium-2-mercaptoethane sulfonate) is used to prevent hemorrhagic cystitis since it binds acrolein. Due to the use of Mesna, ketones are seen in the urine. Protocols differ as to whether Mesna needs to be administered with cyclophosphamide or not. It is usually given together with ifosfamide though. An example of a dosing regimen is: a total dose of Mesna 1.2 times the cyclophosphamide dose in mg is given in divided doses with 24 % of the total dose administered together with the cyclophosphamide dose as a 3 hour infusion and at each of the

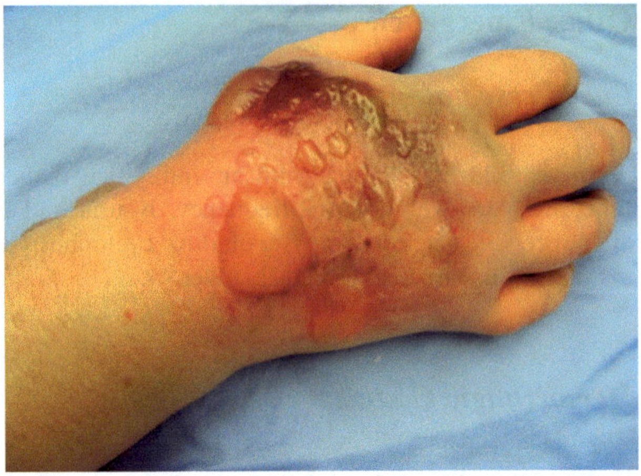

Fig. 5.9 Blistering, erythematous, swollen hand after chemotherapy extravasation

following times: at 3½, 6½, and 9½ h following the cyclophosphamide infusion as 15 minute infusions. It is advised to follow the protocol-specific instructions.

Case Presentation 2

A 7-year-old girl complained of a burning/stinging sensation around her cannula site after receiving doxorubicin. On inspection the area appeared erythematous, blistered and swollen (Fig. 5.9), and it was painful. There was no blood return upon aspiration of the cannula.

Chemotherapy Extravasation

Extravasation is the accidental leakage of the chemotherapeutic agent from the vein to the surrounding tissue with resultant injury, which ranges from a very mild skin reaction to severe necrosis depending on the characteristics of the drug involved (Table 5.2).

Cancer drugs are grouped into three broad categories, based on their potential to cause tissue damage upon extravasation: non-vesicants (non-irritants), which rarely produce an acute reaction or progress to necrosis if extravasated, followed by irritants, which may cause pain, phlebitis, or local hypersensitivity reactions, and thirdly vesicants, which can result in local pain, discomfort, tissue damage, and extensive necrosis if extravasation occurs.

Table 5.2 Potential of drugs for causing local damage

Drugs with high potential to cause damage	Drugs with moderate potential to cause damage
Daunorubicin	Dactinomycin
Idarubicin	Fluorouracil
Mitomycin C	Mitoxantrone
Vinca alkaloids	Paclitaxel
Epipodophyllotoxin (if highly concentrated)	–
Etoposide	–
Teniposide (if highly concentrated)	–
Cisplatinum	–

Mechanism of Action

A chemotherapy agent may cause damage due to DNA binding: the drug is absorbed locally and enters the cells, binds to nucleic acids (i.e., DNA) and usually initiates a protracted course of tissue necrosis and progressive ulceration that can persist for many weeks or months. Doxorubicin, daunorubicin, actinomycin, and mitomycin cause the most severe reactions. Significant levels of doxorubicin can be detected in surrounding tissues weeks and months after extravasation. The continued release of drug from necrotic cells which damages surrounding healthy tissue is the presumed mechanism of action. Extravasation in immunocompromised patients is associated with a high incidence of infection and bacteremia.

Vinca alkaloids are classified as non-DNA binding. Cell death occurs, but tends to be less severe than that associated with the anthracyclines and the damage is not progressive.

Clinical Presentation

The initial symptoms of extravasation occur immediately after the blood vessel has been breached. Depending on the agent, there may be discomfort or pain which ranges from mild to intense to permanent tissue damage and necrosis. If vesicant extravasation is not recognized and dealt with promptly, the tissue damage can become so severe that surgical debridement and plastic surgery may be required. All incidents of extravasation, especially of vesicant agents, should be documented and reported to senior staff.

Table 5.3 Vesicant chemotherapeutic agents and antidotes and that have been recommended

Drug	Antidote	Dose per mL
Actinomycin D	Sodium thiosulfate 10 %	1–4
Daunomycin	Dexamethasone 8 mg/2 mL	1
Doxorubicin	Hydrocortisone 100 mg/2 mL or topical dimethylsulfoxide (DMSO)	2
Mechlorethamine	Sodium thiosulfate 10 %	3
Vinblastine	Sodium chloride 0.9 % or hyaluronidase by injection	3
Vincristine	Hyaluronidase by injection or topical application	1

Source: Adapted from Cox K, Stuart—Harris R, Abdini G et al. The management of antitoxic—drug extravasation. Guidelines drawn up by a working group party for the Clinical Oncologic Society of Australia. Med J Aust 148:185–189, 1988

Treatment

The administration of the cancer drug must be stopped immediately by disconnecting the infusion line, but the cannula should not yet be removed at this point. As much of the offending drug as possible should be aspirated with a 10 mL syringe, after which the cannula should be removed. A loose, dry dressing should be applied. If the extravasated drug is non-vesicant, application of simple cold compresses and elevation of the limb is sufficient to limit the swelling.

If the extravasated drug is vesicant and falls in the group of DNA binding, e.g., anthracyclines, 50–100 mg of hydrocortisone (Solu-Cortef) or 4 mg of dexamethasone (Decadron) should be administered into the undisturbed cannula and by subcutaneous injection. The appropriate antidote (see Table 5.3) may also be injected subcutaneously in a clockwise manner into the extravasated area using 4–5 injections. Note that only anthracyclines, mitomycin C, and mustine have specific antidotes (Table 5.3). The cannula should then be removed and a cold pack should be applied to the affected area for 20 minutes, 4 times daily for 1–2 days. The limb should be elevated.

If the extravasated drug is vesicant and in the non-DNA binding group, e.g., vinca alkaloids, several subcutaneous injections of 150–1500 IU of hyaluronidase diluted in 1 mL sterile water should be given around the extravasated area to allow wider dispersion of the extravasated vinca alkaloid. For the best outcome, hyaluronidase should be administered within an hour of extravasation. The cannula/needle should then be removed and a warm compress applied to the affected area for 20 minutes, 4 times a day for 1–2 days. The limb should again be elevated. A sterile dressing and 1 % hydrocortisone cream should be applied three times per day if the skin is persistently red and inflamed. The use of corticosteroid injections or cold compresses may exacerbate tissue injury with these agents.

Suggested Reading

Ablin AR (1997) Supportive care of children with cancer. Current therapy and guidelines from the children's cancer group. John Hopkins University Press, Baltimore

Anderson AR (2011) Pediatric oncologic emergencies, emedicine. Medscape.com, article/990480. Accessed 13 June 2011

Andıran N, Alikaşifoğlu A, Kupeli S, Yetgin S (2006) Use of bisphosphonates for resistant hypercalcemia in children with acute lymphoblastic leukemia: report of two cases and review of the literature. Turk J Pediatr 48:248–252

Cheng KK, Molassiotis A, Chang AM, Wai WC, Cheung SS (2001) Evaluation of an oral care protocol intervention in the prevention of chemotherapy-induced oral mucositis in paediatric cancer patients. Eur J Cancer 37(16):2056–2063

Cruz LB, Ribeiro AS, Rech A, Rosa LGN, Castro CG Jr, Brunetto AL (2007) Influence of low-energy laser in the prevention of oral mucositis in children with cancer receiving chemotherapy. Pediatr Blood Cancer 48:435–440

Kerdudo C, Aerts I, Fattet S, Chevret L, Pacquement H, Doz F, Michon J, Garabedian M, Orbach D (2005) Hypercalcemia and childhood cancer: a 7-year experience. J Pediatr Hematol Oncol 27(1):23–27

Lee DA, Margolin J (2014) Emergencies in pediatric cancer patients. www.uptodate.com. Accessed 14 May 2014

McKay C, Furman WL (1993) Hypercalcemia complicating childhood malignancies. Cancer 72:256–260

Morris JC, Holland JF (2000a) Oncologic emergencies. In: Bast RC Jr, Kufe DW, Pollock RE et al (eds) Holland-Frei cancer medicine, 5th edn. BC Decker, Hamilton, Chapter 158

Morris JC, Holland JF (2000b) Oncologic emergencies, Chapter 158. Oncologic emergencies. www.ncbi.nlm.nih.gov, NCBI

Özçay F, Kayıran SM, Özbek N (2003) Successful medical management of neutropenic enterocolitis (typhlitis) in a child with acute lymphoblastic leukemia. Turk J Paediatr 45:248–250

Stefan DC, Rodriguez-Galindo C (2014) Pediatric hematology-oncology in countries with limited resources. A practical manual. Springer, New York

Thoeni RF, Cello JP (2006) CT imaging of colitis. Radiology 240(3):623–638

Weiner MA, Cairo MS (2002) Pediatric hematology/oncology secrets. Anley & Belfus, Philadelphia

Wengström Y, Margulies A (2008) European oncology nursing extravasation guidelines. Eur J Oncol Nurs 12(4):357–361

Wong Kee Song L, Marcon NE (2012) Typhlitis (neutropenic enterocolitis). www.uptodate.com. Accessed 14 May 2014

Suggested Reading

Chapter 6
Osteosarcoma

Case Presentation

A 14-year-old girl presented with a painful swollen R leg for 3 weeks. She had difficulty in bending her knee and she had a painful gait. No history of trauma, weight loss, or systemic symptoms were found (Fig. 6.1).

Findings on Examination

Not acutely ill.

She had a swollen distal femur with limited joint effusion. The leg was warm and painful to touch.

The rest of the clinical examination was within normal limits.

What is the differential diagnosis?

Differential diagnosis:
Trauma
Osteosarcoma
Ewing sarcoma
Lymphoma

D.C. Stefan, M. Harif, *Pediatric Cancer in Africa*,
DOI 10.1007/978-3-319-17936-0_6

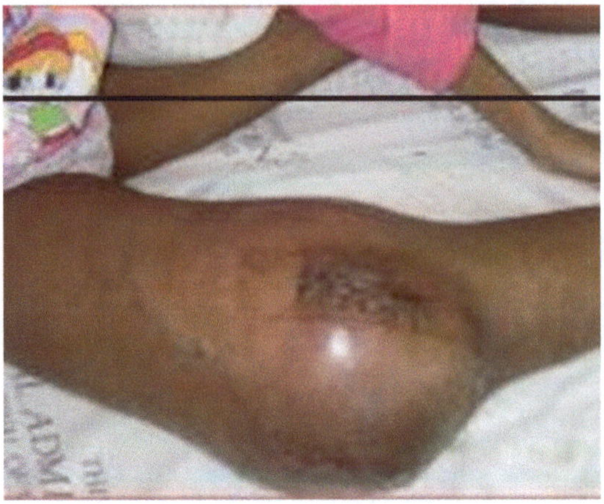

Fig. 6.1 Initial presentation work-up and diagnosis were done by the orthopedic department

What investigations would you like to request?

CB*C*
X-rays of the affected limb
Chest X-ray (PA view and lateral view)
CT scan/MRI if available
Herein listed are available results for your case scenario (Table 6.1):

Diagnosis: based on clinical suspicion and radiography and confirmed by biopsy (pathological examination).

Epidemiology

Osteosarcoma is the most common malignant bone tumor in children and adolescents.

The incidence of osteosarcoma is five per million with less new cases reported in the black population. It is more common in older children and young teenagers.

Most patients present during the second and third decades of life, 70–75 % of patients being between the ages of 15 and 25 years.

The bones with a rapid growth such as the distal femur, proximal tibia, and proximal humerus are the most affected.

Risk factors for the development of osteosarcoma include the presence of a germline mutation in the *RB1* (bilateral retinoblastoma syndrome) or *TP53* genes (Li-Fraumeni syndrome). Survivors of bilateral retinoblastoma are at a significantly increased risk of developing osteosarcoma; this risk is augmented if the patient has received radiation therapy. Patients with Rothmund-Thomson syndrome have also a high chance of apparition of this bone tumor.

Table 6.1 Histopathology classification of osteosarcoma

Wcc	Hb	Mcv	Plt	N	L	Na	K	Ur	Cr
11.1	8.6	85	269	5.5	4.1	139	5	3.5	24

The modern treatment consists in chemotherapy and surgery and the cure rate reaches now more than 70 %. The advanced forms with lung metastases have a poor prognosis.

In Africa

There are very few reports regarding osteosarcoma in Africa as the incidence is not known. It is postulated that osteosarcoma is rarer in black children than in the white population.

Most patients present late with disseminated disease and their prognostic remains reserved. The lack of specialized units and orthopedic surgeons contribute to the challenges of the disease.

Clinical Presentation

The clinical picture of the disease is dominated by pain, which is present in more than 90 % of the patients. The pain is persistent with exacerbation during the night and is not responding to pain medication. The pain also occurs at rest and may be associated with constitutional symptoms such as weight loss, pallor, and anorexia. The pain is related to the tumor itself but can also be caused by nerve or vascular compression depending on the site. The pain is associated in majority of the cases with impressive swelling. The symptoms are usually present for several weeks before the presentation to the clinic or to the general doctor.

On rare occasions a pathological fracture can be associated with the tumor, following a minor trauma.

In Africa

Most African patients with osteosarcoma present with advanced disease. At presentation, a limp or loss of function and/or decreased range of motion may be detected.

The most common sign is a mass that is invariable firm and tender.

Lesions are typically located in the metaphyseal region of long bones, with the distal femur and proximal tibia making up approximately 50 % of all cases.

Diagnosis of Osteosarcoma

The diagnosis is based on the suspicion of persistent bone pain associated with a growth in most of the cases. The radiographic changes contribute to the suspicion but the confirmatory diagnosis is based on the pathological examination of the tissue obtained during a biopsy.

Diagnosis Work-Up

Laboratory Tests

Laboratory tests are usually normal and noncontributing to the diagnosis.
Hematological studies:

Complete blood count (CBC).
In advanced cases the patients may present with chronic anemia following bleeding of the tumor.

Biochemical studies:

Renal function studies (blood urea nitrogen, creatinine, serum electrolytes, urinalysis) and liver function studies are performed prior to the administration of the chemotherapy. LDH and ALP (alkaline phosphatase) are commonly elevated in the setting of large tumor burden.

Viral studies:

Hepatitis B and C serology, HIV antibody, HSV antibody, CMV antibody, varicella antibody (as in any assessment of other cancer).

Radiological studies include the following investigations:

Radiography of the involved limb (Fig. 6.2): Plain X-rays are indispensable for diagnosis, and the clinical suspicion of osteosarcoma is often confirmed by plain radiographs. Typical radiographic findings of an aggressive bone-forming tumor with a periosteal reaction and extraskeletal soft tissue extension are present in 80–90 % of cases.
Early osteosarcoma, however, can often be overlooked or mistaken for benign lesions.
Chest radiograph (posterior, anterior, and lateral) (Fig. 6.3): The chest radiograph is part of the essential investigations and it is necessary in order to look for *possible* pulmonary metastases.
Other radiological investigations in osteosarcoma: Computed tomography, magnetic resonance imaging, bone scintigraphy, positron emission tomography fluorine-18-fluorodeoxyglucose.
CT abdomen (Fig. 6.4) and MRI of the affected limb (Fig. 6.5) are expensive and in most cases not available.

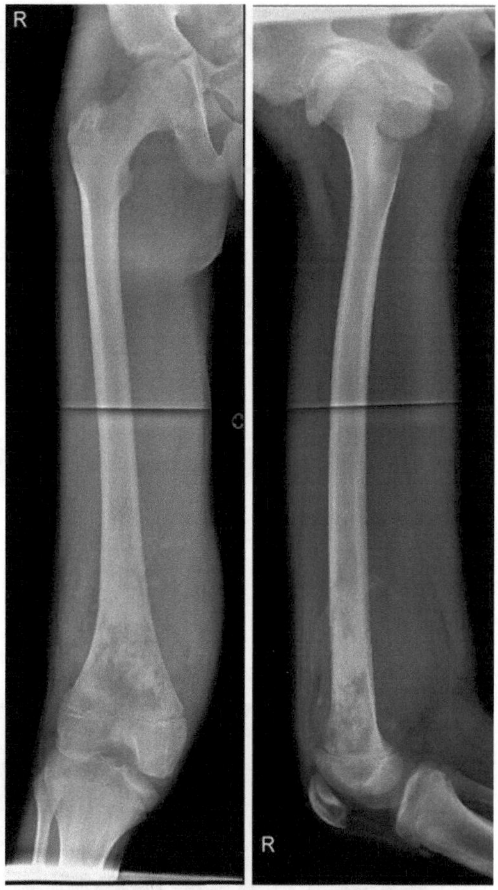

Fig. 6.2 X-ray of limb

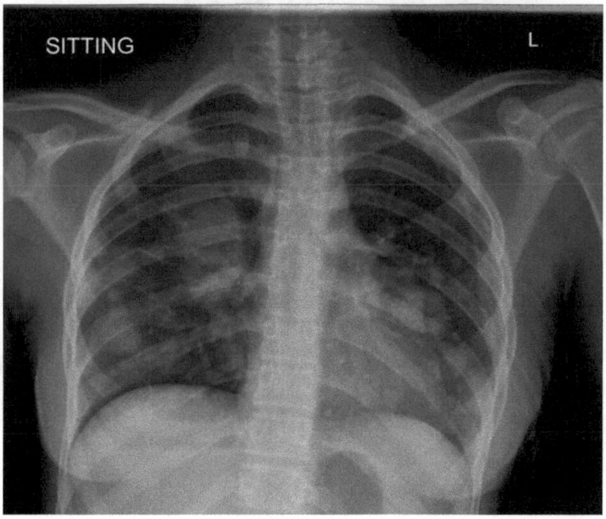

Fig. 6.3 Chest X-ray

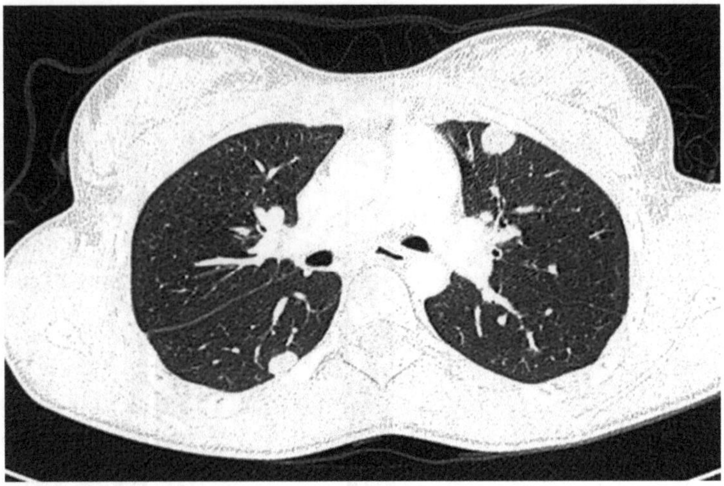

Fig. 6.4 CT chest: (not required)

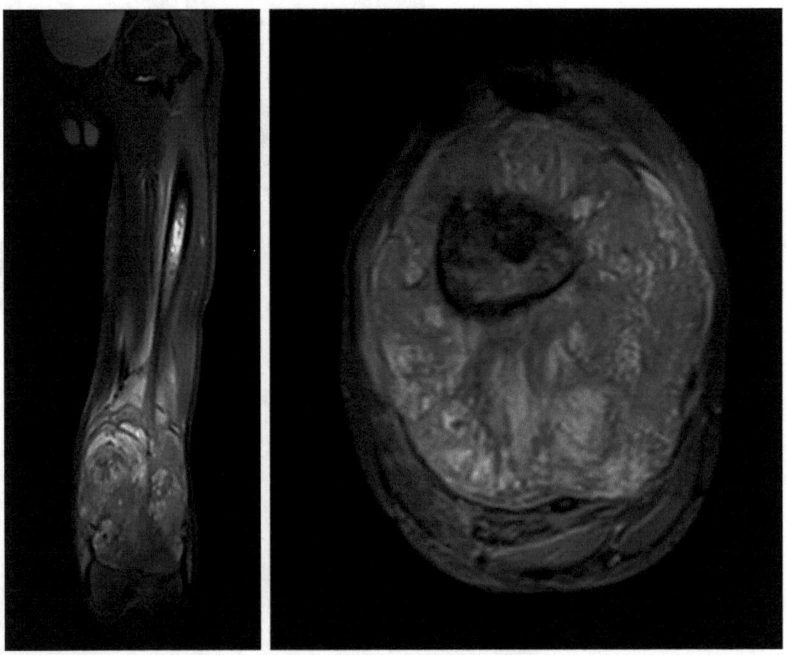

Fig. 6.5 MRI of limb

Computed tomography (CT) or *magnetic resonance imaging* (MRI) is not required in most cases or advanced cases but proved to be useful when there is doubt as to the nature of a bony lesion in a child or adolescent. These modalities can show subtle aggressive features not apparent on plain radiographs.

Most of our African patients present with locally advanced disease and classic radiographic findings.

Bone scintigraphy and occasionally *angiography* used previously for diagnosis and staging purposes are not recommended anymore.

MRI is used to delineate the extent of the tumor, plan biopsy and definitive surgery, and identify any possible skip lesions.

CT scan of the chest and abdomen is performed to identify any visceral metastases, while bone scintigraphy should be done to rule out bony metastases.

Positron emission tomography fluorine-18-fluorodeoxyglucose (PET 18-FDG) may be used as an alternative staging modality but it is not recommended in the routine staging of the patient.

Pathology

To confirm the diagnosis of osteosarcoma, a biopsy is always required.

As with all suspected malignant bone tumors, the biopsy should be done in a specialized unit by the surgeon who will also perform the definitive surgery.

Biopsy is preferably done open, through a longitudinal incision, without jeopardizing possible future limb salvage surgery. The biopsy incision must be placed in an area where it can be totally excised at the time of eventual resection, to allow successful limb salvage surgery. In expert hands, a tru-cut core needle biopsy of the soft tissue component may provide a good diagnostic specimen.

Once confirmed histologically, the definitive treatment decision is based on the stage of disease and prognosis.

Staging is performed based on the histological grade, local extent, and presence of metastases.

Multiple prognostic factors have been proposed including detectable metastases, advanced age, non-extremity location, large tumor volume, elevated LDH and ALP, and poor histological response to neo-adjuvant chemotherapy.

Of these, only metastatic disease, unresectable tumors, and poor response to neo-adjuvant chemotherapy have consistently been associated with poor outcome.

Histological Study

The World Health Organization's histological classification further divides osteosarcoma into medullary and surface tumors, which are each divided into several subtypes. Conventional osteosarcoma (the high-grade medullary variant) is the most common subtype, making up about 90 % of all cases.

Staging: needs to define if the disease is localized or has distant metastases (lungs being the most common).

– Includes radiographies (chest radiography)

Prognosis

If the disease is limited to the bone a combined therapeutic approach including surgery and chemotherapy is associated with survival rates above 80 %.

The presence of lung metastases and/or reduced cardiac function diminishes considerably the cure.

Approach to Therapy

The treatment of osteosarcoma includes administration of chemotherapy preoperative, surgery, and postoperative chemotherapy. Radiotherapy does not contribute to the cure of the disease and is also not used as palliative method.

Osteosarcoma is a chemosensitive tumor. The chemotherapy drugs used for the treatment of osteosarcoma are presented in Tables 6.2 and 6.3.

Surgery

The primary surgical objective is complete resection of tumor tissue. Therefore, limb salvage and prosthetic replacement can only be considered if a viable, functional limb remains after resection and a complete resection with negative margins

Table 6.2 Chemotherapy drugs used in the treatment of osteosarcoma

Cisplatinum	100 mg/m^2 day 1 as 24 h infusion
Doxorubicin	25 mg/m^2 days 1, 2, 3
Methotrexate	8–12 g/m^2/day as 4 h infusion

Table 6.3 Additional drugs used for the treatment of osteosarcoma can be administered according to the following protocols

Drugs used for relapsed disease	ICE (ifosfamide, carboplatin, etoposide) or ICA (ifosfamide, carboplatin, adriamycin)
Ifosfamide	Up to 5–10 g/m^2 (median 7.5)
Etoposide	300–500 mg/m^2 (median 450)
Carboplatin	300–750 mg/m^2 (median 350)
Doxorubicin	50–80 mg/m^2 (median 60)

can be assured. If limb salvage is considered, preoperative neo-adjuvant chemotherapeutic treatment is instituted to facilitate the surgical dissection.

If limb salvage is not possible, ablation of the limb may be performed. For patients with large tumors and those in limited resource settings for whom a limb salvage procedure is not possible, upfront amputation followed by chemotherapy is also an option.

The literature reports limb salvage rates in excess of 80 % in developed countries with localized disease, which is usually not possible for the African patients. However, with appropriate radical surgery and systemic therapy, greater than 50 % of patients with localized disease can be cured in low income settings.

Following surgical tumor excision, either through limb salvage or ablation, all patients are considered for postoperative systemic chemotherapy.

Follow-Up During Treatment

During the chemotherapy CBC and renal functions are required.

An evaluation of the cardiac function and an audiogram are performed at the beginning of the therapy and regular monitoring is part of the protocol. We suggest one initial evaluation and a last one at the end of the protocol.

The preferred treatment protocol in countries with limited resources includes the administration of Cisplatinum and Adriamycin 2–3 cycles before surgery and another 3–4 cycles postoperative.

The administration of methotrexate is extremely toxic and is associated with febrile neutropenia, mucositis, severe vomiting, and dehydration. If blood levels are difficult to obtain the patients should receive large amounts of fluids, diuresis must be monitored carefully, and antiemetics administered regularly.

Supportive care measures should include the availability of blood products and platelets, antibiotics.

Follow-Up After Treatment

The follow-up after treatment includes clinical examination, radiography, and the assessment of cardiac function and hearing test.

Complications Related to Therapy

Complications related to therapy are associated with the toxicity of the drugs: cardiotoxicity and ototoxicity for the administration of cisplatinum and anthracyclines.

The prolonged administration of chemotherapy isolated or together with radiotherapy increases the risk of febrile neutropenia, susceptibility to infection, anemia, and thrombocytopenia.

Relapse of Osteosarcoma

The relapse of osteosarcoma can occur at the initial site or present with metastases.

In most cases the treatment will consist in palliation, as the prognosis in these cases remains reserved.

Summary

Osteosarcoma is the most common bone tumor, which presents usually in older children and young teenagers after a prolonged period of bone pain and not associated with trauma.

Clinical examination should be completed by radiography and a local biopsy.

It is a chemosensitive but not a radiosensitive tumor. The common protocols used in the treatment of osteosarcoma are toxic and special attention should be given to supportive care.

In Africa

Amputation remains the choice of surgery or the only choice of surgical intervention due to lack of skilled expertise of the orthopedic surgeons and increased cost of prosthesis.

Cultural beliefs and tradition contribute to the increased reason of abandonment of surgical treatment of these patients.

Methotrexate levels are difficult to measure and the addition of the drug in the protocol does not provide statistical increase in survival rate.

Early diagnosis with inclusion of radiography of the affected limb, chest radiography, 2 drugs chemotherapy protocols, and surgery could be used with success in Africa.

Owing to its relative rarity, osteosarcoma is unfortunately often missed on the initial visit to a local hospital. To improve the early recognition of osteosarcoma, a high index of suspicion, liberal use of radiographs, and a sound knowledge of the subtle X-ray changes are needed.

When faced with a suspected osteosarcoma, consultation with a referral unit that specializes in these diseases is advisable, as missed or late diagnoses could have catastrophic consequences.

Suggested Reading

Cristina Stefan D, Rodriguez-Galindo C (eds) (2014) Pediatric hematology oncology in countries with limited resources—a practical manual. Springer, New York

Hogendoorn PCW, ESMO/EUROBONET Working group et al (2010) Bone sarcomas: ESMO clinical practice guidelines for diagnosis, treatment and follow up. ANN Oncol 23(suppl 7):vii100–vii109

Chapter 7
Ewing Sarcoma

Case Presentation

A 10-year-old boy, previously well, presents with an 8 month history of right hip pain, which he attributes to a fall. He also reports significant weight loss and complains of fatigue and pallor.

Findings on Examination

The boy appears chronically ill. He is cachectic with no subcutaneous fat and severely reduced muscle bulk. There is a large mass arising from the right hip and extending to the perineum and the right buttock, with resultant swelling of the right leg (Fig. 7.1). The right hip is kept in abduction and the patient does not tolerate any movement of the hip. A 90° flexion contracture of the right knee is present. On abdominal examination the mass is also palpable in the right fossa iliaca. There are no paresthesias and he has normal dorsiflexion of the right foot. There is no hepatosplenomegaly. The respiratory examination is normal. The patient is mildly tachycardic, but otherwise the cardiovascular system is also normal. He appears withdrawn and depressed, but otherwise there are no neurological abnormalities.

What is the possible diagnosis?

D.C. Stefan, M. Harif, *Pediatric Cancer in Africa*,
DOI 10.1007/978-3-319-17936-0_7

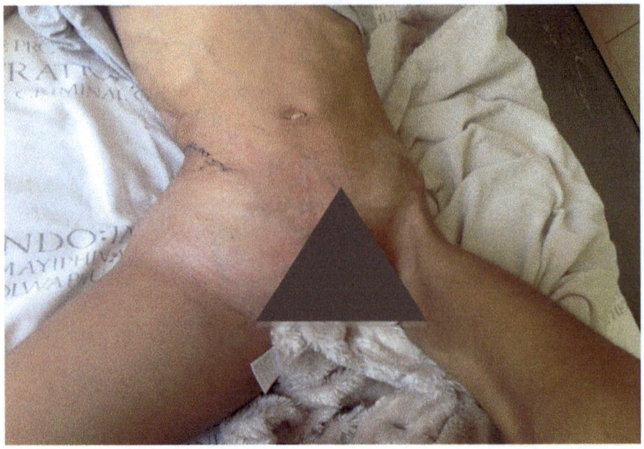

Fig. 7.1 Initial presentation

What Is the Differential Diagnosis?

Differential Diagnosis

Bone tumors (osteosarcoma, Ewing sarcoma, chondrosarcoma), neuroblastoma, rhabdomyosarcoma, nonrhabdomyosarcoma soft tissue sarcoma, germ cell tumor

What Investigations Would You Like to Request in this Case?

- X-ray of right hip and pelvis (Fig. 7.2)
- Chest X-ray (PA view and lateral view) (Fig. 7.3)
- CT scan right hip and pelvis (Fig. 7.4)
- MRI right hip and pelvis (Fig. 7.5)
- CBC, ESR, renal function, LDH, ALP
- Biopsy

A biopsy of the right hip mass was performed and confirmed Ewing sarcoma.

Epidemiology

Ewing sarcoma is a malignant bone or soft tissue tumor that is currently regarded to be a member of the so-called Ewing sarcoma family, which includes tumors of the soft tissues and bones with neuroectodermal differentiation and the same genomic alteration (fusion of *EWS* with a member of the *ETS* family of transcription factors). Ewing sarcoma occurs predominantly in older children and adolescents (10–16 years of age). It includes Ewing sarcoma, Askin tumor, and extraosseous Ewing sarcoma (previously known as peripheral primitive neuroectodermal tumors—the term PNET removed from the 2013 WHO Classification) (Table 7.1).

The annual incidence of Ewing sarcoma is 2–3 cases per million children. It is rare in the Black and Asian populations and it is less common than osteosarcoma.

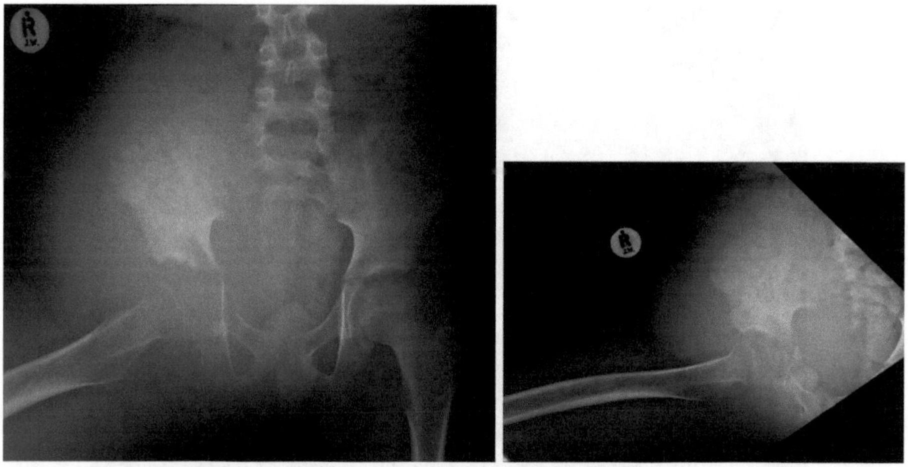

Fig. 7.2 X-ray of right hip and pelvis

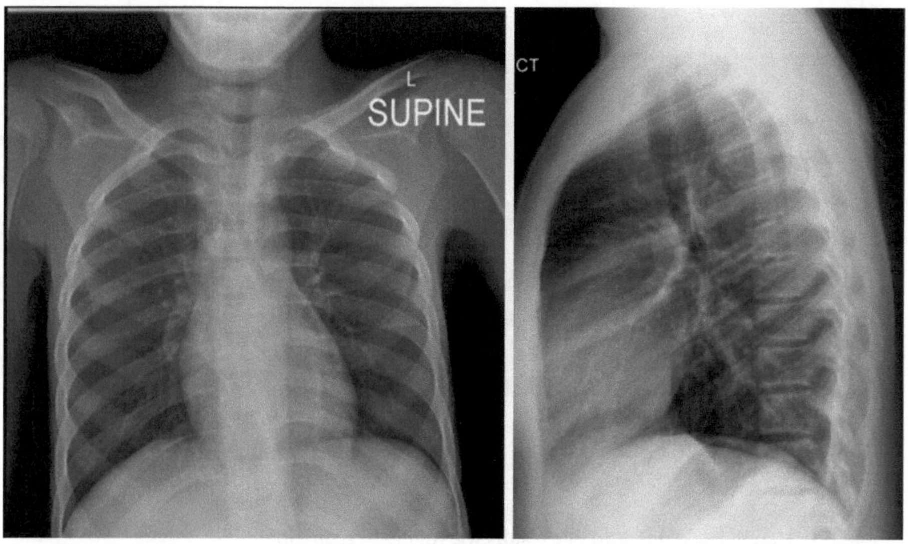

Fig. 7.3 Chest X-ray: AP and lateral

The incidence of these tumors in the Caucasian population is at least nine times higher than in the Black population.

Almost a third of the tumors occurs in the first decade of life and more than half during the second decade.

It differs from osteosarcoma through its location both in long bones and in flat bones as well by frequent involvement of the diaphyseal structure.

Advances in modern therapeutic programs allow cure rates of more than 70 % of patients in localized forms.

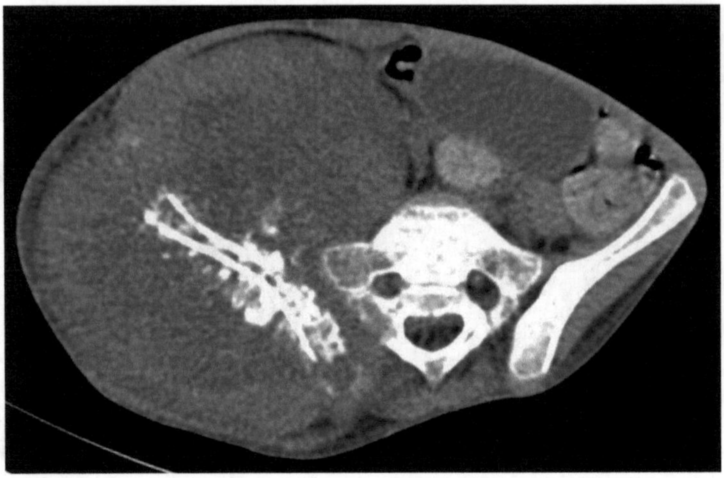

Fig. 7.4 CT scan of the pelvis

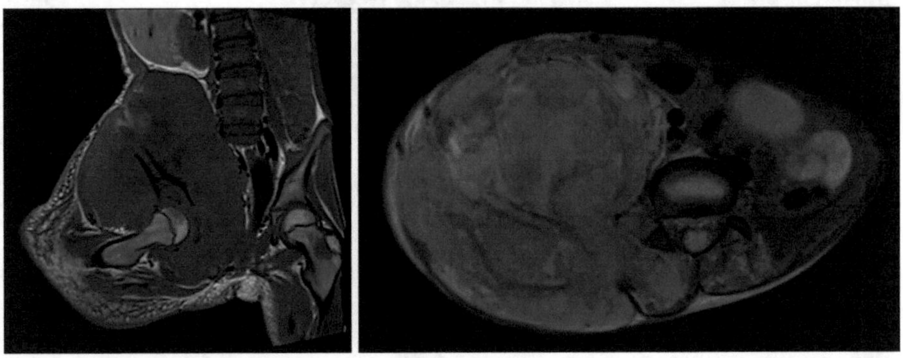

Fig. 7.5 MRI: pelvis and right hip

Table 7.1 Herein listed are available results for your case scenario

Wcc	Hb	Mcv	Plt	N	L	ESR	Na	K	Ur	Cr	Ca	Mg	Pho
12	6.3	78	675	4.5	3.2	141	135	4.4	5	<20	2.0	0.9	1.2

Clinical Presentation

The clinical expression is dominated by pain in 85 % of the patients and often is associated with swelling (in more than 60 % of the cases). The pelvis and ribs are commonly affected and the tumor infiltration of the soft parts can be very large and

Table 7.2 Distribution of Ewing sarcoma

Lower extremities (femur, tibia, fibula, foot)	44 %
Pelvis (iliac bone, sacrum, pubis, ischium)	24 %
Upper extremities (humerus, scapula, radius, ulna, hand)	17 %
Trunk (vertebra, clavicle, mandible, skull)	15 %

sometimes compressing the adjacent structures. Fever is observed in almost one third of cases. Exceptionally, the disease is manifested by paraplegia due to epidural extension more than vertebral involvement.

This expansion of the tumor represents an oncological emergency and the decompression is obtained through surgical intervention in most cases (if diagnosed and intervened within 48–72 h). Ewing sarcoma usually is a chemo-and radiosensitive malignancy, and immediate initiation of chemotherapy and emergency radiation therapy are also valid alternatives in case of acute spinal compression when surgery is not an option.

Ewing sarcoma is localized at the long bones as well as the flat bones, with a special predilection towards the pelvis and ribs (Table 7.2).

Diagnosis Work-Up

The diagnosis work-up includes laboratory tests, imaging, and biopsy.

Laboratory Tests

Laboratory tests are usually normal and noncontributing to the diagnosis.

Hematological studies: Complete blood count (CBC) and erythrocyte sedimentation rate (ESR)

Biochemical studies: Renal function studies (blood urea nitrogen, creatinine, serum electrolytes, urinalysis) are in most cases normal.

The determination of urinary catecholamines may be recommended to distinguish from neuroblastoma if in doubt (however difficult to perform in Africa) so correlation with other possible clinical signs is required.

Viral studies: Hepatitis B and C serology, HIV antibody, HSV antibody, CMV antibody, varicella antibody (as in any assessment of other cancer)

Cytogenetic and Molecular Studies

Cytogenetic studies can be used to confirm the diagnosis of Ewing sarcoma if *t*(11;22) or a related translocation is found. For standard cytogenetics, fresh tissue should be sent in appropriate media to a cytogenetic laboratory.

Cytogenetics tests are most likely not available in Africa and if available are at exorbitant costs. A typical histology in the context of a compatible clinical presentation is usually sufficient for diagnosis.

The priority is to obtain images of the suspected primary lesion or of any region with symptoms. If a bony mass is palpated, plain radiography is indicated Fig. 7.6a, b

The lesions are usually mixed but often predominantly lytic. Cortical disruption, periosteal sometimes a spur Codman appearance and soft tissue infiltration reaction reflect the malignancy.

CT allows a better analysis of the tumor, a more detailed study of the pineal gland and the adjacent joint (Fig. 7.7).

MRI is the modality of choice for the analysis of local extension in a case of Ewing sarcoma. The tumor usually takes contrast, appears hypointense on T1 and hyperintense on T2 (Fig. 7.8). The relationship with the neurovascular structures is well identified in an MRI as well as the possible presence of spinal metastases.

Radiography and CT of the thorax are usually performed in search of pulmonary metastases. In case of small nodules visible only on CT, tumor type should be discussed. If lung metatases are present the disease is disseminated and the prognosis remains reserved.

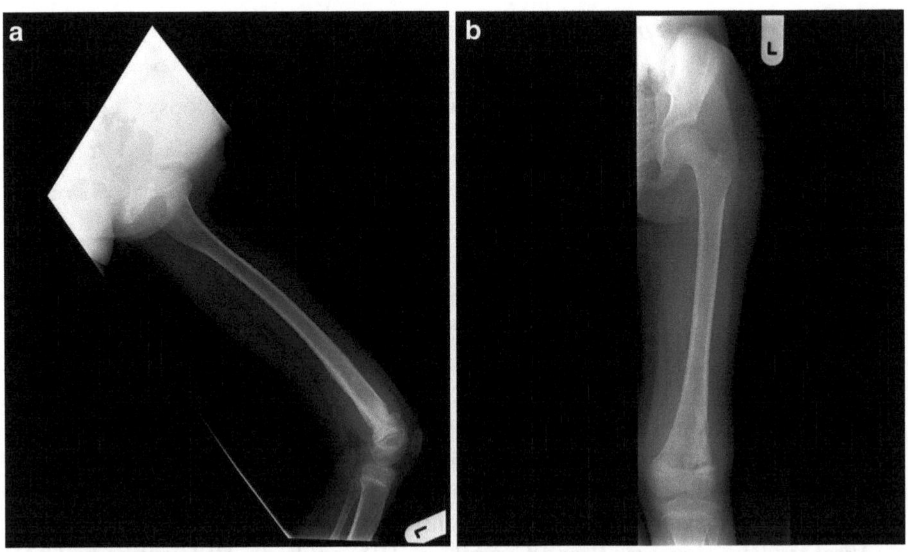

Fig. 7.6 Radiography of long bones

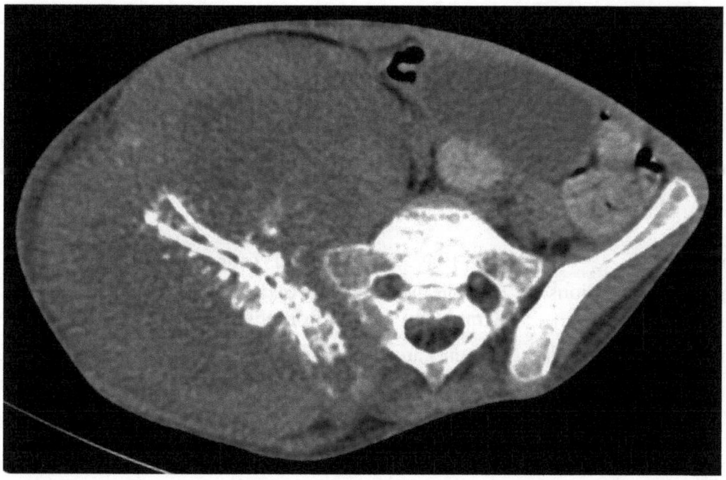

Fig. 7.7 CT scan

Fig. 7.8 MRI of Ewing sarcoma

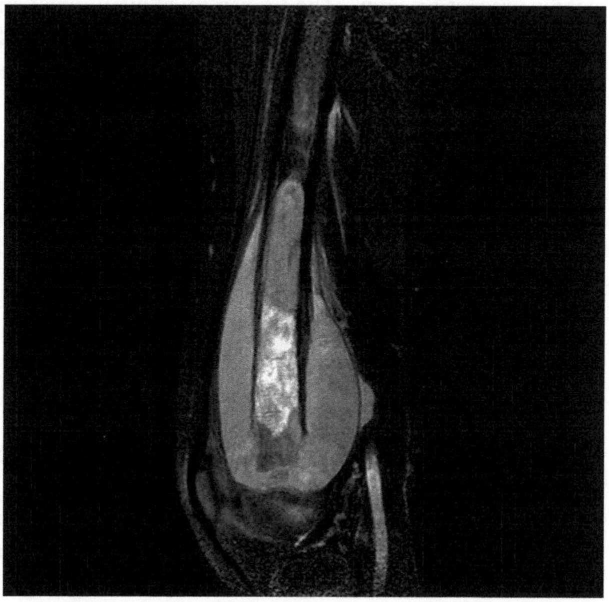

Staging should include the search for bone metastases which is done by the use of Tc99 scintigraphy.

Other investigations performed for the diagnostic work-up of the disease include CT chest and abdomen and MRI which are expensive and in most cases not available in most African countries. In the presence of bone or lung metastases, bilateral bone marrow aspirates and biopsies are recommended to complete staging (Table 7.3).

Table 7.3 Initial assessment of Ewing sarcoma and minimal investigations required for the diagnosis

History	Pain (especially lower extremities, pelvis, trunk) associated with swelling and fever
Clinical examination	Swelling and palpable tumor (not always); signs of neurological involvement
Hematology and biochemistry	Noncontributory
Viral studies	HIV, EBV, CMV, hepatitis (noncontributory)
Radiological investigations	Radiography of the involved limb, CT scan, or/and MRI, chest X-ray (CT chest if affordable)

Involvement of the spinal cord represents an oncological emergency and requires immediate intervention

Pathology

The diagnosis is confirmed after biopsy which follows the same rules as those of the biopsy in osteosarcoma. This should be done by the surgeon who will be required to achieve resection later. The biopsy must avoid weakening of the bone and cause a fracture that may call into question the possibility of conservative surgery. The biopsy ideally should be done at the end of the CT scan and/or MRI at a later stage.

Histology

Ewing sarcoma is characterized by a dense pattern of small, round, blue cells, which can be differentiated or undifferentiated, as reflected in a rosette formation. The mitotic figures are not numerous and iIntracytoplasmic glycogen is found in 75 % of cases. The immunohistochemical markers include membranous staining with MIC2 (12 E7) antigen (CD99) which is characteristic but not pathognomonic. The search for the translocation *t*(11,22) or less often *t*(21,22) helps the diagnosis in cases of atypical histology (Fig. 7.9).

The prognosis of Ewing sarcoma is closely related to the size and site of the tumor as well as the presence or absence of metastases at diagnosis (Table 7.4).

In addition to these initial prognostic factors, the quality of surgical excision and histological response to preoperative chemotherapy also has a high prognostic value.

Approach to Therapy

The treatment of Ewing sarcoma consists in chemotherapy, surgery, and radiotherapy and lasts in general an average of 6–9 months.

Ewing sarcoma is a radiosensitive and chemosensitive tumor.

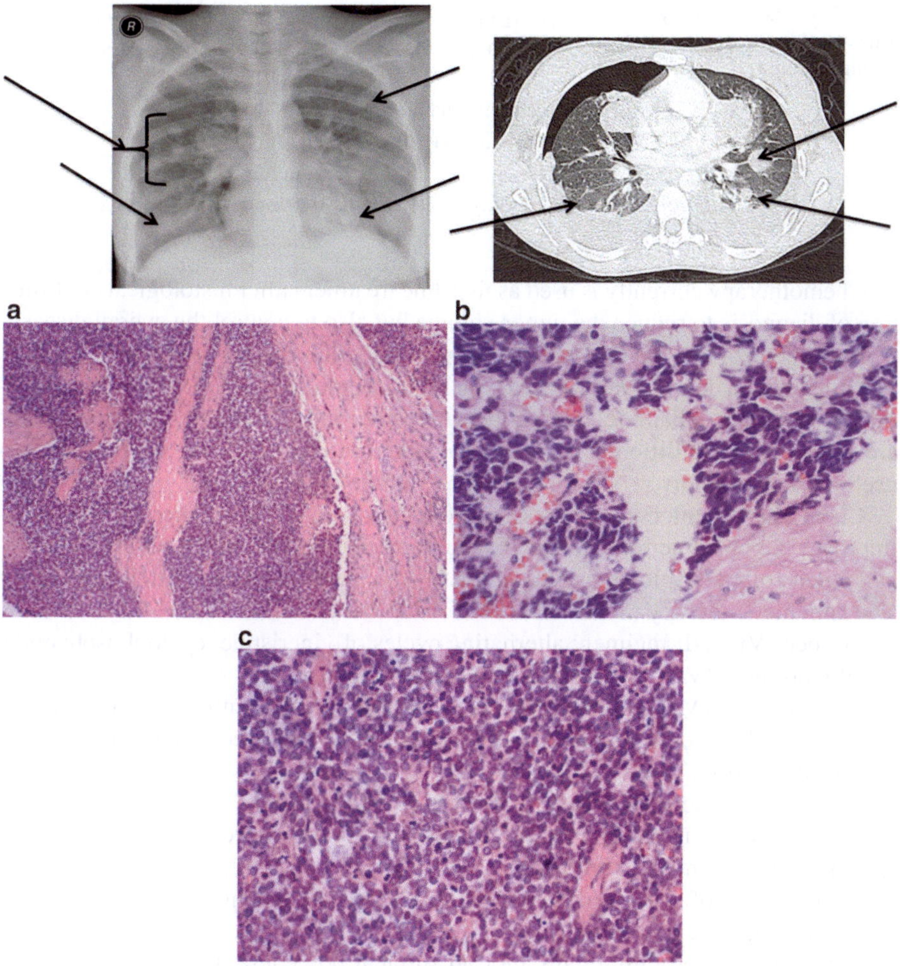

Fig. 7.9 (a–c) Chest X-rays and CT chest pictures

Table 7.4 Prognostic factors

	Poor prognosis	Good prognosis
Site primitive tumor	Axial	Distal
Size of the tumor	Big	Small
Metastases	Present	Absent
LDH	Elevated	Reduced
Response to treatment (histology)	No	Yes

Table 7.5 Chemotherapy drugs used in the treatment of Ewing sarcoma

Vincristine	1.5 mg/m^2 day (max 2 mg/day)
Doxorubicin	75 mg/m^2 over 48 h or 37.5 mg/m^2 bolus day 1 and 2
Cyclophosphamide	1,2 g/m^2 day 1
Etoposide (VP16)	100 mg/m^2/day × 5 days
Ifosfamide	1.8 g/m^2/day × 5 days
Actinomycin D	0.0045 mg/kg day 1 (max 2.5 mg)

Chemotherapy currently is used as first-line treatment after histological confirmation of diagnosis to reduce the tumor volume but also to control the overall disease.

Local control may be obtained by surgery, radiation therapy, or both.

Drugs with a demonstrated efficacy in monochemotherapy are vincristine, doxorubicin, cyclophosphamide, ifosfamide, etoposide, and actinomycin D. These drugs are associated with different regimes. The addition of ifosfamide and etoposide is useful in large tumors.

Chemotherapy interval compression from the standard 3 week therapy to 2 weeks improves the outcome for localized Ewing sarcoma without increased toxicity.

Patients often develop episodes of fever while neutropenic and often need intensive antiemetic therapy (Table 7.5).

Protocol VDC/IE regimen: alternating cycles of vincristine, cyclophosphamide, and doxorubicin (VDC) with ifosfamide and etoposide (IE).

Protocol VDC/VAC regimen: based on the use of VDC with vincristine, actinomycin D, and cyclophosphamide—for patients with localized disease and aggressive local control.

The survival rate in localized forms is from 55 to 70 %.

In patients with metastatic disease survival rates rarely exceed 15–20 % despite a good response to initial chemotherapy.

Management of the primary tumor site is critical for long-term cure. Surgical resection should be functional.

In the absence of a minimally morbid surgical procedure, local control may be achieved with radiation therapy.

Radiotherapy plays an important role in the therapy of Ewing sarcoma..

The recommended dose for radiation is 45–55 Gy but adaptation is recommended according to the seat, volume, and proximity to sensitive organs. Several studies have shown that the risk of relapse is lower in patients who underwent surgical resection.

Follow-Up During Treatment

During the chemotherapy only CBC and renal functions are required.

An evaluation of the cardiac function is performed at the beginning of the therapy.

A special attention must be given to supportive care measures especially in severely malnourished children with prolonged administration of chemotherapy associated or not with radiotherapy.

Follow-Up After Treatment

Primary and metastatic sites are evaluated approximately every 10–12 weeks during therapy and every 3–4 months during the first year after therapy.

Reevaluations are spaced out gradually for 5–6 years after the completion of therapy. After 5 years of disease-free remission, no further scanning is indicated; however, the patient should have annual follow-up visits to monitor the function of the primary site and late effects of therapy, preferably in a late-effects clinical setting.

Complications Related to Therapy

Complications related to therapy are associated with the toxicity of the drugs: cardiotoxicity and renal toxicity.

The prolonged administration of chemotherapy isolated or together with radiotherapy increases the risk of febrile neutropenia, susceptibility to infection, anemia, and thrombocytopenia.

Other complications include recurrence of primary disease in the first 10 years after diagnosis. A second malignancy occurs in approximately 1–2 % of patients beginning 5 years after diagnosis; the most common second malignancy is acute myeloid leukemia, followed by radiation-induced sarcomas.

Therapeutic toxicities to the heart and kidneys, to the nervous and endocrine systems, and to mental status should be monitored in patients who suffered acute toxicity and in those who developed symptoms after therapy.

Relapse of Ewing Sarcoma

The relapse of the disease is associated with a poor prognosis. Considerations need to be made depending on site of disease recurrence and prior therapy.

Chemotherapy combinations such as cyclophosphamide/topotecan, vincristine/irinotecan/temozolomide, and gemcitabine/docetaxel have been considered in recurrent Ewing sarcoma but not applicable to African settings.

Radiation and/or surgery may have a role for local control and disease palliation.

Summary

Ewing sarcoma family is part of the peripheral neuroectodermal primitive tumors.

It is a rare tumor in Africa. Biopsy is needed for diagnosis and the treatment combines chemotherapy with surgery and/or radiotherapy.

The prognosis depends on the tumor mass and the presence or absence of metastasis.

Suggested Reading

Rodriguez-Galindo C, Navid F, Liu T, Ca B et al (2008) Prognostic factors for local and distant control in Ewing sarcoma family of tumors. Ann Oncol 19(4):814–820

Stefan DC, Rodriguez-Galindo C (eds) (2014) Pediatric hematology oncology in countries with limited resources—a practical manual. Springer, New York

Widhe B, Widhe T (2000) Initial symptoms and clinical features in osteosarcoma and Ewing sarcoma. J Bone Joint Surg Am 82(5):667–674

Chapter 8
Nephroblastoma (Wilms Tumor)

Case Presentation

A 2-year old presented to the hospital with a 2-week history of abdominal distension and palpable right flank mass. Informal ultrasound at a peripheral hospital demonstrated a solid mass in the right flank of unknown origin.

No previous medical history of note (Fig. 8.1).

Findings on Examination

Not acutely ill
$W = 9$ kg, $H = 84$ cm
Observations: BP 101/58 mmHg, rest normal Urine Dipsticks: NAD
No pallor. No lymphadenopathy
Cardiovascular, respiratory and central nervous system: Normal examination
Abdominal examination: Distended. Right flank mass extending to the liver edge, not crossing the midline

What Is the Differential Diagnosis?

Abdominal masses: lymphoma, neuroblastoma, hepatoblastoma.
Benign renal conditions: hydronephrosis, cystic renal dysplasia, mesoblastic nephroma, xanthogranulomatous pyelonephritis.
Less common renal tumors: clear cell sarcoma of the kidney, rhabdoid tumor, mesoblastic nephroma, renal cell carcinoma.

D.C. Stefan, M. Harif, *Pediatric Cancer in Africa*,
DOI 10.1007/978-3-319-17936-0_8

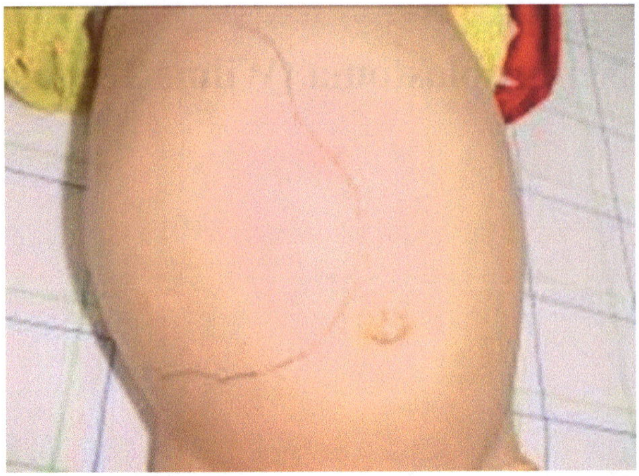

Fig. 8.1 Initial presentation abdominal distension; flank mass delineated by a marker

What Investigations Would You Like to Request?

CBC, renal function.
Abdominal ultrasound.
Chest X-ray (PA view and lateral view).
CT scan abdomen.

Herein listed are available results for your case scenario:

Wcc	Hb	Mcv	Plt	N	L	Na	K	Ur	Cr
11.1	8.6	85	269	5.5	4.1	139	5	3.5	24

A large, capsulated, well-circumscribed, heterogeneous solid mass containing some well-defined cystic areas of various sizes is noted measuring approximately 11.3 × 9.3 × 16.9 cm and which appears to originate from the lower pole of the right kidney (Figs. 8.2, 8.3, 8.4, 8.5, and 8.6).

There is a large mixed solid cystic heterogeneous mass arising from the lower pole right kidney which measures 14.5 × 11.5 cm. The tumor also compresses and displaces the IVC.

The marked atelectasis may relate to elevation of the left and right hemidiaphragm in a patient with a large intra-abdominal mass lesion. No pulmonary metastatic lesions seen.

Histological Diagnosis: made by histopathological examination of tissue obtained during surgical resection (Fig. 8.7).

Epidemiology

Nephroblastoma or Wilms tumor (WT) is the most common renal malignancy in children.

It represents 5–10 % of childhood cancers and its annual incidence is about eight new cases per million children under 15 years.

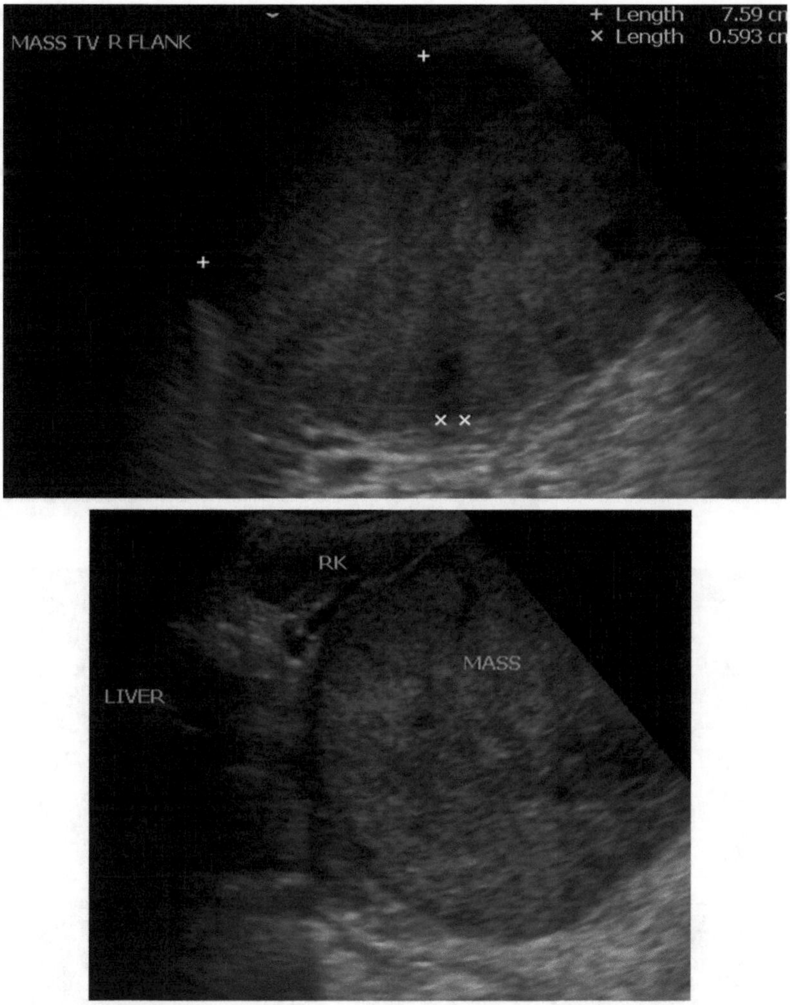

Fig. 8.2 Ultrasound abdomen

More than 2/3 of the cases occur in children under the age of 5 years and 95 % in patients occur under the age of 10 years.

Girls are more affected than boys and in 5–10 % of cases both kidneys can be affected simultaneously. Asynchronous involvement is also possible. The modern multidisciplinary approach will cure more than 90 % of patients.

In Africa

Nephroblastoma remains one of the most common solid tumors in Africa exceeding 10 % of total pediatric cancers in many countries (Rwanda 26.0 %, Senegal 22 %, Ivory Coast 14.5 %, Mali 17.6 %, Congo 15.5 %).

Fig. 8.3 Chest X-ray: AP

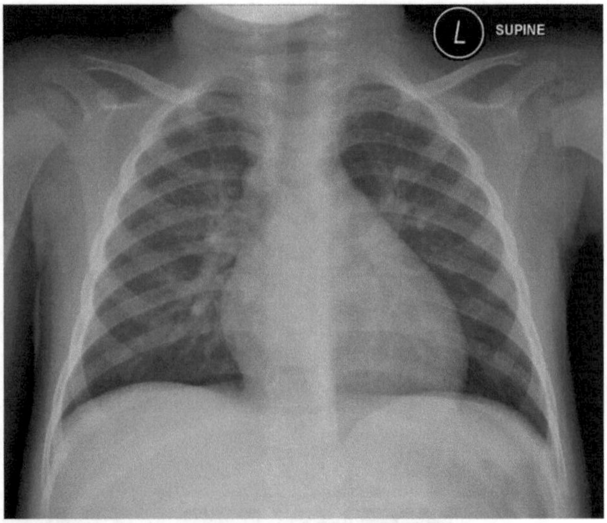

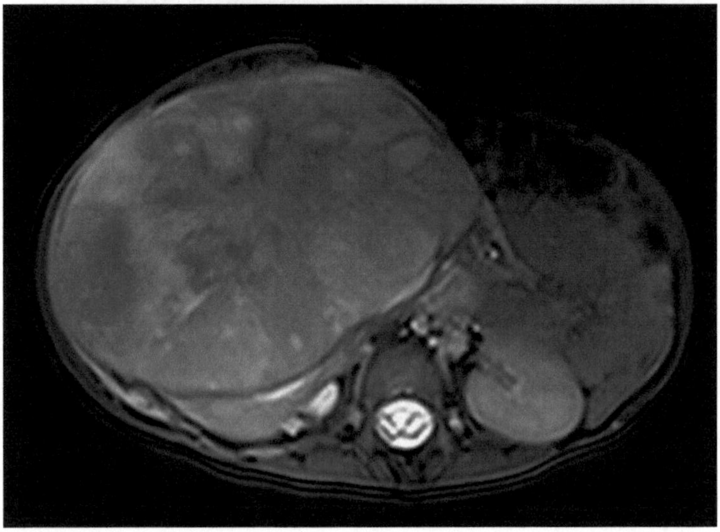

Fig. 8.4 CT scan abdomen (not required if not affordable)

Associated Genetic Abnormalities

The WT1 gene plays an important role in the development of the kidney and gonads. A deletion or mutation of the 11p13 region involving the WT1 gene can be detected in tumor cells in less than 10 % of the sporadic forms.

The abnormalities may be isolated or part of a syndrome predisposing to the occurrence of Wilms tumor. Isolated anomalies are essentially genitourinary resulting

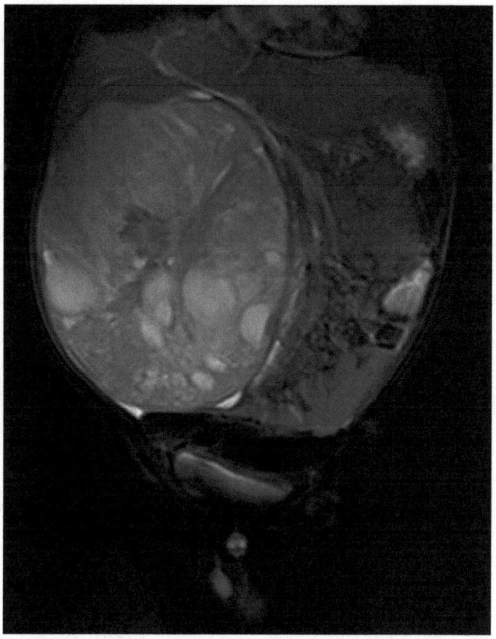

Fig. 8.5 MRI abdomen (not required)

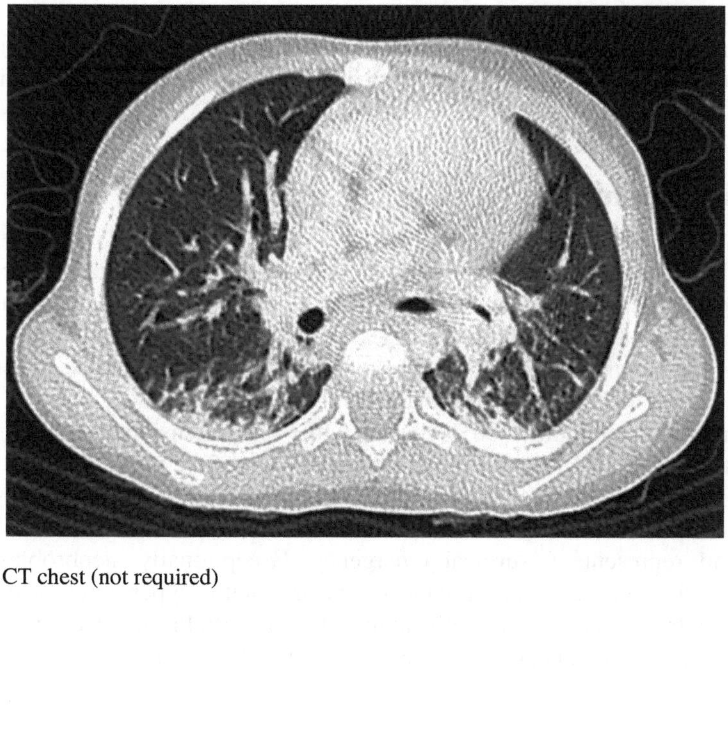

Fig. 8.6 CT chest (not required)

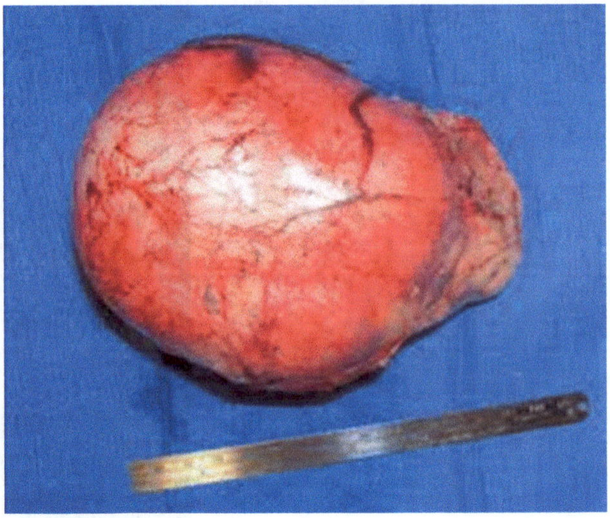

Fig. 8.7 Excised tumor specimen

in a duplication of the urinary tract, a horseshoe kidney, hypospadias, or cryptorchidism. The hemi-body hypertrophy and Wilms tumor have been described. Aniridia is also associated with Wilms tumor and may occur together with genitourinary anomalies and mental retardation (WAGR syndrome). In Denys–Drash a mutation of WT1 is found leading to nephrotic syndrome before developing Wilms tumor. Loss of imprinting (LOI) of 11p15 is found in the Beckwith–Wiedemann syndrome. One percent of Wilms tumors are familial with different known genetic anomalities.

Clinical Presentation

The finding of an abdominal mass by parents or during a consultation for fever or digestive disorders is the most common mode of presentation. The abdominal tumor is located anteriorly and is mobile, painless ,and ballotable (Fig. 8.8). It can be associated with abdominal pain if it becomes voluminous and should raise the suspicion of intratumoral hemorrhage if trauma is involved.

Hematuria is found in 15–20 % of cases while a hypertension due to renin release by the tumor cells or less frequently by compression of the renal artery is observed in 30–40 % of cases. The finding of a profound anemia or anemia developing quickly, with or without abdominal pain, must fear a rupture or abdominal hemorrhage and represents a surgical emergency. Exceptionally, nephroblastoma is associated with polycythemia related to erythropoietin hypersecretion or hemorrhagic syndrome associated with acquired von Willebrand disease. In young children hypercalcemia can be associated with a rhabdoid tumor of the kidney.

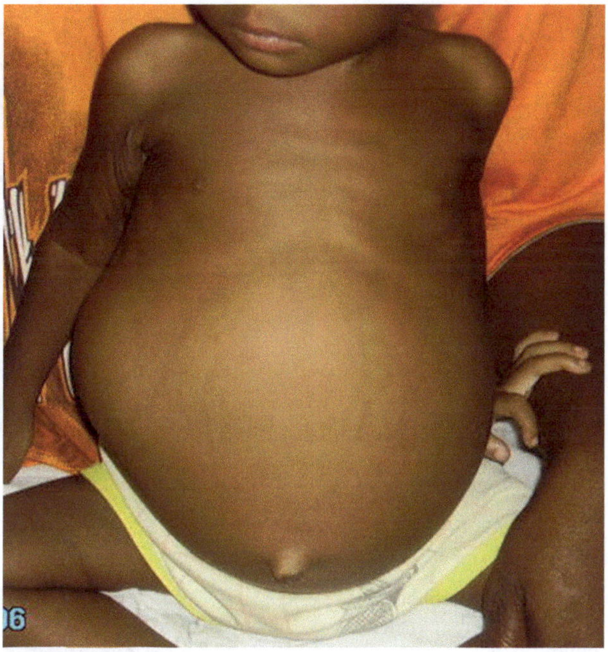

Fig. 8.8 Abdominal anterior visible tumor associated with abdominal pain in a 3-year-old child from Ivory Coast

In Africa

In Africa nephroblastoma is one of the most common and easy to diagnose tumors.

Most children present with advanced disease, huge tumors, severe malnutrition (Figs. 8.9 and 8.10), and with associated comorbidities. A complete nutritional evaluation is required as well as exclusion of other associated infections.

Diagnosis of Nephroblastoma

The confirmatory diagnosis is based on the pathological examination of the tissue after surgical resection or biopsy.

Diagnostic Work-Up

Laboratory Tests

Laboratory tests are usually normal and noncontributory to the diagnosis.

Hematological Studies

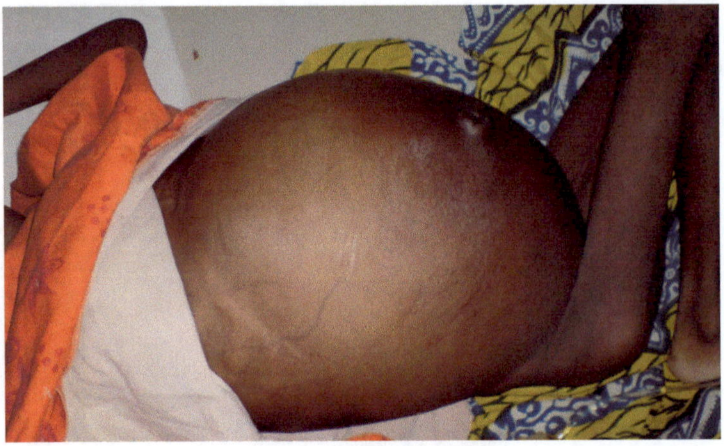

Fig. 8.9 Nephroblastoma with massive abdominal distention in a severely malnourished African child

Fig. 8.10 Nephroblastoma in an older malnourished child

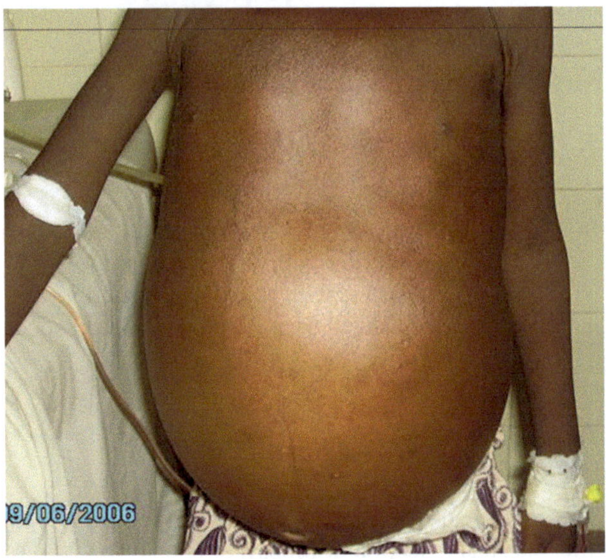

Complete blood count (CBC).
Erythrocyte sedimentation rate (ESR).

Biochemical Studies

Renal function studies (blood urea nitrogen, creatinine, serum electrolytes, urinalysis).

Renal function is normal in most of the cases and maintained even in bilateral nephroblastoma.

The determination of urinary catecholamines may be recommended to distinguish from neuroblastoma if in doubt (however difficult to perform in Africa), so correlation with other possible clinical signs is required.

Viral studies: Hepatitis B and C serology, HIV antibody, HSV antibody, CMV antibody, varicella antibody (as in any assessment of other cancer).

Radiological studies include the following investigations:

Ultrasound examination of abdomen.

Chest radiograph (anterior and lateral).

Other investigations used for the diagnostic work-up of the disease include CT chest and abdomen and/or MRI which is expensive and in most cases not available.

Abdominal ultrasound examination is the first investigation in a patient with an abdominal mass.

It specifies the renal tumor site and specifies its characteristics: solid, cystic, or mixed. The tumor size must be specified in three dimensions to assess treatment response after chemotherapy.

A complete ultrasound report needs to give information about possible hepatic involvement or bilateral kidney involvement, presence of abdominal lymphadenopathy, or renal vein or inferior vena cava thrombosis.

Abdominal CT is not always necessary and affordable. In some cases, it helps to study the mass and eliminate another etiology or reveal nephrogenic rests in the contralateral kidney.

The diagnosis is usually made based on the presentation correlated with the clinical exam and ultrasound findings.

A fine needle aspiration might be requested but will not establish a final diagnosis and requires a skilled cytologist.

An open biopsy is never performed as it upgrades the stage of the tumor and might contribute to the rupture of the mass.

The chest radiograph is part of the essential investigations and it is necessary to look for *possible* pulmonary metastases. CT of the chest will contribute further if the suspicion of disseminated disease exists.

Other investigations used for staging in clear cell sarcoma (difficult to diagnose in Africa) are the scintigraphy with Tc99 for bone metastases and CT or brain MRI which are recommended in the case of rhabdoid tumors (RTK) and clear cell sarcoma (CCSK) of the kidney (Table 8.1).

Pathology

Histologically, nephroblastoma/Wilms tumor consists of three components including blastemal, epithelial, and stromal components (Fig. 8.11). In addition, each component may show a number of different histological patterns, and they may show different lines and degrees of differentiation resulting in a huge number of histological appearances. All three components may be represented in any proportion, and tumors with only two or even one component are not rare. In tumors that received no

Table 8.1 Initial assessment of nephroblastoma and minimal investigations required for the diagnosis

History	Abdominal distension and pain, constipation, hematuria
Clinical examination	Abdominal distension, palpable flank mass, hypertension, hematuria, signs of an associated syndrome may be present
Hematology and biochemistry	Noncontributory
Viral studies	HIV, EBV, CMV, hepatitis (noncontributory)
Radiological investigations	Abdominal ultrasound, chest X-ray (CT chest and abdomen or MRI abdomen if affordable)

Pay attention to blood pressure

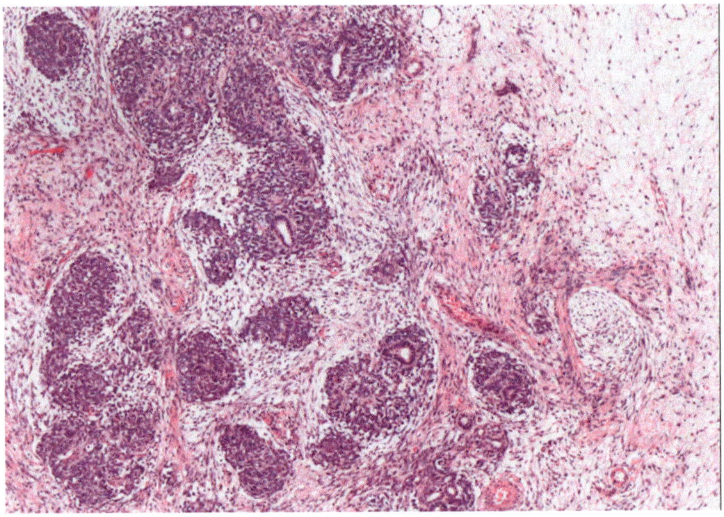

Fig. 8.11 Triphasic/mixed nephroblastoma showing blastemal, epithelial, and stromal components

preoperative chemotherapy, the only unfavorable histological feature is anaplasia which is defined as the presence of atypical, multipolar mitoses, marked nuclear enlargement, and nuclear hyperchromasia. Anaplasia can be either focal or diffuse. It is important to bear in mind that each component may show anaplasia, but the diagnosis should be made only if all three criteria are met. In cases treated with preoperative chemotherapy, tumors with a predominant blastemal component (blastemal subtype) are also regarded as high risk tumors and require more aggressive treatment.

Table 8.2 Staging criteria developed by the SIOP 2001 Trial

Stage I	Tumor is limited to the kidney and is completely excised. The capsule is intact; no tumor rupture
Stage II	Tumor infiltrates the renal sinus or extends beyond the tumor capsule into the perirenal fat but is completely excised
Stage III	Tumor excision incomplete; tumor rupture (pre- or intraoperative); regional lymph nodes contain tumor; open ('wedge') biopsy
Stage IV	Distant metastases (lungs, liver, bone, lymph nodes beyond the abdominopelvic region)
Stage V	Bilateral renal involvement at diagnosis (each side has to be staged separately)

Staging

There are two different staging criteria including the International Society of Paediatric Oncology (SIOP) and the Children's Oncology Group (COG) (formerly known as NWTS-Wilms Tumor National Study Group).

The full staging of the patient requires imaging studies (pulmonary radiography) in search for lung metastases (which are by far the most frequent metastases) and the examination of the contralateral kidney in order to exclude bilateral disease (Table 8.2).

Prognosis

The prognosis is excellent with a survival rate above 90% in early stages in most developed countries.

The two most important factors in determining the prognosis is the stage and the histology: the more advanced the disease the more reserved the outcome.

In Africa the 5-year survival for localized tumors was reported at 76% and 71% for all study patients for the GFAOP (2012) but in many other countries remains much lower due to contributing factors such as malnutrition, sepsis, and delay or omission of chemotherapy.

Approach to Therapy

Progress in the cure of children diagnosed with nephroblastoma recorded survival which is exceeding 90% in resourced countries. These results have been achieved through the appropriate use of chemotherapy, surgery, and radiotherapy.

There are two major therapeutic protocols used internationally: the COG (used mainly in the United States) and SIOP (used worldwide) protocols. The SIOP pro-

Table 8.3 Chemotherapy drugs used in the treatment of nephroblastoma

Vincristine	1.5 mg/m^2 IV bolus (max 2 mg)
Doxorubicin	50 mg/m^2 IV infusion over 6 h
Actinomycin D	45 µg/kg IV bolus (max 2000 µg) > 30 kg: 600 µg/m^2
Cyclophosphamide	450 mg/m^2 IV infusion over 1 h
Carboplatin	200 mg/m^2 IV infusion over 1 h
Etoposide (VP16)	150 mg/m^2 IV infusion over 1 h

Weight < 12 kg: reduction of the dose to 2/3 for each drug
Major intolerance: 2/3 of the prescribed dose for the following course

tocol recommends preoperative chemotherapy while the COG proposes surgery up front.

Nephroblastoma is a chemosensitive tumor, and preoperative chemotherapy reduces its volume and diminishes the risk of tumor rupture leading to down staging of the tumor resulting in less treatment after surgery.

The chemotherapy drugs used for the treatment of nephroblastoma are presented in Table 8.3.

The use of these drugs has been designed to provide maximum therapeutic benefit and minimal side effects in the short and long terms.

The treatment of nephroblastoma is a multimodal therapy and includes surgery, chemotherapy, and in advanced stages radiotherapy.

Radiotherapy is given only for advanced stages (stages 3 and 4) or in stage II in case of anaplastic tumors and with a longer period of chemotherapy. Radiotherapy can be given to the local renal bed or combined with the treatment of the distant metastases.

The choice of treatment is based on the stage, associated comorbidities, and availability and affordability of therapy.

Each patient should receive the treatment, which optimizes her/his chance to be cured based on risk assessment and response adapted.

The choice of treatment is dependent on the availability of the drugs avoiding delays in administration of the chemotherapy.

Follow-Up During Treatment

During the chemotherapy only CBC and renal functions are required.

An evaluation of the cardiac function is performed at the beginning of the therapy. Not more than 250 mg/m^2 cumulative dose of doxorubicin should be given.

A special attention must be given to supportive care measures especially in severely malnourished children with prolonged administration of chemotherapy associated with or without radiotherapy.

Follow-Up After Treatment

The follow-up after treatment includes clinical examination, the assessment of renal function, and kidney ultrasound. In advanced disease, pulmonary radiography is indicated.

Complications Related to Therapy

Complications related to therapy are associated with the toxicity of the drugs: cardiac toxicity and renal toxicity. Acute hepatotoxicity can occur with actinomycin (or is it vincristine as well???) as venous occlusive disease (VOD).

The prolonged administration of chemotherapy isolated or together with radiotherapy increases the risk of febrile neutropenia, susceptibility to infection, anemia, and thrombocytopenia.

The delayed complications are associated with one single functional kidney, apparition of secondary cancers following the use of chemotherapy and radiation.

Relapse of Nephroblastoma

The relapse of nephroblastoma can occur at the initial site, involving the contralateral kidney or presenting with distant metastases: lungs and liver metastases are the most common.

The treatment involves the addition of new drugs such as ICE protocol, combined with surgery and radiotherapy.

The prognosis in these cases remains reserved.

Summary

Nephroblastoma is the most common renal tumor in childhood and one of the commonest childhood cancers in Africa. It usually presents with an abdominal mass, or in other cases parents discover it incidentally.

Clinical examination together with an abdominal ultrasound is in most cases sufficient to diagnose the tumor. The confirmation of the diagnosis is obtained by pathological examination of tissue obtained after surgical resection.

It is a chemo- and radiosensitive tumor with excellent survival rates if diagnosed early.

An awareness program about nephroblastoma should be included in all IMCI (Integrated Management Childhood Illnesses) books.

Suggested Reading

Benchekroun S, Madani A, Zafad S, Harif M, Yaakoubi M, Zamiati S, Sahraoui S, Benjelloun A, Fehri M (2006) Treatment of Wilms tumor according to SIOP 9 protocol in Casablanca, Morocco. Pediatr Blood Cancer 46:472–475

Metzger M, Dome JS (2005) Current therapy for Wilms' tumor. Oncologist 10:815–826

Moreira C, Nachef MN, Ziamati S, Ladjaj Y, Barsoaoui S, Mallon B, Tournade MF (2012) Treatment of nephroblastoma in Africa: results of the first French African pediatric oncology group (GFAOP) study. Ped Blood Cancer 58(1):37–42

Smith MA, Seibel NL, Altekruse SF et al (2010) Outcomes for children and adolescents with cancer: challenges for the twenty-first century. J Clin Oncol 28(15):2625–2634

Sonn G, Shortliffe L (2008) Management of Wilms tumor: current standard of care. Nat Clin Pract Urol 5(10):551–560

Chapter 9
Hepatoblastoma

Case Presentation

Radouane, a 13-month-old boy, who was previously healthy, was brought to the hospital by his parents with a 2-week history of abdominal pain. The mother also noted an abdominal mass when she was giving him a bath. There was no vomiting or any stool changes.

Findings on examination:

Radouane did not look acutely or chronically ill.
Weight = 13 kg, height = 81 cm.
Observations: normal.
No pallor, lymphadenopathy, jaundice, clubbing, or edema was present.
The cardiovascular, respiratory, and neurological examinations were normal.
On examination of the abdomen, the following were found: distension and a large painless mass occupying the right hypochondrium and epigastrium (10 × 15 cm). The mass could not be distinguished from the liver and was not ballotable. No other masses or organomegaly were noted.

What Is the Differential Diagnosis?

Abdominal masses: nephroblastoma and other renal tumors, neuroblastoma, hepatoblastoma, lymphoma, benign renal mass.

D.C. Stefan, M. Harif, *Pediatric Cancer in Africa*,
DOI 10.1007/978-3-319-17936-0_9

What Investigations Would You Like to Request?

- CBC, renal function, bilirubin, liver enzymes.
- Alpha fetoprotein (AFP).
- Abdominal ultrasound.
- Chest X-ray (PA and lateral).
- CT or MRI scan of the abdomen.

Herein listed are available results for your case scenario:

Wcc	Hb	MCV	Pl	Neutro	Lymph	Na	K	Urea	Creat
9.8	11.5	75	385	2.8	5.5	138	4.2	3	35

Bili	AST	ALT	LDH	AFP
7	22	24	157	800,564 ng/mL

The ultrasound showed a massively enlarged liver with heterogenous areas (Figs. 9.1, 9.2, and 9.3).

A large multilobulated heterogenously enhancing mass (135 × 98 × 132 mm) was seen in the right liver lobe. Multiple areas of necrosis present. The majority of the liver is involved; only segment 6 is spared. Hemorrhage within the mass is noted. No vascular involvement seen. Radiological features are in keeping with hepatoblastoma (Fig. 9.4).

Liver tumors are rare in children. Two major types occur, namely hepatoblastoma and hepatocellular carcinoma, of which hepatoblastoma is far more common.

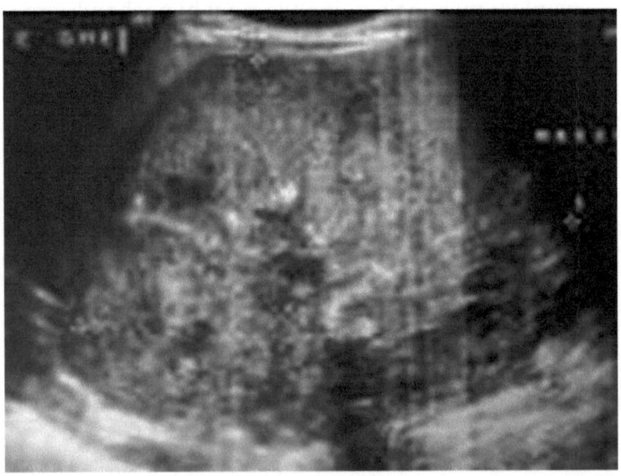

Fig. 9.1 Abdominal ultrasound

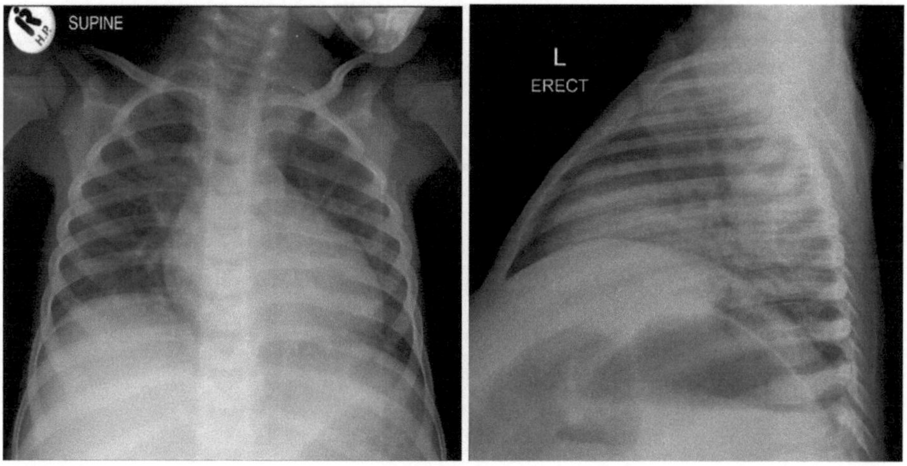

Fig. 9.2 Chest X-ray (normal)

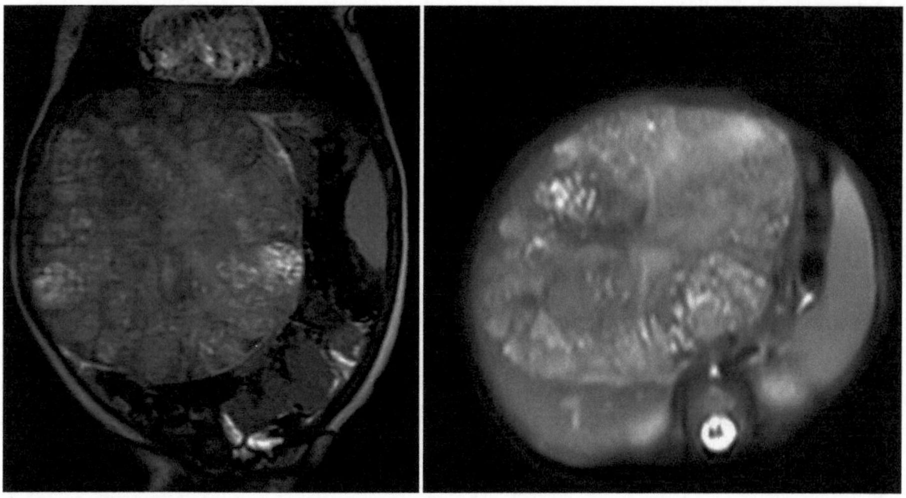

Fig. 9.3 MRI abdomen

Epidemiology

Hepatoblastoma (HB) is a rare tumor, representing only about 0.5–2 % of all childhood cancers. It has a male predominance. The incidence of HB has increased significantly in the United States and it is thought that the ever increasing survival of

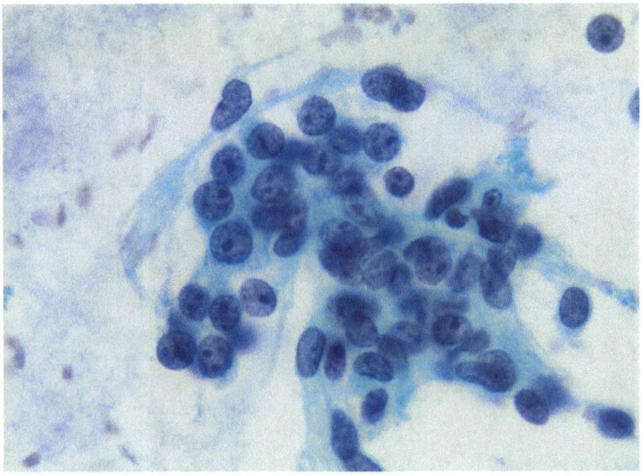

Fig. 9.4 Fine needle aspiration of liver mass

Table 9.1 Risk factors/associated conditions associated with hepatoblastoma and hepatocellular carcinoma

Malignancy	Risk factors/associated conditions
Hepatoblastoma	Aicardi syndrome, hemihypertrophy, Beckwith–Wiedemann, familial adenomatous polyposis, glycogen storage disease, trisomy 18 (and other trisomies), low birth weight
Hepatocellular carcinoma	Alagille syndrome, glycogen storage disease, hepatitis B & C, progressive familial intrahepatic cholestasis, tyrosinemia

very low birth weight babies has contributed to this, since there is a strong association between a low birth weight and HB. A Japanese study reported the risk of HB to be 15 times higher in babies with a birth weight below 1000 g. Most cases of HB occur in children younger than 3 years of age; about 90 % of all liver tumors in children under 4 years are hepatoblastomas.

In addition to a low birth weight, the following are also associated with an increased incidence of HB (Table 9.1): Aicardi syndrome, hemi-hypertrophy, Beckwith–Wiedemann syndrome, familial adenomatous polyposis (FAP), glycogen storage disease, trisomy 18 (and other trisomies).

Histology

Hepatoblastoma is derived from hepatocyte precursors. There are two main pathological subtypes: epithelial (56 %) and mixed epithelial/mesenchymal (44 %). The epithelial group includes the pure fetal type (31 %), as well as the embryonal (19 %), macrotrabecular (3 %), and small cell undifferentiated (3 %) types. The presence of mesenchymal elements such as osteoid and cartilage is associated with a better outcome in advanced disease. The small cell undifferentiated type predicts a poor outcome, while the presence of pure fetal histology in a completely resected tumor is associated with an improved outcome.

Clinical Presentation

The usual clinical presentation is that of an asymptomatic, enlarging abdominal mass situated mainly in the right hypochondrium, but could also extend into the epigastrium or other areas depending on the size of the tumor. The right liver lobe is involved more often than the left. Less frequently, abdominal pain, weight loss, anorexia, and nausea and vomiting may be present. Rarely, jaundice related to bile duct compression may be observed or even signs of an acute abdomen due to tumor rupture. The tumor metastasizes to the lungs and sometimes the bladder or diaphragm may be involved contiguously.

Diagnostic Work-Up

Laboratory Tests

Hematological

A baseline hematological evaluation should be performed: complete blood count and clotting profile. Thrombocytosis is observed in 20 % of cases due to production of thrombopoietin by the tumor.

Biochemistry

Renal function studies (electrolytes, urea, and creatinine) should be performed, as well as liver function studies (bilirubin, albumin, AST, ALT, LDH, GGT). The liver function is most often preserved, even in large tumors. Alpha-fetoprotein (AFP) is the most important laboratory test and is increased in 90 % of cases. This finding is not pathognomonic however. An increased AFP level is also found in two-thirds of hepatocellular carcinoma cases, as well as in patients with infantile hemangioendothelioma and mesenchymal hamartoma. A low AFP level is associated with a very poor outcome. AFP, physiologically produced by the fetal liver, is increased at birth, after which it decreases gradually to reach normal values at 1 year (Table 9.2). The half-life is 5–7 days and it is extremely useful and reliable in the monitoring and follow-up of patients. Following treatment, the level normalizes within a few days or weeks. Rarely, beta-HCG may also be elevated.

Table 9.2 Normal values of AFP birth to 8 months

Age	AFP level (ng/mL)
Premature	134,734 ± 41,444
Newborn at birth	48,406 ± 34,718
Newborn—first 2 weeks	33,113 ± 33,503
Newborn—2 weeks to 1 month	9,452 ± 12,610
2 months	323 ± 278
3 months	88 ± 87
4 months	74 ± 56
5 months	46.5 ± 19
6 months	12.5 ± 9.8
7 months	9.7 ± 7.1
8 months	8.5 ± 5.5

Radiological Studies

A chest radiograph should be performed as a screening test for pulmonary metastases, as well as for pulmonary tuberculosis in areas with a high incidence of tuberculosis. A CT scan of the chest, if available, may be performed to further investigate the extent of pulmonary involvement. A lesion of >10 mm or several lesions with at least one >5 mm seen on chest X-ray or CT scan is regarded as definite metastatic disease. Lesions not meeting these criteria may be biopsied.

An abdominal X-ray is not helpful. An abdominal ultrasound should be performed to confirm the hepatic origin of the mass, as well as the extent of the mass. Ideally, a CT or MRI scan of the abdomen should be performed in order to obtain more anatomical information. This is especially helpful when surgery is being planned.

Histology

It is strongly recommended that the diagnosis should be confirmed by histology in all cases, except in patients with hemangiomas or hemangioendotheliomas (diagnosed by imaging alone) and infantile hepatic choriocarcinoma (diagnosed by imaging and a high beta-human chorionic gonadotropin (beta-HCG)). A percutaneous sonar-guided biopsy is a simple and safe procedure.

Staging

Two surgical staging systems are used: the PRETEXT system, which is used after neoadjuvant chemotherapy but before surgery, designed by the International Society of Paediatric Oncology (SIOP) and the postsurgical staging system of the Children's Oncology Group (COG).

PRETEXT (Pretreatment Extent) Staging System

An ultrasound or CT with/without MRI is required for this system. The liver is radiographically divided into four sectors, and involvement pertaining to these sectors is described. Infiltration of the inferior vena cava, hepatic and portal veins are reported, as well as extrahepatic involvement and metastatic lesions, but this does not affect the PRETEXT stage. The more sections of liver are involved by tumor, the higher the stage and the poorer the outcome. This staging system is now used by all study groups worldwide (Table 9.3).

Postsurgical Staging System

Stage I indicates a completely resected tumor, while stage II is assigned when there is residual microscopic tumor after resection. If the tumor is unresectable at diagnosis or it is resected with gross residual tumor remaining, it is stage III disease. If tumor cells are found in resected lymph nodes, stage III is also assigned to the tumor. Stage IV disease is of course when distant metastases are present, irrespective of the liver involvement.

Prognosis

The overall survival rate of hepatoblastoma has improved considerably over the years and has reached 70–80 % in developed countries. For limited disease (stage I and II), the survival rate is more than 90 %. The 3 year overall survival, however, for metastatic disease has been much poorer, but has also improved. The 3 year overall survival was reported to be 62 % in the SIOPEL-3 study, which included intensive chemotherapy and aggressive surgery.

The prognosis varies according to several factors: the resectability of the tumor (PRETEXT stage) (Table 9.4), response to neoadjuvant chemotherapy, vascular invasion, extrahepatic involvement, and the stage of disease, which includes the presence of metastases at the diagnosis. An AFP level of less than 100 ng/mL predicts a very poor prognosis and may indicate small cell undifferentiated histology. Tumor rupture is also considered to be a high risk event.

Treatment

The treatment of hepatoblastoma comprises systemic chemotherapy and most importantly surgical resection. At diagnosis, the minority of patients have resectable tumors (less than a third of patients), thus neoadjuvant chemotherapy plays an important role in shrinking the tumor in order to attain resectability. In some cases of advanced disease, a liver transplant is the only surgical option.

Table 9.3 The PRETEXT staging system

PRETEXT stage	Extension	
I	Only 1 liver sector is involved	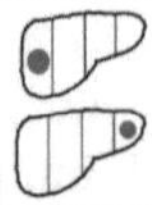
II	One or two sectors involved and two adjoining sectors uninvolved	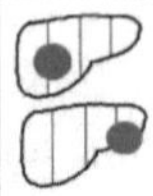
III	Three sectors involved and one sector uninvolved OR two sectors involved and two non-adjoining sectors uninvolved	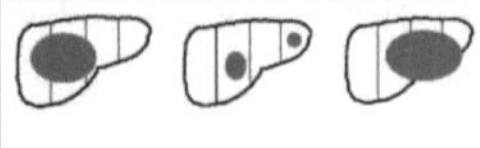
IV	All four liver sectors involved	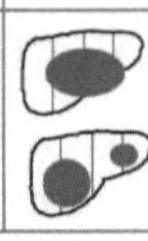
Designations of any stage	Infiltration of the inferior vena cava or all three hepatic veins (V), infiltration of main portal or portal bifurcation vein (P), infiltration of caudate (C), extra-hepatic involvement (E) and distant metastases (M)	

Table 9.4 Prognosis according to the PRETEXT staging system

Stage	3 year overall survival (SIOPEL-2) (%)
I	100
II	95
III	84
IV	61
Intra-abdominal extra-hepatic disease	58
Metastatic disease	44

Chemotherapy

Hepatoblastoma is a chemosensitive tumor. The chemotherapeutic agents that have been used in different protocols are cisplatin, doxorubicin, carboplatin, vincristine, 5 fluorouracyl, ifosfamide, etoposide, and cyclophosphamide. The European SIOP protocol is named SIOPEL. SIOPEL-1 showed the success of preoperative chemotherapy (PLADO–cisplatin and doxorubicin). SIOPEL-2 successfully employed stratification for standard and high risk disease. In SIOPEL-3 standard risk disease was treated with cisplatin monotherapy, which proved to be as effective as PLADO and less toxic. High risk disease was addressed in a SIOPEL-4 feasibility study, where dose-intense cisplatin-based chemotherapy (cisplatin, doxorubicin, and carboplatin) proved to be efficacious. Patients receiving cisplatin-based chemotherapy will develop toxicity, e.g., hematological and renal toxicity, as well as hearing loss, and need adequate supportive care and monitoring.

See Table 9.5 for a summary of the SIOPEL treatment guidelines.

Table 9.5 Risk stratification and advised treatment

Risk group	Criteria	Treatment
Standard	PRETEXT I, II, or III with no additional adverse features, e.g., low AFP level, vascular involvement (V3 or P2), extrahepatic spread, tumor rupture, metastatic disease	Cisplatin monotherapy arm of the SIOPEL-3 study: 4 cycles preoperative chemotherapy, followed by surgical resection and 2 postoperative courses of chemotherapy
High	Any tumor not meeting the standard or very high risk criteria	Super-PLADO arm of SIOPEL-3 study (cisplatin alternating with carboplatin/doxorubicin) Refer to a specialized surgical center
Very high	Metastatic disease or AFP level <100 ng/mL	Dose-intense SIOPEL-4 protocol for high risk disease Refer to a specialized surgical center

A pilot-adapted SIOPEL protocol for developing countries, namely the RCN (resource challenged nations) protocol, consists of cisplatin monotherapy as per the SIOPEL-3 study. It has been developed with the aim of providing a simple, more affordable, and less toxic treatment regimen, yet which is still effective.

Surgery

A complete surgical resection is crucial in the successful treatment of hepatoblastoma. As mentioned, the European SIOPEL approach favors preoperative chemotherapy, followed by resection, similar to the nephroblastoma approach. The North American study group (COG) advises upfront surgery, followed by chemotherapy.

The surgical excision should be planned carefully, using the best available radiological investigations. Ideally, it should take place in a center with expertise in liver, as well as transplant surgery. A multidisciplinary team should be involved and postoperatively patients should be cared for in an intensive care unit, with easy access to blood products. The liver surgery may entail partial or total hepatectomy or liver transplant in cases where resection is still not possible after preoperative chemotherapy. Suspicious para-aortic or celiac lymph nodes should be resected and sent for histology.

Most pulmonary lesions will respond completely to chemotherapy, but metastasectomy should be performed for any remaining lesions.

SIOPEL Studies

In the first SIOPEL study, the resection rate was 53 and 8 % of patients with unresectable tumors underwent a liver transplant. The outcome of these patients was similar to patients who had had a partial liver resection. In SIOPEL-2 and -3, the rates of successful resection increased to 67 % and 74 %, respectively; the corresponding number of liver transplants increased to 12 and 21 %. In SIOPEL-4, the resection rate improved even further to 85 % with 26 % transplants performed.

In Africa

Almost all cases of hepatoblastoma in Africa present late, often with metastatic disease, thus preoperative neoadjuvant chemotherapy is essential. Advanced radiological investigations (CT and MRI scans) may not be available, thus making staging and surgical planning/resection more challenging. Pediatric surgeons, skilled in liver surgery and transplant, are a scarce resource and even in developed countries, patients with advanced disease are referred to centers with experience in this type of surgery. All these factors, as well as a lack of availability of chemotherapy and adequate supportive care, unfortunately lead to poor survival rates.

Relapsed Disease

Risk factors for relapse are PRETEXT stage IV, metastases at primary diagnosis, older age, low AFP level, vascular involvement, and small cell undifferentiated histology. The sites of relapse may be the liver, lungs, peritoneum and the central nervous system. Most patients have an elevated AFP level at the time of relapse. When surgically feasible, the new lesion(s) should be resected. Salvage chemotherapy regimens include carboplatin/etoposide, carboplatin/doxorubicin, irinotecan, high dose cyclophosphamide, and others. About half of patients may be salvaged with second-line combined treatment.

Summary

Hepatoblastoma is a rare tumor, but remains the most common childhood liver tumor.

The diagnostic work-up should include baseline blood tests, as well as an AFP level and at least an abdominal ultrasound and chest X-ray. If available, a CT or MRI scan of the abdomen and a CT scan of the chest should be performed. In most cases, a biopsy should be performed to confirm the diagnosis.

Treatment is based on preoperative chemotherapy, followed by surgical resection and postoperative chemotherapy. Surgical resection may be very challenging and complicated cases should be referred to a center with expertise in the treatment of hepatoblastoma.

Suggested Reading

Agarwala S, Ronghe MD, Aronson DC, Czauderna P, Brock P, Roebuck D et al (2009) Pilot of treatment guidelines for hepatoblastoma (BH) in resource challenged nations (RCN). PBC 53:717

Aronson DC, Czaudema P, Maibach R, Perilongo G, Morland B (2014) The treatment of hepatoblastoma: its evolution and the current status as per the SIOPEL trials. J Ind Assoc Pediatr Surg 19(4):201–207

Herzog CE, Andrassy RJ, Eftekhari F (2000) Childhood cancers: hepatoblastoma. Oncologist 5:445–453

Perilongo G, Shafford E, Maibach R et al (2004) Risk-adapted treatment for childhood hepatoblastoma: final report of the second study of the International Society of Paediatric Oncology—SIOPEL 2. Eur J Cancer 40(3):411–421

Roebuck DJ, Perilongo G (2006) Hepatoblastoma: an oncological review. Pediatr Radiol 36(3):183–186

Roebuck DJ, Aronson D, Clapuyt P et al (2007) 2005 PRETEXT: a revised staging system for primary malignant liver tumours of childhood developed by the SIOPEL group. Pediatr Radiol 37(2):123–132

www.cancertopics/pdq/treatment/childliver/healthprofessional/page1. Accessed 12 April 2015

www.siopel.org. Accessed 12 April 2015

Zsíros J, Maibach R, Shafford E et al (2010) Successful treatment of childhood high-risk hepatoblastoma with dose-intensive multiagent chemotherapy and surgery: final results of the SIOPEL-3HR study. J Clin Oncol 28(15):2584–2590

Zsiros J, Brugieres L, Brock P et al (2013) Dose-dense cisplatin-based chemotherapy and surgery for children with high-risk hepatoblastoma (SIOPEL-4): a prospective, single-arm, feasibility study. Lancet Oncol 14:834–842

Chapter 10
Retinoblastoma

Case Presentation

A 4-year-old girl came for consultation because her parents noticed a growing white reflection in her left eye 6 months before (Fig. 10.1).

1. What would you call this symptom?
2. Eye ultrasound (Fig. 10.2) and CT-Scan (Fig. 10.3) showed a calcified mass. What diagnosis would you consider?
3. What would be your diagnostic approach?
4. What would be your treatment options?

Retinoblastoma is the most frequent intraocular tumor in childhood. This tumor occurs mainly in infants and small children. The tumor can be unilateral or bilateral, uni- or multifocal, sporadic, or hereditary. Children with a hereditary form have a high susceptibility of developing a second tumor. In developed countries, the rate of survival exceeds 95 %, while in Africa, this tumor is very frequent and is usually diagnosed at a later stage.

D.C. Stefan, M. Harif, *Pediatric Cancer in Africa*,
DOI 10.1007/978-3-319-17936-0_10

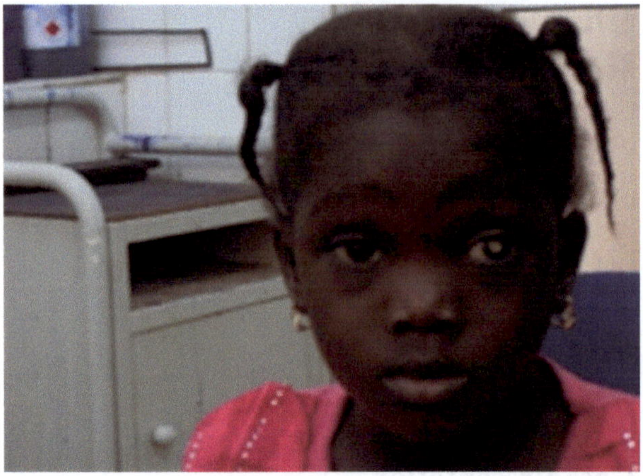

Fig. 10.1 Initial presentation

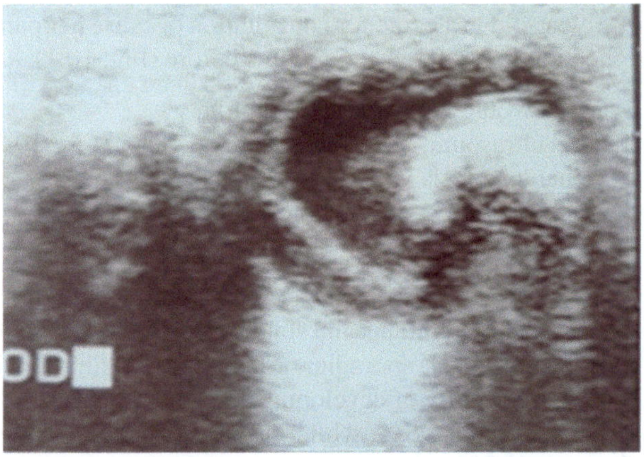

Fig. 10.2 Eye ultrasound

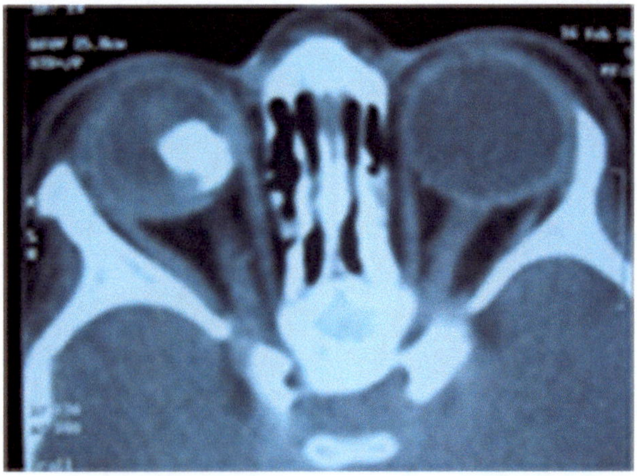

Fig. 10.3 CT Scan of the same patient

Epidemiology and Genetics

The incidence delete of retinoblastoma is 1 per 15,000–30,000 live births. In one-third of cases, retinoblastoma occurs in both eyes and is considered hereditary. These forms occur usually at a lower age compared to sporadic cases. Unilateral forms are usually not hereditary and is usually diagnosed around the age 2 years.

Hereditary forms are typically bilateral or multifocal and are usually diagnosed much earlier, even in the first year of life. Transmission is autosomal dominant with a high risk of occurrence in the siblings and offspring. The risk of transmission to children is 50 %. In 15–20 % of unilateral forms there are mutations in germ cells, with a risk of transmission to the offspring of 50 %.

According to Knudson's theory, two genetic lesions are necessary for the occurrence of retinoblastoma. The first mutation is inherited at the level of the germ cells, while the second mutation occurs spontaneously at the level of the somatic retinal cells and other body tissues. In both mutations, somatic retinal cells are involved in the nonhereditary form. This hypothesis explains the significant higher risk of second cancers in the hereditary forms.

The retinoblastoma gene has been identified and cloned as a tumor suppressor gene located at 13q14 chromosome. The loss of both alleles is required for oncogenesis process of retinoblastoma. Deletion shown in the karyotype, but more often a point mutation leads to mRNA incomplete or absent transcript of retinoblastoma gene. In 5 % of cases, there is an association with other abnormalities and particularly those related to a deletion of chromosome 13 (Table 10.1).

Retinoblastoma seems more frequent in Africa representing the second or third most frequently seen tumor in some pediatric cancer units. No particular predisposing factor has been demonstrated in this setting so far.

Table 10.1 Chromosome 13q deletion syndrome

In chromosome 13q deletion syndrome, a portion of the long arm (q) on chromosome 13 is missing or deleted. The most frequent reported anomalies are:
• Microcephaly
• Widening of naso-frontal bones
• Hypertelorism
• Microphthalmia
• Ptosis
• Micrognathia
• Hypoplasia or absence of the thumb
• Rarely: mental retardation, growth retardation, cleft palate, supernumeraries' fingers or toes

Mode of Spread

Most tumors have an endophytic development (toward vitreous) and exophytic (toward subretinal space). Exophytic extension can cause a retinal detachment. Glaucoma can also occur following occlusion of the trabecular neovascularization network, Iris or invasion to the optic nerve.

If extraocular extension is present, it can reach the orbit or optic nerve; the tumor can also reach preauricular or maxillary lymph nodes through lymphatic pathway, and via the bloodstream of the brain, bones, bone marrow, and other organs. Retinoblastoma can invade the optic nerve and extend along the axons to the brain or across the subarachnoid space and extend to the brain or cerebrospinal fluid. The presence of anorexia, vomiting, headache, or weight loss is usually a manifestation of cerebrospinal metastases.

In the trilateral retinoblastoma, there is an intracranial median most often with pineal involvement, which is associated with the bilateral form. Evolution towards spinal metastases is frequent and has a poor prognosis.

Clinical Characteristics

In developed countries, the tumor is mostly diagnosed as intraocular retinoblastoma, while in developing countries, most patients attend hospital long after the cancer has spread beyond the eye and extraocular disease is present.

The most common symptoms of retinoblastoma in developed countries are leukocoria and strabismus. Leukocoria is a white reflection of the pupil (derived from Greek *leukos* meaning "white" and "*kore*" meaning "pupil"). Leukocoria is an early sign of retinoblastoma, but unfortunately irregular, and is sometimes noticed only after a photoflash. Strabismus is also frequently noted in the early stages.

These signs should raise parents' attention to have their child's eyes examined as soon as possible. In rare cases, the disease presents as red eye as a result of intraocular inflammation, and chemosis, which is more or less associated with eyelid edema. Eye pain is unusual, whereas buphtalmia or exophthalmia reflect a late stage of the disease.

In Africa, most cases are diagnosed at late stages, and exophthalmia is the most common clinical manifestation. Delay in diagnosing retinoblastoma is not only because of difficult access to care, but also because of inadequate education of primary care providers. Nurses or physicians not being aware of early manifestation of retinoblastoma may consider this a benign condition and thereby contribute to the delay in diagnosis (Figs. 10.4 and 10.5).

Because of a high incidence of this tumor in Africa, and the excellent prognosis in early diagnosed cases, the team should introduce early diagnostic campaigns including a public awareness program which also addresses education for caregivers.

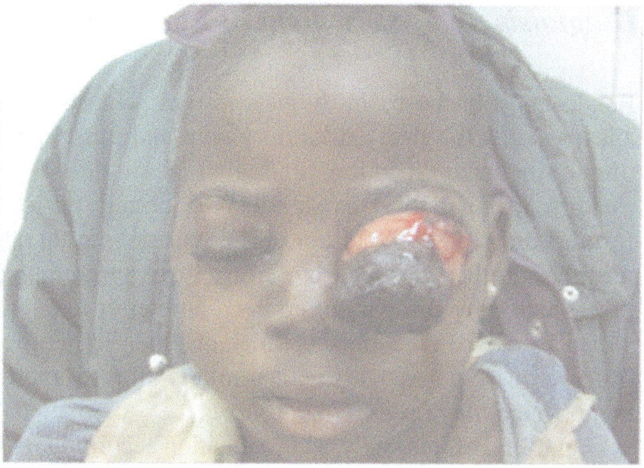

Fig. 10.4 Late stage retinoblastoma with massive optic nerve infiltration

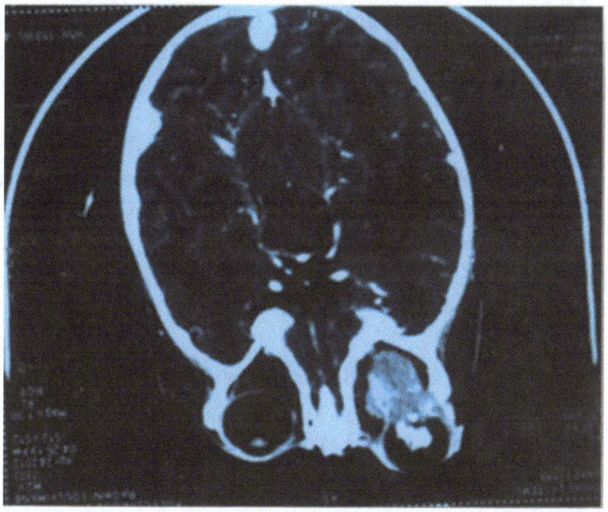

Fig. 10.5 Late stage retinoblastoma with massive optic nerve infiltration (CT Scan)

Differential Diagnosis

The most common differential diagnoses are Coats' disease, cataract, toxocariasis, and retinopathy of prematurity. In Africa, orbital Burkitt's lymphoma may be considered in patients presenting with exophthalmia.

Diagnosis and Assessment of Extension

Fundoscopy is the main diagnostic tool. This is done under sedation or general anesthesia as the first exploratory step and must specify the characteristics of the tumor, the size, location, and also if single or multiple lesions are present. Fundoscopy of both eyes should be routinely performed to rule out the bilateral form. A drawing of the tumor or if possible a digital photo of the lesion may be very useful for follow-up in case of conservative treatment. The size of the tumor must be estimated by comparison to the diameter of the optic nerve head.

On fundoscopy, a pink creamy mass or sometimes a yellowish-white mass is observed associated with neovascularization. Sometimes a retinal detachment or hemorrhage may obscure the tumor.

At the end of this study, a classification according to the criteria of Reese-Ellsworth (Table 10.2) or ABC (Murphree) classification (Table 10.3) must be established. It is important to know that these classifications predict ocular salvage and are not corelated with the patient survival.

Tumor analysis study is also completed with eye ultrasound usually showing a hyper-echoic mass and calcifications in more than 90 % of cases. Retinal detachment may also be highlighted. CT-scan shows a calcified mass and explores possible extension to optical nerve, orbit, and any cerebral extension. MRI is not available in most African countries, though allows for a better evaluation of the optic nerve and the CNS.

The goal of these examinations is to evaluate the overall intraocular, intraorbital, intracranial presence of disease, and search for metastases distances. Analysis of CSF and blood-borne (lungs, liver, bones, bone marrow) metastases is recommended only in cases of extraocular extension or in the case of massive choroidal involvement.

Table 10.2 Reese-Ellsworth classification for retinoblastoma

Group I: Very favorable	(a) Solitary tumor, less than 4 disc diameters (DD) in size, at or behind the equator (b) Multiple tumors, none over 4 DD in size, all at or behind the equator
Group II: Favorable	(a) Solitary tumor, 4–10 DD in size, at or behind the equator (b) Multiple tumors, 4–10 DD in size, behind the equator
Group III: Doubtful/possible	(a) Any lesion anterior to the equator (b) Solitary tumors larger than 10 DD behind the equator
Group IV: Unfavorable	(a) Multiple tumors, some larger than 10 DD (b) Any lesion extending anteriorly to the ora serrata
Group V: Very unfavorable	(a) Massive tumors involving more than one-half of the retina (b) Vitreous seeding

Table 10.3 International intraocular retinoblastoma classification (ABC classification)

Group A: Very low risk Eyes with small discrete tumors away from critical structures	Tumors 3 mm or smaller, confined to the retina >3 mm from the foveola and 1.5 mm from the optic nerve No vitreous or subretinal seeding
Group B: Low risk Eyes with no vitreous or subretinal seeding and discrete retinal tumor of any size or location	Tumors not in Group A No vitreous or subretinal seeding Subretinal fluid >5 mm from the base of the tumor
Group C: Moderate risk Eyes with only focal vitreous or subretinal seeding and discrete retinal tumors of any size and location	Seeding local, fine, and limited Treatable with a radioactive plaque Tumors discrete and of any size and location Up to one quadrant of subretinal fluid
Group D: High risk Eyes with diffuse vitreous or subretinal seeding and/or massive, nondiscrete endophytic or exophytic disease. Eyes with more extensive seeding than Group C	Massive and/or diffuse intraocular disseminated disease More than one quadrant of retinal detachment Fine greasy vitreous seeding or avascular masses Subretinal seeding, plaque-like
Group E: Very high risk eyes Eyes that have been destroyed anatomically or functionally by the tumor. Eyes with one or more than the following:	Irreversible neovascular glaucoma Massive intraocular hemorrhage Aseptic orbital cellulitis Tumor anterior to anterior vitreous face Tumor touching the lens Diffuse infiltrating retinoblastoma Phthisis or prephthisis

Pathology

The goals of pathological study are to confirm the diagnosis of retinoblastoma, to specify the topography of the lesions, and to evaluate the quality of resection. The positive diagnosis is usually made on the standard staining. According to differentiation of retinoblastoma cells, there are immature forms of retinoblasts, well-differentiated forms with rosettes (Flexner–Wintersteiner rosettes) and intermediate forms with the two contingents.

Depending on the topography of the lesions, the analysis distinguishes exophytic, endophytic, and mixed characteristics. Pathology should precise the extension to the eye tunics and possible extension in the anterior chamber. Analysis of the optical nerve is of crucial importance for prognostic evaluation. In the case that this has been reached, the pathologist should specify if the involvement is pre- or retrolaminar.

Cases of the so-called retinocytoma or retinoma, and benign forms with a high degree of differentiation are reported.

Treatment

Retinoblastoma treatment requires a well-coordinated multidisciplinary team. This is the function of the extent of intraocular tumor mass, orbital extension, and the presence of metastases to the level of the central nervous system or elsewhere. If the tumor is intraocular, the likelihood of cure is very high. Treatment should be adapted to each case with continuous dialogue between the pediatric oncologist and the ophthalmologist.

Surgery

Enucleation is recommended when no vision can be preserved. This is the case of most unilateral forms. Acceptance of enucleation is usually a problem in Africa. Appropriate information and also prosthesis should be proposed. Exenteration must be avoided. During the surgery, it is necessary to ensure to include a minimum length of 10–15 mm of the optic nerve and make orbital biopsies in the event of suspicious lesions.

An orbital implant should be placed in the cavity at the end of intervention; its size must allow closure of the eyelid without traction. The ocular prosthesis can be placed within postoperative weeks (Fig. 10.6).

Radiotherapy

Radiotherapy is not available in most African countries. When possible, external radiation is indicated after enucleation in case of microscopically incomplete resection. The usual dose is 45–50 Gy. External radiation is also recommended in the cases of small tumors with potential saved vision. This can be associated with the photocoagulation or cryotherapy.

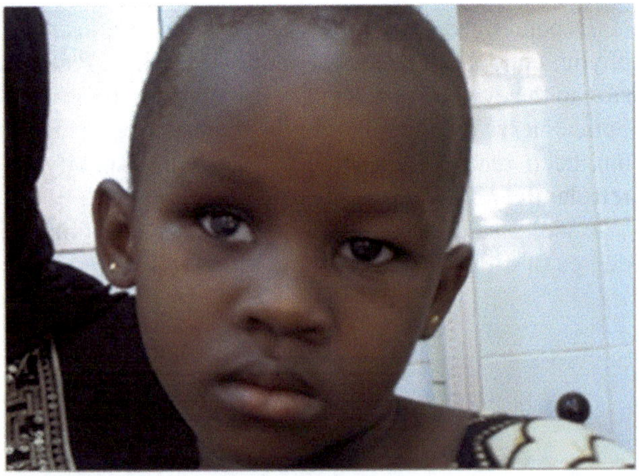

Fig. 10.6 Prosthesis after enucleation for retinoblastoma

Radiotherapy can be complicated by radiation choroidal or retinal vasculitis, vitreous hemorrhage or a secondary glaucoma, cataract, atrophy of temporal or orbital bones and is also associated with an increased risk of secondary cancer and particularly osteosarcoma. Modern techniques of radiation therapy and particularly conformational radiotherapy allow for better targeting of the tumor and can be an alternative to brachytherapy.

Thermotherapy

This technique uses Argon or Xenon laser photocoagulation, which is recommended in small tumors (less than 10 mm) not invading the optical disc, the macula, or the vitreous parts. In very small tumors (less than 2 mm), thermotherapy is associated with chemotherapy (thermochemotherapy) by administration of IV carboplatin 2 h before the course of thermotherapy to avoid the use of an external beam radiotherapy. The size of the laser, its power spot, and the duration of exposure are adapted to each case. More than 90 % of the eyes can be preserved by this technique without radiation therapy. However, it can be complicated by retinal detachment, hemorrhage or dissemination of the tumor, and loss of vision if used at the level of the optical way or the fovea.

Cryotherapy

Cryotherapy may be recommended in small peripheral tumors, alone or in combination with brachytherapy, or external beam radiotherapy in the event of remaining tumor mass. Electrodes are directly applied by placing these on the conjunctiva and sclera. Usually three cycles allow tumor control. This must not be recommended in the case of vitreous involvement. The more frequent complications are vitreous hemorrhage and retinal detachment.

Chemotherapy

Chemotherapy is used for extraocular or metastatic retinoblastoma. Indications have recently been extended to some intraocular tumors in order to reduce their size and make them amenable for focal treatments. Neoadjuvant chemotherapy may be proposed to reduce tumor volume and make it accessible to conservative treatment. The use of additional local treatment is mandatory. The most used medications are carboplatin, etoposide, and vincristine.

In case of an extraocular tumor, association of chemotherapy and irradiation of orbit allows for control of the disease. Usually, the treatment uses vincristine, cyclophosphamide, doxorubicin, cis-platinum, and the carboplatin. The prognosis is poor in cases of central nervous system or bone marrow metastases.

Secondary Cancers

After 5 years, the main cause of death of patients on treatment is caused by metastases. These secondary tumors are in the form of osteosarcomas, and less frequently soft tissue tumors, brain tumors, leukemia, or epithelial tumors. More than two-thirds of these tumors develop at the site of initial radiation.

Suggested Reading

Chantada G, Luna-Fineman S, Sitorus RS et al (2013) SIOP-PODC recommendations for graduated-intensity treatment of retinoblastoma in developing countries. Pediatr Blood Cancer 60:719–727.

Dimaras H, Kimani K, Dimba EAO et al (2012) Retinoblastoma. Lancet 379:1436–1446

Sow AS, Ndoye Roth PA, Moreira C et al (2014) Thérapeutique du rétinoblastome: expérience sénégalaise. J Fr Ophtalmol 37:381–387

Togo B, Sila F, Traore F et al (2010) A 30-month prospective study on the treatment of retinoblastoma in the Gabriel Toure Teaching Hospital, Bamako, Mali. Br J Ophthalmol 94(4):467–469

Chapter 11
Neuroblastoma

Case Presentation

A 4-year-old girl (Figs. 11.1 and 11.2) presented with abdominal mass. Ultrasound showed retroperitoneal mass without other specifications. During her stay at the hospital, a faint eyelid bruising was noticed which was more evident after 5 days.

1. What diagnostic tests would you propose?
2. How would you confirm the diagnosis?
3. How would you estimate the prognosis in this case?
4. What would your treatment approach be?

Neuroblastoma originates from the neural crest giving rise to the adrenal medulla and the sympathetic ganglia. This tumor occurs mainly in infants and young children, and the abdomen is the most frequent location. The tumor has great heterogeneity features ranging from spontaneous regression to resistance to intensive therapies. Furthermore, it is also characterized by the secretion of catecholamine (vanillylmandelic acid VMA or homovanillic acid HVA). Biological characterization of these tumors have made a tremendous progress towards a more accurate diagnosis and prognosis evaluation and opening the era of targeted therapy. This tumor seems very rare in Africa and usually diagnosed at an advanced stage.

D.C. Stefan, M. Harif, *Pediatric Cancer in Africa*,
DOI 10.1007/978-3-319-17936-0_11

Fig. 11.1

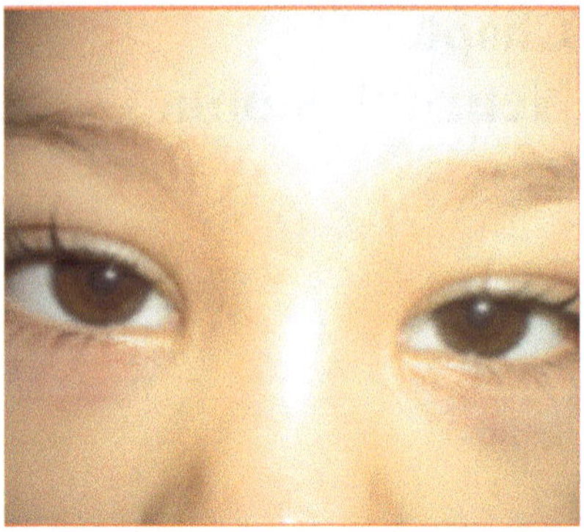

Fig. 11.2

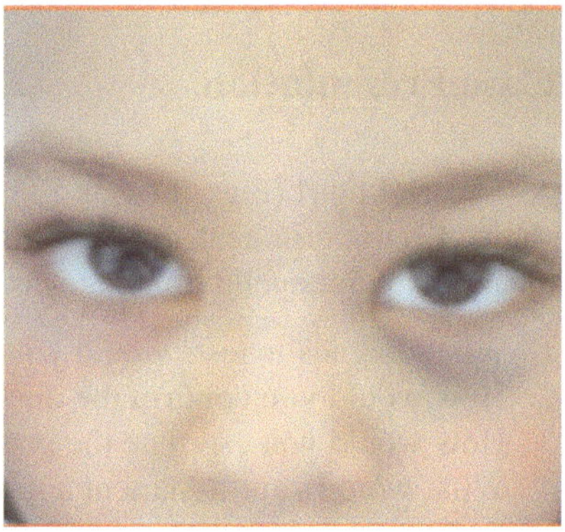

Epidemiological Features

Neuroblastoma represents 8–10 % of cancers in children. Annual incidence is 10 new cases per million children younger than 15 years old. This disease seems less frequent in the African population presenting at late stages in most cases. Diagnostic difficulties contribute in these factors.

In Western industrialized countries, this tumor is the most common extracranial solid type. More than 50 % of neuroblastomas are diagnosed before the age of 2 years and more than 90 % before the age of 5 years. Screening determination of urinary catecholamine found a higher incidence of biologically favourable neuroblastoma with good clinical outcomes. However, cases found have been associated with benign clinical features and therefore with spontaneous regression.

Some neural crest derived diseases particularly Hirschprung disease are associated with increased incidence of neuroblastoma. Familial forms are reported occuring at an early age and generally with favourable outcome.

Pathology and Genetic Characteristics

Neuroblastoma or peripheral neuroblastic tumors are derived from sympathetic, progenitor cells of the sympathetic nervous system. Depending on the level of maturation, these tumors can be described as the immature and malignant neuroblastoma, ganglioneuroblastoma, a mixed form, and the ganglioneuroma, a completely differentiated tumor. These tumors can originate anywhere along the path where neural crest cells migrate, including the adrenal medulla, paraspinal sympathetic ganglia, and sympathetic paraganglia.

Neuroblastoma is a homogeneous small round cellular tumor, with a hyperchromatic nucleus and reduced cytoplasm. Pseudo-rosette figures are observed in nearly 50 % of cases.

In immunohistochemistry, the tumor expresses neural cell markers including Neuron Specific Enolase (NSE), synaptophysin, chromogranin A, and ganglioside GD2.

The international neuroblastoma pathology classification (INPC) based on the Shimada classification takes into account age, the level of neuroblastic differentiation, richness in Schwannian stroma, and mitosis-karyorrhexis index (MKI) (Table 11.1).

Besides pathological features, molecular biology contributed significantly in improving characterization of these tumors and prognostic evaluation. MYCN amplification has been found as an important prognostic marker and is associated with advanced stages, rapid tumor progression, and poor outcome. The 1p deletion also carries a bad prognosis, and is however associated with MYCN deletion.

Clinical Features

Clinical manifestation includes symptoms related to the primary tumor, or to metastasis, and rarely to a paraneoplastic syndrome. The most common site of the tumor is the abdomen, especially the adrenal gland. Mediastinal locations and in the neck are associated with better outcomes. The localized forms are usually asymptomatic, and sometimes fortuitously discovered.

Table 11.1 International neuroblastoma staging system (modified Shimada) pathology classification of neuroblastic tumors (MKI: Mitosis-Karyorrhexis Index)

Stroma features	Age	Favorable histology	Unfavorable histology
Stroma-rich appearance	All	Well-differentiated (ganglioneuroma) Ganglioneuroblastoma Intermixed	Ganglioneuroblastoma, nodular
Stroma-poor appearance (i.e., neuroblastoma)	<18 months	MKI <4 %	MKI >4 % or undifferentiated
	18–60 months	MKI >2 % and differentiated	MKI >2 % or undifferentiated or poorly differentiated
	>60 months	None	All

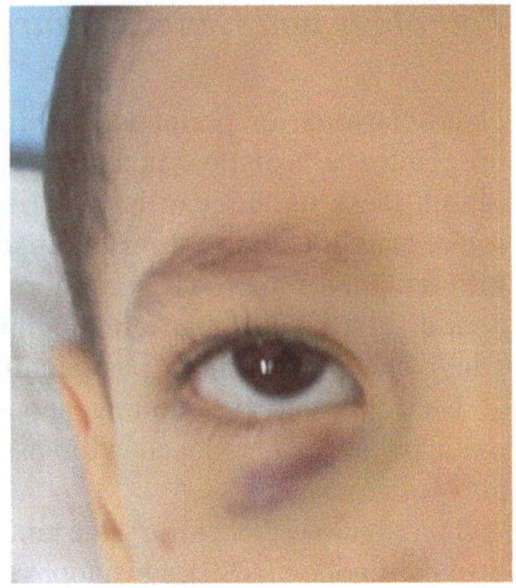

Fig. 11.3 Orbital metastases in abdominal neuroblastoma

General signs include fever, anorexia, lethargy, pallor, weight loss, or irritability. They may also be the main manifestation of the disease and are usually associated with aggressive characteristics.

In the abdomen, the tumor is usually present as an abdominal mass associated with pain, anorexia, and more rarely vomiting.

In the pelvis, signs of compression including constipation or urinary retention is present. On rectal examination, the mass is found in the presacral area.

In the thorax, the appearance varies according to the main location. In the thorax, the tumor appears in the posterior mediastinum, in the paraspinal region. At the upper mediastinum, the tumor can induce dyspnea, dysphagia, or pulmonary infectious complications or lymphatic compression. Lower chest locations are usually not symptomatic.

In the neck, the tumor is usually present as a palpable mass, sometimes associated with the Claude Bernard Horner syndrome (ptosis, myosis, enophthalmia), iris heterochromia or anisocoria.

In the paraspinal spaces, epidural or intradural extension with spinal compression is observed in 5–15 % of cases. This may be associated to a localized pain, lameness, weakness in the lower extremities, hypotonia, sphincter control disorders, muscular atrophy, areflexia, or hyperreflexia, or in most compressive tumors paraplegia. Central nervous system and lung dissemination are exceptional at diagnosis.

Metastasis can be locoregional through lymphatic vessels or blood stream. Liver and bone marrow or bone metastasis are the most frequent metastatic sites. Bone metastasis gives rise to intense pain or a limp. In infants they may be manifest as an irritability. Orbital metastasis is usually present as a periorbital hematoma called also "raccoon eyes" (Fig. 11.3) as a result of retro-orbital venous plexus tumor spread. Orbital infiltrations can induce exophthalmia, edema of the eyelids, and the conjunctiva or ptosis.

Liver infiltration is especially observed in the newborn, and usually present as huge hepatomegaly that may cause a digestive or respiratory compression and could be life threatening.

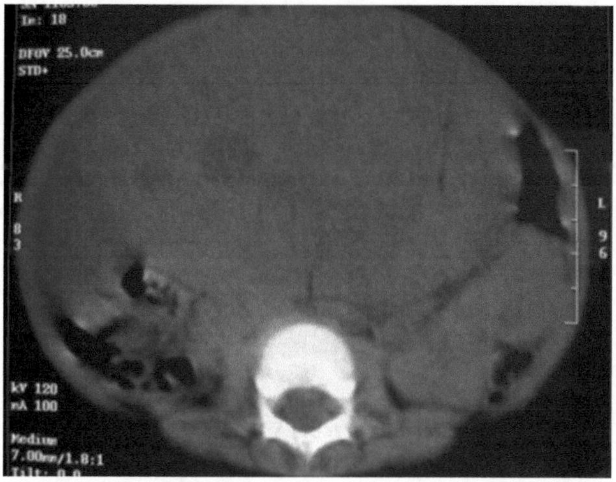

Fig. 11.4 Massive liver infiltration in stage 4 s neuroblastoma

Central nervous system infiltration is rare, though presents with papillary edema, retinal hemorrhage, optic atrophy, or strabismus.

Neonatal Neuroblastoma

Neonatal neuroblastoma is often associated with a favourable outcome evolving to maturation or spontaneous regression. In very young infants, however, there is a risk of lung compression that may be life threatening. At this age, it is most often stage 4s, also known as Pepper's syndrome neuroblastoma, combining massive hepatomegaly (Fig. 11.4), skin nodules, and adrenal medulla infiltration. This is often of benign behavior evolving to a maturation and spontaneous regression. In infants younger than 2 months, there is a risk of compression that may be life threatening. Breathing compression can lead to hypoxia and acidosis with return to the fetal circulation (opening of the oval foramen or arterial canal). The compression of the inferior vena cava and renal vasculature can also induce renal failure.

Paraneoplastic Syndromes

These are rare characteristics of neuroblastoma.

- Hypersecretion of catecholamine can cause physiological changes such as a sweating, flushes, headache, palpitations and arterial hypertension. Arterial hypertension is exceptional in neuroblastoma and may be related to hypersecretion of related of renin (renal–vascular hypertension) because of the tumor mass compressing the renal vessels.
- Hypersecretion of vasoactive peptides causes diarrhea, abdominal distension, and hypokalemia. This is attributable to secretion of the entero-hormone vasoin-

testinal peptide (VIP), known as the Kerner-Morrison syndrome. This syndrome is usually associated with a favorable histology.

- Opsomyoclonus syndrome, with episodes of anarchic eye movements (dancing eye syndrome) and uncontrolled movements of the trunk and the limbs. These seizures like syndrome may persist even after tumor resection. Chronic progression may lead to neurological deficit, mental retardation, and behavioral disorders. This syndrome is caused by the production some autoantibodies that cross-react against neurons (Purkinje cells) and white matter axon cells. This syndrome occurs more often in neuroblastomas presenting in the mediastinum and are usually of favourable oncological outcome.

Diagnosis and Prognosis

An assessment of the tumor mass and its locoregional and distance extension is necessary for evaluating the prognosis and adapting the treatment. The primary tumor can be studied according to its location by standard X-ray, ultrasound or when possible, computed tomography (CT) or magnetic resonance imaging (MRI).

Abdominal radiography can be useful in showing finely stippled tumor calcification. Paraspinal widening may also be found. On chest radiographs paraspinal widening is also an indicator of thoracic tumor or extension of an abdominal tumor. The ultrasound examination may show calcifications. In the African setting, ultrasound may be sufficient in the diagnostic approach.

Bone marrow evaluation should be done by bone marrow aspiration and biopsy. In a patient with clinical manifestation of metastases, bone marrow biopsy should be done only if bone marrow aspiration did not show metastases. Scintigraphy with MiBG (meta-iodo-benzyl-guanidine) is specific and very sensitive in the search for bone marrow and bone metastasis (Fig. 11.5). This examination is not available in

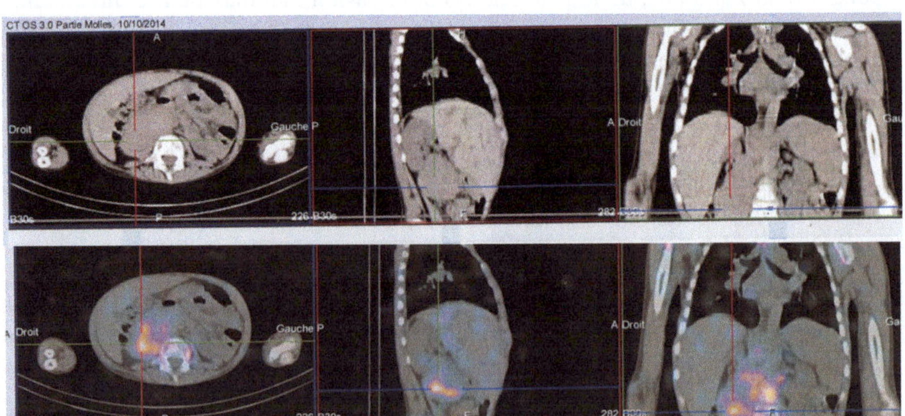

Fig. 11.5 CT/MIBG scintigraphy in abdominal neuroblastoma in a 3-year-old boy

most African countries. Technetium bone scan is useful, though inferior to MiBG in detecting metastases. MIBG (meta-iodo-benzyl-guanidine) is the most specific and sensitive test for neuroblastoma. Technetium bone scan is required for bone assessment despite the use of MIBG. For other sites evaluation is clearly inferior to MIBG.

Neuroblastoma tumor cells are characterized by their capacity to produce catecholamines. This is an interesting marker for diagnosis and also follow-up. The catecholamines, vanillylmandelic acid (VMA), and homovanillic acid (HVA) has been detected in the urine of more than 90 % of patients. Catecholamine secretion can be performed in one urine sample but most frequently is performed in a 24 -h urine collection. In rare instances (5–10 %), however, the tumor does not secrete excessive catecholamine.

Diagnostic criteria have been established by the INSS (International Neuroblastoma Staging System) and most recently by the International Neuroblastoma Risk Group (INRG, 2009). Neuroblastoma should be confirmed on an unequivocal pathologic diagnosis made on biopsy of the tumor (with or without immune-histochemistry) or cytology smears of the bone marrow associated with urinary catecholamine elevation. In Africa, when clinical characteristics are suggestive of the diagnosis of neuroblastoma, the diagnostic test can be accepted if bone marrow aspiration shows metastatic cells. This risk of error is very low, though every effort should be done to get a urinary catecholamine level.

Stages of Extension

The INSS classification is postsurgical (Table 11.2) and the INRG pre-surgical, mostly radiological. In the case of multifocal location (e.g., bilateral adrenal medulla involvement), the larger mass should be considered adding the letter M. In stages 4 s, bone marrow involvement is minimal, but in stage 4 there is a massive bone marrow infiltration.

Prognostic Factors

The prognosis of neuroblastoma varies according to age, location, stage of extension, and biological characteristics of the tumor. Age at diagnosis has an independent and major prognostic value. Thus, children under 18 months usually have a favorable outcome. The abdominal locations are often associated with a higher stage and biological characteristics indicating a poor prognosis. Elevated serum LDH, NSE, and ferritin levels are also an indication of a bad prognosis, as is a HVA/VMA ratio lower than 1.

Significant progress in the prognostic characterization of neuroblastoma has been achieved when cytogenetic studies and molecular biology have been used. A hyperdiploid or almost triploid number is associated with localized stages and has a favorable prognosis. MYCN oncogene amplification is associated with a poor outcome in all stages. It is amplified in 20–30 % of all neuroblastomas. This is amplified in

Table 11.2 International neuroblastoma staging system criteria

Stage	Criteria
1	Localized tumor with complete gross excision, with or without microscopic residual disease; representative ipsilateral lymph nodes negative for tumor microscopically (nodes attached to and removed with the primary tumor may be positive)
2A	Localized tumor with incomplete gross excision; representative ipsilateral non-adherent lymph nodes are negative for tumor microscopically
2B	Localized tumor with or without complete gross excision, with ipsilateral non-adherent lymph nodes positive for tumor. Enlarged contralateral lymph nodes must be negative microscopically
3	Unresectable unilateral tumor infiltrating across the midline, with or without regional lymph node involvement OR: Localized unilateral tumor with contralateral regional lymph node involvement OR: Midline tumor with bilateral extension by infiltration (unresectable) or by lymph node involvement
4	Any primary tumor with dissemination to distant lymph nodes, bone, bone marrow, liver, skin, and/or other organs (except as defined for stage 4 s)
4 s	Localized primary tumor (as defined for stages 1, 2A, or 2B), with dissemination limited to skin, liver, and bone marrow (limited to infants younger than 1 year) Marrow involvement in this stage should be minimal (i.e., <10 % of total nucleated cells identified as malignant on bone marrow biopsy or on marrow aspirate). More extensive marrow involvement would be considered to be stage 4. The meta-iodo-benzyl-guanidine scan (if performed) should be negative in the marrow

30–40 % of stages 3 and 4 neuroblastoma cases and in 5 % of the localized forms and stage 4 s keeping its pejorative meaning. Losses of putative tumor suppressor genes in chromosomal regions 1p,3p,11q,and 14 q have also shown an impact on the prognosis. However, these anomalies in most cases corelate with ploidy changes.

In Africa, like everywhere else in the world, patients older than 18 months of age with bone marrow metastases have an unfavourable prognosis. No other prognosis evaluations are needed. In localized neuroblastoma, the LDH level may be helpful and correlate with N-Myc. It is important to remember that most patients who are younger than 18 months have a very good prognosis.

Treatment

The treatment takes into account age at diagnosis, stage, and biological prognostic factors.

Treatment of Low-Risk Patients

INSS Stage 1 neuroblastoma has an excellent prognosis with a survival rate close to 95 % after treatment with surgery alone. When resection is incomplete (stages IIA or B) with favorable biological characteristics, survival rates are also more than 95 % without additional chemotherapy.

Chemotherapy is reserved for progressive forms, relapses, or cases of functional or vital threat. Chemotherapy for biological favourable tumors should be reserved for cases with functional (paraspinal) or vital (lung compression) threat.

In the case of stage 4 s, spontaneous regression is the rule in most cases. Chemotherapy or low-dose radiotherapy is reserved for large tumors or to the massive hepatomegaly with respiratory or gastrointestinal compression. The recommended radiotherapy dose is 4.5 Gy administered in 3 fractions of 1.5Gy on 3 consecutive days (British Journal of Cancer 2003). Chemotherapy may be recommended (like the CO regimen of Cyclophospamide 5 mg kg1 day 1, days 1–3 and vincristine 0.05 mg kg1, day 1, day1) administered every 2 weeks for a total period of up to 9 courses). In Africa, special attention should be given and treatment with low-dose chemotherapy implemented at the first clinical sign of compression.

Treatment of Intermediate-Risk Patients

The prognosis of stages 3 and 4 in children younger than 18 months old is usually good and should be adapted to histopathological criteria and biological characteristics. In the favorable forms, the surgical treatment and chemotherapy allow for similar survival of the low-risk group. Effective medications are vincristine, cyclophosphamide, etoposide, doxorubicin, cisplatinum, and carboplatin.

Treatment of High-Risk Patients

Although neuroblastoma is a chemosensitive tumor, high-risk forms have long-term survival rates of less than 50 %. The treatment combines an induction phase chemotherapy, local treatment, an intensification phase with high-dose chemotherapy and autologous hematopoietic stem cell rescue, followed by maintenance treatment for residual disease.

Induction treatment aims for the maximum reduction of tumor burden and control of metastases. The usual treatment combines vincristine, cyclophosphamide, doxorubicin, etoposide, and platinum.

The local tumor control is usually ensured by the combination of surgical resection and external radiation. This control allows reducing the risk of recurrence and improving survival of patients. Radiation at 20–40 Gy is usually recommended. Maintenance treatment with cis-retinoic acid combined with anti-GD2 immunotherapy has demonstrated its effectiveness. This treatment aims at maturation of residual cell tumor while building a long term immune reactivity.

In African areas, where these resources are not available it is better to propose a good supportive care program.

Treatment of Patients with Spinal Cord Compression

This is a neurological emergency. The medical treatment is effective in 80–85 % of the cases. This includes chemotherapy according to disease risk factors associated with corticosteroids (Dexamethasone). The response to treatment is sometimes late. Laminectomy must be done in case of ineffectiveness of chemotherapy. Radiation is not recommended.

Treatment of Opsomyoclonus Syndrome

In this rare syndrome, the addition of corticosteroids (Dexamethasone) to chemotherapy adapted to the risk factors is recommended. In case of persistence of abnormal movements, the early use of high doses of IgG or immunosupressive medications like cyclophophamide or Rituximab should be considered.

Practical Recommendation in Limited Resources Setting

Diagnosis

- Situation 1: Abdominal mass, with orbital involvement with/without bone pain. Bone marrow aspiration shows metastases in most cases. If urinary catecholamine testing is available, this should be ruled out.
- Situation 2: Infant with hepatomegaly, skin nodule, and adrenal mass on ultrasound examination. Bone marrow aspiration may show metastases. If urinary catecholamine testing is available, this should be ruled out. Skin biopsy may be useful if bone marrow is normal.
- Situation 3: In the case of a mass without evidence of metastases, biopsy or if possible resection should determine the diagnosis.

Prognosis

- Low-risk group
  - Age up to 18 months
- Intermediate-risk group
  - Age older than 18 months
  - Nonmetastatic
  - Normal LDH level

- High-risk group
  - Age older than 18 months
  - Metastases
  - High LDH level

Treatment

- Low-risk group: surgery, Wait and see, low-dose cyclophosphamide if no spontaneous regression.
- Intermediate-risk group: Complete surgery if possible, if not chemotherapy using cyclophosphamide, vincristine, and doxorubicin.
- High-risk group: Palliative care.

Suggested Reading

Stefan DC, Rodriguez-Galindo C (2014) Pediatric hematology oncology in countries with limited resources—a practical manual. Springer, New York

Chapter 12
Germ Cell Tumors

Case Presentation

A 5-year-old girl complained of diffuse abdominal pain for several months. Since then, her parents found an abdominal mass. Plain radiography of the abdomen showed unstructured pelvic calcifications. Abdominal ultrasound and CT scan found a voluminous abdominal and pelvic mass, heterogeneous, with components cystic components and calcifications. The level of alpha-fetoproteins was 159 ng/mL, while the beta gonadotropin hormone was lower than 2 ng/mL (Fig. 12.1).

1. What complementary diagnostic strategy do you propose?
2. What do you think of this tumor's prognosis?
3. What do you suggest as therapy?

Germ cell tumors (GCT) are neoplasms which develop in the embryo (fetus) from primordial germ cells that would normally give rise to sperm (in males) or ova (in females). GCT are a rare and heterogeneous group of diseases. In the black population, they seem to occur less frequently. They can be located in the gonads, throughout the axial region of the trunk and also in the brain (extragonadal sites). Their clinical manifestations are very heterogeneous. Moreover, these germ cells have a broad potential for differentiation in various tissues. However, the diagnostic approach is relatively simple and the survival rate exceeds 90 % when appropriate treatment is applied.

D.C. Stefan, M. Harif, *Pediatric Cancer in Africa*,
DOI 10.1007/978-3-319-17936-0_12

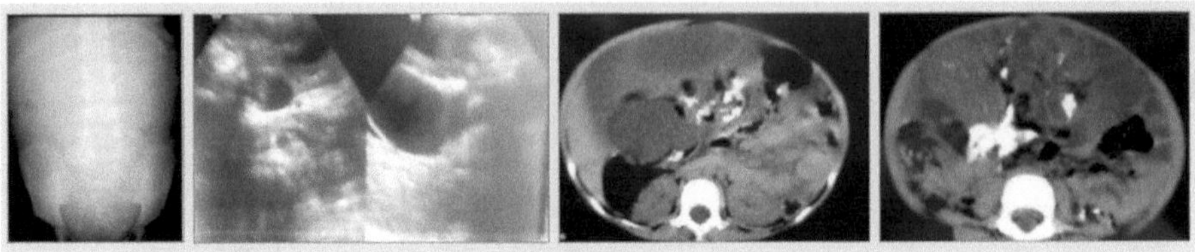

Fig. 12.1

Embryogenesis

Primordial germ cells originate at the level of the yolk sac and migrate toward the posterior via the abdomen yolk channel and the mesentery then towards the gonadal ridges as early as the fifth week of gestation (Fig. 12.2). Aberrant migration is at the origin of extragonadic tumors.

Epidemiology

GCTs are seen in 2–3 % of childhood cancers in western populations with a slight female predominance. The main locations are gonads and sacrococcygeal area (Table 12.1). Gonadal tumors are observed more frequently in adolescents, whereas extragonadal tumors usually occur in the newborn and infant. Extragonadal tumors are mostly arising from the sacrococcygeal area.

Patients with sex chromosome abnormalities are at higher risk of developing GCT. In Klinefelter syndrome (47, XXY), there is a high risk to develop extragonadal GCT. Mediastinal GCT associated with the Klinefelter syndrome is found in almost half of these patients. On the other hand, in the gonadal dysgenesis (45, X/46, XY) and in the case of ectopic testes, a high risk for developing a gonadal GCT exists.

Pathology

GCTs may have various characteristics of benign or malignant behavior according to the histopathology, the site, and the age of the patient. These tumors may be undifferentiated or engage in ways of differentiation to the various tissues (Fig. 12.3). The pathological study should search for malignant components.

Teratomas contain at least a differentiation in two of the three embryonic layers (ectoderm, endoderm, and mesoderm). They can be mature or immature, and with or without malignant germ cells. In the mature forms, tissues are well differentiated,

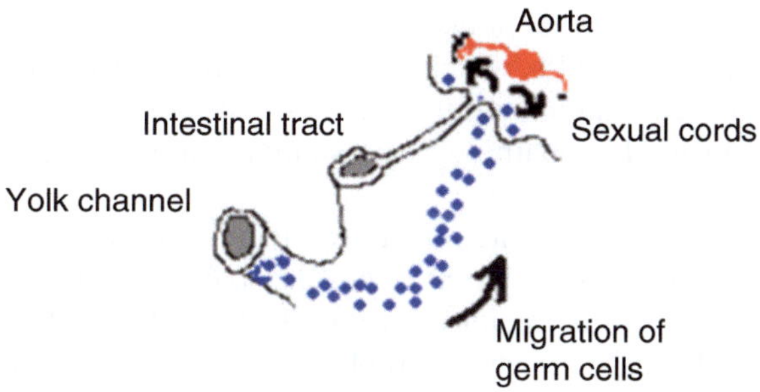

Fig. 12.2 Migration of germ cells around the fifth week of gestation

Table 12.1 Locations of germ cell tumors

Sacrococcygeal region	42 %
Ovary	24 %
Testicle	9 %
Mediastinum	7 %
Pineal region	6 %
Retroperitoneal	4 %
Other	8 %

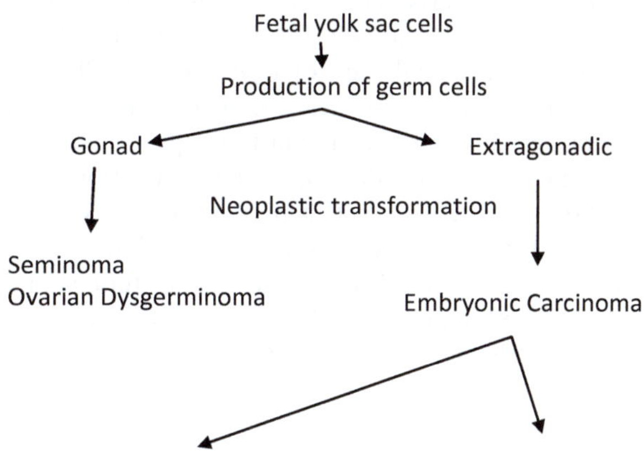

Fig. 12.3 Histogenesis of germ cell tumors

and the tumor may have organoid structures present (teeth, hair, bone, skin). Immature tissues contain suggestive elements of fetal or embryonic structures. Malignant characteristics may show endodermal sinus qualities, but also neuroblastoma, neuroepithelioma, and sometimes sarcoma characteristics, evoking a rhabdomyosarcoma or an angiosarcoma. Risk of recurrences or metastases is linked to the presence or not of the malignant component.

The germinomas also known as dysgerminoma, are the most frequent pure GCTs of the ovaries and the central nervous system. In the case of testicular origin, they are called seminoma. They are frequently found in patients with chromosomal aberrations or cryptorchidism. They may be difficult to distinguish from other round-cell tumors, and may also include choriocarcinoma foci.

Endodermal sinus tumors called also yolk sac tumors originate from totipotent germ cells, which differentiate into extraembryonic structures. These are the most common malignant GCTs in infants and are usually located in the testicles. During histopathological examination, they are identified by the Schiller-Duval bodies.

Embryonal carcinomas are aggressive histological forms and characterized by the presence of figures of anaplasia, frequent mitoses, and necrosis.

Choriocarcinomas have a histological aspects pattern to the placental chorion and consist of syncytiotrophoblasts or cytotrophoblasts.

Tumor Markers

GCTs have tumor markers. These tumor markers are of great importance for diagnosis, prognosis, and follow-up of. Those markers are alpha-fetoproteins (α-FP) and beta subunit of gonadotropin hormone (β-HCG). These markers also called oncofetoproteins are elevated in the serum but can also be highlighted by immunohistochemical staining of tumor tissue.

The α-FP is produced by embryonic liver, yolk sac, and at a lesser degree by the digestive tract. During the first months of life, this rate declines gradually to reach adult stage around the age of 1 year (<10 ng/dL) (Table 12.2).

A high level of α-FP can occur in other clinical circumstances which include neoplastic diseases (hepatoblastoma, gastrointestinal, pancreatic, or lung tumors), viral infection (hepatitis B, C, HIV infection), other liver diseases (cholestasis, cirrhosis) or medication (Phenytoin Methotrexate).

The β-HCG is produced by syncytiotrophoblast cells, and is increased in embryonal carcinoma, endodermal sinus tumors and choriocarcinoma. β-HCG can be increased in tumors of the liver, pancreas, digestive tract, breast, lung or bladder too and has a half-life of 24–36 h.

Table 12.2 Serum levels of alpha-fetoprotein in the first year of life

Age	Level in ng/mL	
Premature	134,734	+/−41,444
Newborn	48,406	+/−34,718
Newborn to 2 weeks	33,113	+/−33,503
Newborn 2 weeks to 1 month	9,452	+/−12,610
2 months	323	+/−278
3 months	88	+/−87
4 months	74	+/−56
5 months	46.5	+/−19
6 months	12.5	+/−9.8
7 months	9.7	+/−7.1
8 months	8.5	+/−5.5

In teratomas, an increase of α-FP or β-HCG is an expression of a malignant subset. Noteworthy is that an increase in α-FP and β-HCG levels at initiation of treatment can be related to tumor cell lysis.

Clinical and Prognostic Characteristics

Clinical manifestation is related to the tumor site. These tumors are most often expressed by compression signs of surrounding structures.

The diagnosis is made by histopathology of the tumor. However, when clinical manifestation is consistent with GCT, the diagnosis can be accepted only if α-FP and/or β-HCG are elevated. In all cases, determination of α-FP and β-HCG should be ruled out before initiation of treatment.

Sacrococcygeal Teratoma

This location represents almost 40 % of GCTs and nearly 80 % of extragonadic locations. Sacrococcygeal teratomas (SCTs) are observed with higher frequency in the female and can be associated with musculoskeletal or neurological abnormalities. SCTs, in their vast majority, are diagnosed during the neonatal period. They can also be discovered during pregnancy and induced heart failure or hydrops fetalis because of a vascular shunt. Intrauterine debulking surgery may be recommended. Type 1 neonatal SCTs are usually benign (Table 12.3).

Ovary Tumors

These tumors most commonly occur during adolescence. Their clinical expression is usually abdominal pain with or without palpable mass. Ovary torsion can be the mode of revelation. An isolated abdominal or abdominopelvic mass may also reveal the disease. Extraordinarily, the tumor can be discovered following an abdominal ultrasound or CT scan carried out to evaluate amenorrhea, genital bleeding, or precocious puberty.

Plain abdominal radiograph may show calcifications that may be suggestive of the disease. An ultrasound or a CT scan may primarily suspect teratoma in the pres-

Table 12.3 Anatomical classification of sacrococcygeal teratomas

Type I	Essentially exopelvic tumor
Type II	Tumor exopelvic with significant endopelvic component
Type III	Endopelvic predominant and sometimes abdominal tumor
Type IV	Exclusively endopelvic tumor

ence of a well-limited tumor, with areas of calcifications, fat, and/or cystic structures. The prognosis will depend on the histopathology type and stage (Table 12.4).

Tumor of the Testicles

The risk of cancer of the testicles is 10–50 % more important in children with ectopic testicles. Non-painful testicular mass is the most frequent revealing symptom. The pain may be a manifestation of testicular torsion. Trans-illumination can be positive because of a reactive hydrocele associated with the tumor. Testicular ultrasound shows the tumor in most cases. The prognosis varies according to the histopathological type and stage (Table 12.5).

Mediastinal Tumors

These tumors have an anterior mediastinal location, are more frequent among boys and can be associated with the Klinefelter syndrome. Symptoms and signs are usually mild. More or less severe respiratory signs, sometimes with hemoptysis, are the main clinical manifestations.

Intracranial Tumors

They are usually located at pineal gland and at the level of the suprasellar region. Clinical expression may include visual disturbances, Parinaud syndrome, diabetes insipidus, precocious puberty, a hypopituitarism or anorexia.

Table 12.4 Classification of the children oncology group of germ cell tumors of the ovary

I	Tumor confined to the ovary completely removed
	Regression then negativity of tumor markers
II	Microscopic residue or adenopathy ≤2 cm
III	Macroscopic residue or biopsy
	Locoregional extension (peritoneum, bladder, intestine)
	Metastatic lymph nodes >2 cm
	Tumor cells in peritoneal lavage fluid
IV	Distant metastases

Table 12.5 Classification of the children oncology group of tumors of the testicles

I	Tumor limited to the testicle, orchidectomy resected through inguinal or trans-scrotal way without tumor dissemination. Regression then negativity of tumor markers
II	Trans-scrotal orchiectomy with tumor dissemination
	Microscopic spread of the disease to the scrotum or spermatic cord (<5 cm from the end proximal)
	Retroperitoneal lymph (≤2 cm)
III	No regression of the tumor markers
	Lymph node metastatic retroperitoneal >2 cm
IV	Distant metastases

Spinal cord metastases are frequent. To rule up those metastases spinal MRI and CSF analysis are recommended.

Other Locations

The retroperitoneal locations are rare. Orbital locations were described, as well as cases of hepatic choriocarcinoma of gestational origin.

Treatment

Treatment options depend on the tumor site, age, histopathological type, and extension of the disease. Surgical excision should be made whenever possible without major sacrifice. Surgical removal may be done upfront or after chemotherapy. Survival rates exceed 90 % in these tumors, with a treatment modulated according to the risk of relapse. The main antimitotic drugs used are vinblastine, actinomycin D, bleomycin, doxorubicin, cis-platinum, and etoposide, which are linked to various protocols (Table 12.6).

In SCT, surgery is the first therapeutic option. The surgery should remove the tumor and the coccyx. If the coccyx is not removed there is a risk of relapse in 30–40 % cases. Additional treatment with chemotherapy is necessary in the malignant forms.

In ovarian tumors, conservative surgery (ovarosalpingectomy) with palpation and biopsy of the contralateral ovary and analysis of peritoneal liquid lavage is recommended. In the case of ovarian dysgerminoma, complementary irradiation may be recommended, targeting a tumor residue.

In testicular tumors, the recommended approach is inguinal orchidectomy with removal of the spermatic cord. In stage I, no further treatment is necessary. Chemotherapy is indicated in other cases. In mediastinal tumors chemotherapy is added to the surgical treatment. Usually these tumors have a poorer prognosis.

In the brain locations, chemotherapy may be sufficient to control the disease. The association with radiotherapy may be recommended.

Table 12.6 Main chemotherapy regimens used in malignant germ cell tumors

Schema I: PVB/3 weeks	
Cis-platinum	20 mg/m^2 D1–J5
Vinblastine	0.2 mg/kg D1, J2
Bleomycin	30 mg/m^2 D2, D9, D16
Schema II: PEB/3 weeks	
Cis–Platinum	100 mg/m^2 D1
Etoposide	100 mg/m^2 D1–J3
Bleomycin	15 mg/m^2 D2
Schema III: JEB/3 weeks	
Carboplatin	600 mg/m^2 D1
Etoposide	120 mg/m^2 D1–J3
Bleomycin	15 mg/m^2 D2, D9, D16

Practical Recommendation in Resources-Limited Settings

Diagnosis

GCTs are usually easily diagnosed when:

- A tumor in the gonadal or sacrococcygeal region is associated with a high level of α-FP or β-HCG. Other locations are less frequent.
- Plain radiographs may be helpful in showing organoid calcifications.
- US and CT scan may be helpful in better characterizing these tumors.

Pathology examination is necessary for diagnosis and to identify histological components.

Treatment

- Complete resection should be considered either upfront or after chemotherapy. No other treatment may be needed if surgery is complete and tumor marker negative.
- Combination chemotherapy of cis-platinum, vinblastine, bleomycin, and etoposide is usually used.
- Radiotherapy is not needed in most cases.

Suggested Reading

Echevarría ME, Fangusaro J, Goldman S (2008) Pediatric central nervous system germ cell tumors: a review. Oncologist 13(6):690–699

Ma IT, Cullen MH, Hussein SA (2011) Biology of germ cell tumors. Hematol Oncol N Am 25:457–471

Rescorla FJ (2012) Pediatric germ cell tumors. Semin Pediatr Surg 21:51–60

Valteau-Couanet D, Dubrel M, Dufour C, Couanet D, Hartmann O, Patte C (2008) Les tumeurs malignes de l'ovaire dans l'enfance. Arch Pediatr 15(5):781–782

Chapter 13
Malignant Soft Tissue Tumors

Objectives

- To learn about the clinical presentation of the main malignancies of soft tissues in children and in particular the rhabdomyosarcoma.
- To be able to diagnose the tumors of soft tissues.
- To know the prognosis of malignancies of soft tissue.
- To learn about the principles of the treatment of soft tissue tumors and in particular of rhabdomyosarcoma.

Malignant soft tissue tumors are heterogeneous entities whose origin is the mesenchyme. They often have a high potential of local relapse and of blood-borne metastases. Rhabdomyosarcoma is distinguished by its frequency and its particular response to chemotherapy and radiotherapy.

Rhabdomyosarcoma

The rhabdomyosarcoma (RMS) is the most frequently encountered soft tissue tumor. The modern multidisciplinary approach allows for a better characterization of the different entities and for tailoring the treatment accordingly.

Epidemiology

This is a tumor of striated muscle that represents nearly 50 % of soft tissue tumors in children and 10–12 % of childhood cancers. The average age of onset is 6 years. However, the RMS of the limbs are more often encountered in adolescence and are mostly of alveolar type, while head and neck locations are rather embryonic and occur with greater frequency in infants and small children.

A genetic predisposition is reported in the context of neurofibromatosis and Li-Fraumeni syndrome. In the latter, there is a mutation in the suppressor gene p53. The RMS can also be associated with the syndrome Beckwith-Wiedemann with a

D.C. Stefan, M. Harif, *Pediatric Cancer in Africa*,
DOI 10.1007/978-3-319-17936-0_13

Image

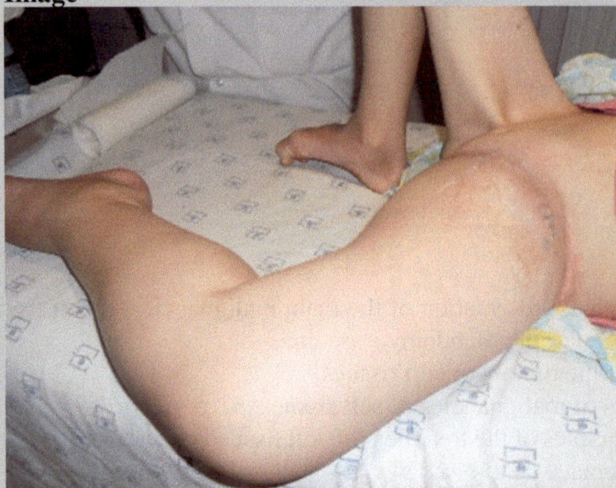

Child 5 years old with swelling of the left lower limb

Fatima, 5 years old, is admitted for a swelling of the left lower limb gradually installed over 2 months and the recent finding of a left inguinal mass. On examination, a functional impairment of the left lower limb is found; the edema is soft and pitting. The inguinal mass has a firm consistency, is fixed, painless, and measures 5×3 cm. Ultrasound and CT show a mass in the iliac and inguinal areas on the left, of 12×7 cm. The biopsy of the inguinal mass indicates a rhabdomyosarcoma of the alveolar type.

What complementary assessment do you propose?
What is the prognosis in this case?
What strategy of management would you adopt?

chromosomal abnormality at the level of the 11p15 region. The RMS is also common as part of the syndrome of Castello. Finally, the consumption of marijuana or cocaine by the mother and also by the father seems to increase the risk of development of a RMS.

Anatomical Pathology

The RMS is included among the round cell tumors. The diagnosis and its classification are usually possible by optical microscopy studying the tumor cells and tissue architecture. It may be necessary to resort to immuno-histochemistry to look for muscle markers: actin, myosin, desmin, and myoglobin. The expression of myogenin is also common.

The embryonic type represents almost two-thirds of cases. It takes the appearance of fetal muscle at 7–10 weeks of pregnancy with a rich stroma and fusiform, non-alveolar cells. The preferential location of the embryonic type is the head and neck and genitourinary apparatus. Two variants of this type are described, the botryoidal form and the fuso-cellular form. In the botryoidal form, the proliferation has a polypoid aspect with a sub-epithelial layer of dense tumor cells (cambial layer). The location in this case is naso-pharyngeal, vaginal, or in the urinary bladder, while in the fuso-cellular type, the preferred location is para-testiculaire.

In *the alveolar type*, representing almost 25 % of the cases, round tumor cells are densely grouped within an architecture resembling the pulmonary alveoli. A variant is described known as "alveolar solid", in which the alveolar architectural organization is not found, but the genetic study connects it to the alveolar RMS. The usual locations of the RMS of alveolar type are the extremities, trunk, and the perineum.

Undifferentiated sarcoma is made of round cells whose morphological appearance, architecture, and antigenic markers expressions do not classify it. It is a diagnosis of exclusion.

Genetic Abnormalities

Genetic studies allow us to better characterize the RMS. Thus, the translocation t(2; 13) (q35; q14) is characteristic of the alveolar RMS. This translocation leads to the juxtaposition of the PAX3 gene involved in neuromuscular differentiation and FKHR (or FOXO1a) gene. Testing by PCR, the merging of PAX3 and FKHR genes is very sensitive for the identification of alveolar RMS. Embryonic RMS cases have a recurring loss of heterozygosity 11p15. In addition, the ploidy assessment by flow cytometry shows that hyperdiploidy (>51 chromosomes) has a better prognosis than the diploidy.

Clinical Signs

The clinical presentation varies according to the anatomical location (Table 13.1). It's usually an asymptomatic mass sometimes associated with organ dysfunction related to the location of the tumor. Initial metastases, mainly to the lung, have no clinical signs.

In almost 40 % of the cases, the tumor *involves the head and neck*. The distinct locations are orbital, para-meningeal (nasopharynx, middle ear, para-nasal sinuses, the temporal and pterygo-maxillary fossae), and others (larynx, oropharynx, oral cavity, parotid, cheek, scalp). The orbital location is usually rapidly diagnosed due to the exophthalmos. Metastases are rare in this location. In the para-meningeal locations, patients present with signs of oral or nasal obstruction or symptoms related to the ears. Headache, vomiting, or paralysis of one or more cranial nerve pairs already reflect a brain invasion by infiltration of the base of the skull. In other locations, the tumor often remains localized.

Genitourinary localization is dominated by bladder and prostate lesions. The tumor is usually of the embryonic botryoidal type and develops at the trigone. Its clinical expression is often noisy in the form of a dysuria or retention of urine or acute hematuria and more rarely as a pelvic mass. Sometimes muco-sanguinolent fragments of tumor are eliminated in urine. Vaginal or uterine tumors are usually botryoidal and also manifested themselves by elimination of tumor fragments. The para-testicular RMS appears as a painless scrotal or inguinal mass.

Table 13.1 Clinical signs of rhabdomyosarcoma based on location

Location		Clinical signs
Head and neck	Neck	Mass of the soft parts
		Dysphonia
		Dysphagia
	Nasopharynx	Sinusitis
		Pain
		Epistaxis
		Dysphagia
	Para-nasal sinus	Sinusitis
		Unilateral rhinorrhea
		Pain
		Epistaxis
	Middle ear	Otitis media
		Polyp of the ear canal
		Facial paralysis
	Orbit	Exophthalmos
		Strabismus
		Oculo-motor paralysis
		Conjunctival mass
Genitourinary	Vagina-uterus	Vaginal bleeding
		Mass like "bunch of grapes"
	Prostate	Dysuria, urinary retention
		Hematuria
	Bladder	Retention of urine
		Hematuria
		Repeated urinary infection
	Para-testicular	Painless para-testicular mass
Limbs		Asymptomatic mass
Retroperitoneal		Abdominal pain
		Abdominal mass
		Bowel obstruction
Pelvis		Constipation
		Genitourinary obstruction

RMS of the members and the trunk is usually a non-inflammatory painless mass increasing in volume. A history of trauma may be found, evoking a hematoma. In some cases with rapid evolution, the tumor may be painful or present signs of inflammation that suggest an abscess. These tumors are often of the alveolar type and have a tendency to locoregional and distant extension.

The other locations are rare and often diagnosed late. The RMS can be retroperitoneal, intrathoracic, hepatic, perianal, and even more rarely in the biliary tract, brain, breast, ovaries, or the heart. Cases of metastatic RMS whose primary tumor was not found were also reported.

Diagnosis and Assessment of Extension

The strategy varies depending on location. As soon as the diagnosis is suspected, a biopsy or excisional biopsy should be envisaged. In cases of cavitary tumors, the pathological examination of tumor fragments, either eliminated or obtained by endoscopy, enables the diagnosis. Any suspicious lymphadenopathy should be biopsied to specify its nature.

Particular care must be given to the clinical evaluation, indicating the tumor mass and clinical signs of metastases particularly in the regional lymph nodes. In the head and neck location, it is recommended to do a specialist ENT consultation and possibly an ophthalmic examination. Radiological examinations are required for a proper assessment of the tumor mass and search for metastasis. This assessment will allow monitoring of response to treatment and a better definition of the tumor mass for a possible local treatment by surgery or radiotherapy. Echography is a good first approach, but in the majority of cases a CT scan is necessary. MRI is a better choice in the locations of the head and neck, at the level of the limbs, and in the case of pelvic tumors. The search for lung metastases is done by radiographs and especially by the CT scan. The ^{99}Tc scintigraphy is very sensitive in the search for bone metastases. The place of the PET scan in the initial assessment and to monitor the response to treatment is a subject of study. Although isolated metastases in the bone marrow are exceptional, it is recommended to do this research by myelogram and bilateral bone marrow biopsy even when the blood count is normal.

Classification and Prognosis

The prognosis is closely related to the tumor mass and the presence or absence of metastases. Localized forms whose complete excision is possible have a better prognosis, as well as the occurrence at an age between 1 and 10 years. The embryonic histological type is also of better prognosis than the alveolar type. The orbital locations, those on eyelids, head, and neck (not para-meningeal) or genitourinary para-testiculaires, vulvo-vaginal, or uterine are favorable (Table 13.2). Elsewhere,

Table 13.2 Rhabdomyosarcoma TNM classification

Stage I: Localized disease involving orbit, head, and neck (not para-meningeal) or genitourinary (not vesical or prostatic)
Stage II: Tumor localized in unfavorable site, less than 5 cm, no regional lymphadenopathy
Stage III: Tumor localized in unfavorable site, greater than 5 cm and/or regional lymphadenopathy
Stage IV: Distant metastasis

Table 13.3 Prognostic groups according to Intergroup Rhabdomyosarcoma Study

Group I: Complete resection
A: Localized, complete resection, confined to the site of origin
B: Localized, complete resection, exceeding the original site
Group II: Microscopic residue
A: Tumor with microscopic residue
B: Lymph node extension, complete resection
C: Lymph node extension, resection with microscopic residue
Group III: Macroscopic residue
A: Biopsy or removal of less than 50 %
B: Removal of more than 50 %
Group IV: Metastases at diagnosis

the location is considered unfavorable. The prognosis is also unfavorable for tumors greater than 5 cm or in the presence of tumoral lymph nodes.

The classification of the Intergroup Rhabdomyosarcoma Study (Table 13.3) is post-surgical groups depending on the quality of excision.

Treatment

The treatment combines surgery, radiotherapy, and chemotherapy, depending on the case. The surgical aim is complete tumor resection. Radiation therapy complements local control, while chemotherapy aims to control the obvious metastases or the microscopic ones, or to reduce tumor volume to facilitate the local therapy.

Surgical resection should be envisaged from the outset when it is feasible without functional sequelae or major cosmetics. This is usually possible in the locations on the limbs and the trunk, in the absence of distant metastases. A revision surgery may be considered when the resection proved to be incomplete. The place of second-look surgery is questionable. It should be considered in case of residual tumor after chemotherapy and irradiation, to clarify the nature of the residue and to complete local control. This surgery is function of the tumor site and the quality of the response to treatment with chemotherapy and/or radiation (Table 13.4).

Table 13.4 Type of usual surgery according to the location of rhabdomyosarcoma

Location		Type of surgery
Head and neck		No surgical resection
Genitourinary	Vagina-uterus	Conservative surgery after chemotherapy
	Vesico-prostatic	Resection if bladder tumor on the fundus. Also conservative treatment except poor response
	Para-testicular	Initial orchiectomy via the inguinal canal removing the spermatic cord
Limbs		Complete removal with lymph node exploration
Thorax-pelvis-retroperitoneal		Full resection if wall tumor

In the para-testicular locations, orchidectomy by inguinal route with removal of the spermatic cord in its entirety must be the rule. The systematic exploration of the retroperitoneal lymph nodes is discussed in various study groups. On the other hand, when lymph nodes are highlighted by the radiological exploration, biopsy should be performed. In the vulvo-vaginal or uterine involvement, surgery is usually done after reductive chemotherapy. Hysterectomy is rarely required for local control, and excepting obvious invasion, oophorectomy should be avoided. In the vesico-prostatic location, resection surgery is advocated in the involvement of the bladder dome, after initial chemotherapy. The urethro-prostatic function should be preserved as much as possible. Radical total cystectomy and anterior pelvic exenteration are reserved for forms, which did not respond to the combination of chemotherapy and radiation.

When the head and neck are involved, surgery is often limited to diagnostic biopsy.

With limb locations, complete tumor resection with regional lymph node exploration is recommended, without major functional sacrifice. Amputation must be restricted to forms with significant neuro-vascular or bone invasion or when radiation therapy might originate major sequelae.

At the level of the trunk, complete excision is usually possible. It is recommended in the chest locations to perform a rib resection on both sides of the lesion. In pelvic, retro-peritoneal or intrathoracic localizations resection surgery is rarely possible due to locoregional spread.

Radiotherapy is a major therapeutic weapon of the RMS. It allows to control the tumor in inaccessible locations to conservative surgery and complete the latter in the case of inoperable residue. Usual doses are 40–45 Gy for the microscopic disease control and 50–55 Gy in case of macroscopic residue. Trials are attempted to reduce the dose in order to minimize the consequences without compromising the survival. The North American Intergroup Rhabdomyosarcoma Study (IRS) recommends a systematic irradiation to 36 Gy in the alveolar forms where excision was complete.

Radiation therapy comes in the majority of cases after chemotherapy of tumor reduction. In the invasive para-meningeal locations at the base of the skull or in neurological involvement, radiation therapy is recommended as soon as possible.

Brachytherapy is advocated in the case of small tumors of difficult access, particularly in the bladder, prostate, vagina, head, and neck or limbs. This technique has fewer sequelae when compared to external radiation therapy.

Chemotherapy has transformed the prognosis of these tumors. Drugs that have demonstrated their effectiveness are actinomycin D, cyclophosphamide, vincristine, cis-platinum, the carboplatin, the dacarbazine (DTIC), and doxorubicin. More recently, ifosfamide and etoposide were added to the therapeutic arsenal. These products are always used in combination according to protocols. The duration and intensity of treatment vary depending on the initial prognosis and response to treatment. In the IRS studies, ifosfamide does not seem to bring additional therapeutic benefit compared to cyclophosphamide.

The survival depends on stage, location and quality of excision. In the low-risk group, the survival is 90 %. This group includes the cases of RMS of embryonic type, complete resection in favorable locations (orbital, para-testicular, etc.). In other cases of nonmetastatic RMS, the survival is 60–80 %, while in metastatic forms it does not exceed 20–30 % (Table 13.5).

Other Tumors of Soft Parts

This group of tumors is characterized by its rarity and its heterogeneity. They are most often observed in adults.

Epidemiologically, these tumors occur, in contrast with the RMS in older children and adolescents. Etiological factors are found in less than 5 % of cases. A greater susceptibility is found in the Li-Fraumeni syndrome, neurofibromatosis, and Gardner syndrome (desmoid tumors).

The clinical expression is usually quiet and limited to the presence of a painless and non-inflammatory mass involving the limbs or trunk. The increase in volume is variable depending on the aggressiveness of each type of tumor. The spread to regional structures can cause pain or other signs of compression or invasion.

The anatomopathologic study is of major importance in the characterization of these tumors and in the assessment of the quality of resection. The characterization of these tumors often requires studies of immuno-histochemistry and genetics.

The prognosis is closely related to the tumor mass, the presence or not of metastases, and the quality of surgical excision. A high risk of local relapse is observed in the case of tumor more than 5 cm, incomplete resection, or abdominal tumor. A risk of metastasis is also found in invasive tumors, greater than 5 cm, or histologically high-grade.

The treatment aims initially at local control. Excision surgery must be carried out if it is possible without sacrifice. Preoperative treatment with chemotherapy and/or radiotherapy could make these tumors amenable to resection surgery. Survival is closely linked to the quality of resection. Thus, it reached 90 % with complete resection and only 50 % in non-resected tumors and 35 % in case of metastases.

Radiation therapy may be recommended preoperatively to reduce the tumor volume and allow conservative surgery and also reduces the risk of locoregional intraoperative contamination. In these cases, it is given at a dose of 45–50 Gy. Usually more than 99 % of the tumor cells are destroyed at these doses. Postoperative radiation therapy requires a wider field at a dose of 45 Gy. The local relapse risk is significantly reduced.

Table 13.5 Main associations of Chemotherapy in Rhabdomyosarcoma

Protocol	Administration
VA	
Vincristine	1.5 mg/m²/day, IVD, D1, D8, D15
Actinomycin D	1.5 mg/m²/day, IVD, D1
VAC	
Vincristine	1.5 mg/m²/day, IVD, D1
Actinomycin D	1.5 mg/m²/day, IVD, D1
Cyclophosphamide	250 mg/m², D1–D5 or 1.2 g/m², D1
VACA	
Vincristine	1.5 mg/m²/day week 1 to week 4
Actinomycin D	1.5 mg/m²/day, week 4
Cyclophosphamide	1.2 g/m² D1, week 1, 4, 7
Adriamycin	30 mg/m², D1 and D2, weeks 1, 7
IVA	
Ifosfamide	3 g/m² D1 and D2 (+ Uromitexan)
Vincristine	1.5 mg/m², D1
Actinomycin D	1.5 mg/m²,D1
VACA	
Vincristine	1.5 mg/m²/day weeks 1–7
Actinomycin D	1.5 mg/m²/day week 1 and week 7
Ifosfamide	2 gr/m² D1–D3 or D1–D5 (+ Uromitexan) week 1, 4, 7
Adriamycin	40 mg/m² D1 and D2 week 4
CEVAIE	
Carboplatin	500 mg/m²/day, week 1
Epirubicin	150 mg/m²/day, week 1
Vincristine	1.5 mg/m²/day, weeks 1–7
Actinomycin D	1.5 mg/m²/day, week 4
Ifosfamide	3 gr/m² D1–D3 (+Uromitexan) weeks 4, 7
Etoposide	200 mg/m² D1–D3 week 7
IVADo	
Vincristine Has ctinomycine	1.5 mg/m² D1
Doxorubicine	1.5 mg/m² D1
Ifosfamide	30 mg/m² D1, D2
	3 g/m² D1, D2

The benefit of chemotherapy in the improvement in survival is not demonstrated. However, preoperative chemotherapy in unresectable forms can reduce the tumor volume and facilitate local treatment. Chemotherapy combining vincristine, cyclophosphamide, doxorubicin, and actinomycin D does not benefit survival. However, chemotherapy with ifosfamide and doxorubicin combined with preoperative radiotherapy is recommended in most high-risk forms.

Infantile Fibrosarcoma

It is a tumor of infant of less than a year. The histopathologic appearance is similar to that of the adult fibrosarcoma, but is distinguished by the presence of the t(12;15) translocation. It is a tumor with rapid development and may be neonatal. It usually is located on the limbs or trunk. It is rarely metastatic.

A wide surgical excision is the treatment of choice for these tumors. Survival exceeds 90 %. Spontaneous regression is reported in the case of partial resection. Chemotherapy combining vincristine, cyclophosphamide, and actinomycin D and ifosfamide can be indicated in inoperable forms at the outset.

Synovial Sarcoma

It is a relatively frequent tumor, occurring mostly in the adolescent. The histopathology reveals cells of fusiform aspect, fibrosarcomatous, and epithelioid, organized in pseudo-glandular structures. Monophasic forms and biphasic forms can be distinguished. The synovial sarcoma is characterized by the expression of EMA, Cytokeratin, BCL2, and CD99 markers.

It is also characterized by the presence of the translocation t(X;18) (q11; Guide 11) in more than 90 % of cases.

The synovial sarcoma is located mainly at the level of the lower limbs and especially at the level of the thighs and knees. The prognosis is a function of tumor mass, the presence or not of metastases, histological aggressiveness, and the quality of surgical excision. Survival is close to 90 % in the case of small tumors, non-metastatic, and completely resected. Radiation therapy is reserved for the case of non-oncological resections. In inoperable forms or with a macroscopic postoperative residue, chemotherapy is recommended. It usually combines the cis-platinum, doxorubicin, and ifosfamide.

Tumors of the Peripheral Nerve Sheaths (Malignant Schwanoma, Neuro-Fibrosarcoma)

These tumors are associated in 20–50 % with neurofibromatosis type 1. They may complicate the evolution of plexiform neurofibroma. The histopathological study may pose a problem of differential diagnosis with fibrosarcoma. The protein S100, Cytokeratin, and CD57 markers are usually found.

These tumors are situated on limbs or trunk and less frequently on the head and neck. The tumor presents as a painless mass.

The treatment of choice is complete tumor resection. Radiotherapy is indicated in cases where resection limits are not large enough. The survival rates in these cases are 65–80 %. Otherwise, the survival is poor. Chemotherapy does not seem to bring additional benefit.

Hemangiopericytoma

The hemangiopericytoma is a unique tumor in childhood. It originates in the pericyte cells adjacent to vascular endothelial cells.

Clinically, it is described as the infantile form occurring in infants less than 1 year and usually has a mild course, unlike the forms in older children which are more aggressive. In infants, the tumor is localized in the dermis and in the oral cavity. Spontaneous regressions are reported. In older children, the tumor is located in the limbs. It is metastatic in 20 % of cases. It can be accompanied by hypoglycemia due to the secretion of an insulin-like factor or hypophosphatemia regressing after resection of the tumor. On the histopathological, immuno-histochemical and ultrastructural level, the proliferation has a fibroblastic aspect.

The genetic study may highlight translocations t (12; 19) (q13; q13.3) and t(13; 22) (q22; q11) or sometimes complex abnormalities.

In childhood forms, the treatment is surgical excision. Various protocols used in inoperable forms with vincristine, cyclophosphamide, doxorubicin, actinomycin D, methotrexate, and mitoxantrone showed an objective response. Survival is almost 90 %. In the forms of adult type, the role of chemotherapy is not established. The survival rate varies from 30 to 60 %, depending on the tumor volume and quality of resection.

Alveolar Sarcoma of Soft Parts

Exceptional tumor of the adolescent, it is mainly located on the lower limbs. Histologically, the tumor does not show signs of cell differentiation. The architecture is pseudo-alveolaire. The genetic study shows in some cases a translocation t(X;17) (p11.2; q25), which produces the fusion the ASPL-TFE3 gene. It is notable that the same fusion gene is found in the renal adenocarcinoma. It is a tumor of indolent evolution. The treatment consists of surgical excision. Irradiation is reserved for forms leaving a tumor residue. Survival is more than 90 % in the localized forms located, while it is less than 20 % in cases with metastases.

Leiomyosarcoma

Smooth muscle tumors are very rare in children. They often complicate an immune deficiency (HIV, transplant). They occur more rarely as a second tumor, and in particular, in the case of bilateral retinoblastoma. These tumors may have various locations with a predominance at the level of the digestive tract, and in particular, the stomach in children. Regarding their histopathology, smooth muscle tissue tumors have cells with myofilaments. There are markers of EBV in the tumor tissue. The translocation t(12;14) (q14–15; q23–24) is reported.

The treatment of these tumors is wide surgical excision. The role of chemotherapy and radiotherapy is not shown. Apart from colorectal lesions, the digestive locations are of poor prognosis.

Liposarcoma

These tumors can occur in the teenager. The main locations are the lower limbs and the retro-peritoneal area. Its histopathology describes clearly differentiated forms, myxoid forms, round cells forms, or pleomorphic of increasing aggressiveness. Translocations t(12; 16) (q13; p11) and t(12; 22) (q13; q12) are found in the myxoid and round cells liposarcomas.

These tumors rarely develop metastases. Wide tumor resection can usually control the disease. In the retro-peritoneal locations, complementary irradiation is recommended as complete excision is rarely possible.

Desmoplastic Round Cell Tumors

These are adolescents' and especially males' tumors. The usual location is retro-peritoneal, associated with ascites. More rarely, they are located at para-testicular or chest level. This is a very aggressive tumor, often infiltrating the adjacent structures. Histopathologically, the tumor comprises a fibrous, dense stroma ("desmoplastic") with small round cells that can show epithelial, neuroendocrine, neuroblastique, rhabdomyoblastique, or rhabdoid differentiation. Immuno-histochemical study reflects this diversity of differentiation by finding epithelial markers (cytokeratin, EMA), myogenic markers (desmin), mesenchymal (vimentin), or neural (neuron-specific enolase). Genetically, we find the translocation t(11; 22) (p13;q12) that can help in the diagnosis of these tumors.

Therapeutically, locoregional infiltration does not allow for a carcinological satisfactory surgery. A complement of chemotherapy is recommended by various associations including the anthracyclines. These tumors often continue to progress despite intensive treatment.

Desmoid Tumors

They consist of an invasive fibromatosis. This is observed with greater frequency in the context of Gardner syndrome, in familial adenomatous polyposis associated with a mutation in the level 5 q21. Its histopathology found fibroblasts in an abundant collagenous matrix expressing the vimentin and actin.

The most common locations are the shoulder, chest, head and neck, and the abdomen. The location can be multicentric. The abdominal disease is asymptomatic, but mesenteric involvement can generate digestive hemorrhage or perforation.

When the resection was complete, no further treatment is necessary. Additional irradiation is recommended if resection margins contain tumor. In inoperable forms, chemotherapy combining vincristine, actinomycin D and cyclophosphamide or low dose of vinblastine and methotrexate allows partial or complete response. However, the response to chemotherapy is relatively slow.

What You Should Remember

- Soft tissue tumors are dominated by rhabdomyosarcoma which represents almost 50 % of these tumors.
- Their clinical expression is usually an asymptomatic mass or signs of compression or bleeding, particularly in head and neck or genito-urinary locations.
- The diagnosis requires the anatomopathological study of a biopsy, excisional biopsy for small tumors, or more rarely by the study of tumor fragments spontaneously eliminated, either in urine in the bladder locations or nasally in ENT locations.
- The prognosis is dependent on tumor volume, histological type, and distant extension.
- Local treatment involves a surgical resection with or without radiotherapy according to the quality of excision.
- Rhabdomyosarcoma is a chemosensitive tumor. It can be indicated before surgery to reduce the tumor volume and to facilitate the surgical act.

Suggested Reading

Kagome H, Kili A et al (2010) Pediatric rhabdomyosarcoma in Morocco. Pediatr Blood Cancer 54:25–28

Stevens MCG, Rey A, Bouvet N et al (2005) Treatment of nonmetastatic rhabdomyosarcoma in childhood and adolescence: third study of the International Society of Paediatric Oncology—SIOP Malignant Mesenchymal Tumor 89. J Clin Oncol 23:2618–2628

Winston WH, Stephen XS (2010) Childhood rhabdomyosarcoma: new insight on biology and treatment. Curr Oncol Rep 12(6):402–410

Chapter 14
Hodgkin Lymphoma

Case Presentation

A 14-year-old girl presented to the hospital with fever, sweating, loss of weight for the last 6 months and lower back pain for a week. On physical examination the patient was not acutely ill, had moderate pallor and lymphadenopathy along the left jugular chain, small, not tender and mobile palpable lymph nodes. Two firm tender lymph nodes (5×2 cm diameter) in the right inguinal area were noted. The lower lumbar spine was tender to palpation but no deformity noted. Rest of the exam was unremarkable (Figs. 14.1 and 14.2).

What Is the Differential Diagnosis?

Differential diagnosis.

Infections: EBV, HIV, tuberculosis, toxoplasmosis, cat scratch disease, histoplasmosis.

Lymphomas: NHL, Hodgkin lymphoma.
Metastatic adenopathy from solid tumors.

Autoimmune disorders: lupus, autoimmune lymphoproliferative disorder, Rosai Dorfman disease.

D.C. Stefan, M. Harif, *Pediatric Cancer in Africa*,
DOI 10.1007/978-3-319-17936-0_14

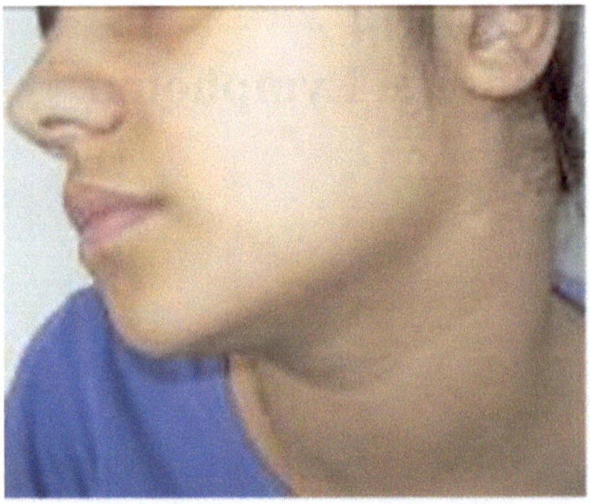

Fig. 14.1 Lymphadenopathy

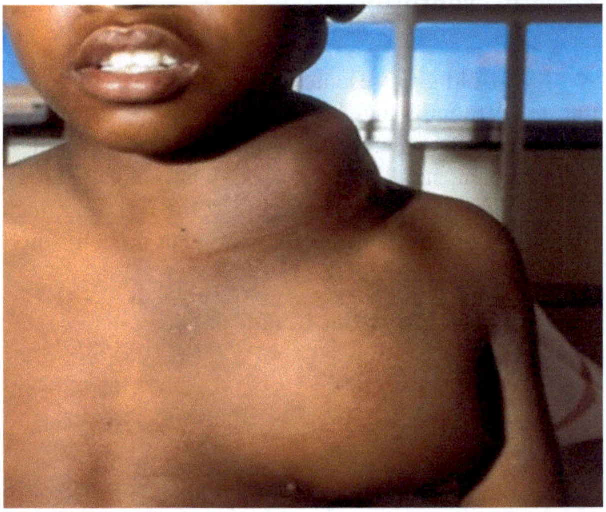

Fig. 14.2 Lymphadenopathy

What Investigations Would You Like to Request?

- CBC, ESR, CRP, peripheral smear, LDH, biochemistry
- Chest X-ray PA view and lateral view and spine
- CT scan of the neck, chest, abdomen, and pelvis
- Lymph node biopsy
- HIV, EBV, CMV

Herein listed are available results for your case scenario:

WBC	HB	MCV	PLT	N	L	Na^+	K^+	Ur	Cr	Ca^{++}	Mg^{++}	PO_4	UA	HIV
6.3	9.9	83	219	3.5	1.7	136	3.6	2.7	46	2.2	0.7	0.9	0.35	Neg

Peripheral blood film: No abnormal cells (Figs. 14.3 and 14.4).

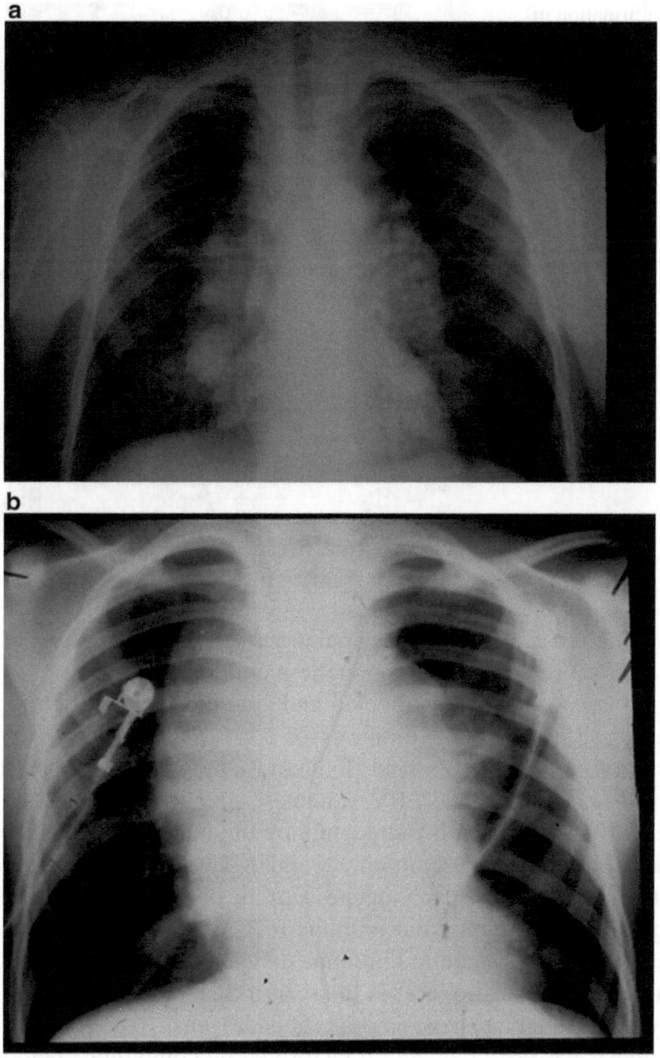

Fig. 14.3 Chest X-ray (**a** and **b**)

Epidemiology and Etiology

Hodgkin lymphoma amounts to around 10 % of all childhood cancers and roughly 17 % of all cancers in adolescents.

This disease is predominantly present in boys (ratio M/F = 3:4) and primarily affects the lower socioeconomic class.

This is the most common childhood cancer in 15–19-year-olds and has a bimodal distribution with peaks in the late teens and then later above age 55 years.

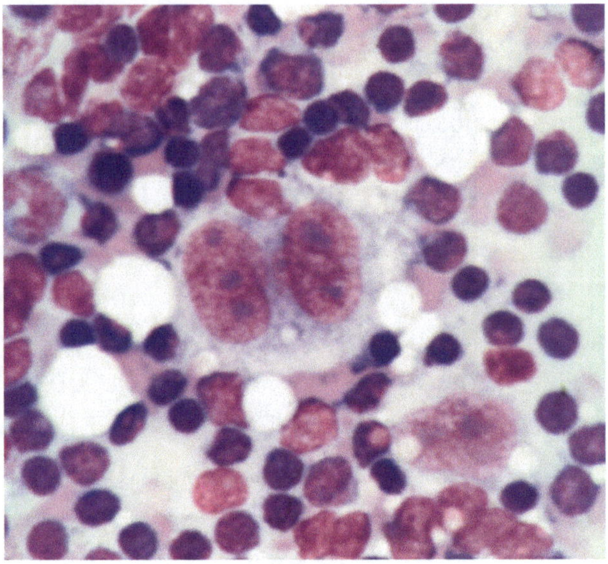

Fig. 14.4 Confirmation of diagnosis by biopsy with the presence of Reed-Sternberg cells

In young children in Westernized populations this disease is rare, but in developing countries it is more prevalent among these children.

The lymph nodes are mainly affected and are characterized by the presence of Reed-Sternberg (RS) cells in the tumor tissue.

The Epstein–Barr virus (EBV) and Hodgkin Lymphoma often coexist but causality is not well understood. The EBV genome is frequently found (up to 50 %) in tumor tissue. This association is more common in young children and in the mixed cellularity type which is more commonly found in developing countries (up to 90 %). However, its exact role in the carcinogenesis of the disease is not established.

The hypothesis of an abnormal immune response was also raised. The higher incidence in patients with acquired immune deficiency or constitutional (ataxia telangiectasia syndrome Purtillo) argues in favor of this hypothesis. Other risk factors are a family history and late exposure to oral pathogens.

The prognosis has been radically transformed by combining chemotherapy and radiation treatments that allow a survival rate of 90 %. New therapeutic approaches aim at maintaining high survival rates with minimal sequelae.

In Africa

The real incidence of HL on the African continent is not known because of lack of data and registries. A study looking at the patterns of distribution of childhood cancer showed that HL represented 9 % of the total childhood cancers in Senegal, 8.4 % in Mali, and 7.6 % in Kenya. Other studies reported an incidence of 6.8 % in Benin and Nigeria, and 7 % in Morocco and Namibia.

Clinical Presentation

Hodgkin lymphoma is characterized by progressive lymph node enlargement. More than 95 % of cases present at a site above the diaphragm.

This disease is unicentric in origin and begins in one node or group of nodes. Subsequently, it spreads in a predictable way to contiguous nodes which is more likely associated with the nodular sclerosing subtype. Whereas noncontiguous spread is more likely involved with mixed cellularity and lymphocyte depletion.

The disease can present with general signs: pruritus, fever, anorexia, weight loss, and/or night sweats.

Taking down history is important and involves looking for the symptoms that would classify the disease as A (patients without symptoms) or B (patients with symptoms). The presence of symptoms of heavy night sweating (drenching), fever (>38 °C for 3 days or more), and weight loss of >10 % in the preceding 6 months are specifically important aspects to ask about.

Other history is the presence of nodes, which is important if these have been present for a long time and may have increased or decreased in size over time.

The lymph nodes, especially in the neck are the most affected and represent the usual mode of revelation of the disease. The lymph nodes are usually painless, mobile, and in groups.

Of special interest is the presentation of the patients with signs and symptoms suggestive of tuberculosis. The misdiagnosis, in these cases, can lead to a delay in the diagnosis and treatment of the lymphoma. In countries with a high incidence of tuberculosis, the coexistence of the two diseases may present a challenge for the administration of the therapy and the management of added side effects.

Deep mediastinal lymphadenopathy can be present and is initially asymptomatic. These lymph nodes can transform in the rapidly evolving compressive forms which will then cause coughing or true compression: the superior vena cava syndrome.

In the mediastinal location, the bulky form is defined by a mass exceeding 33 % of the diameter of the thorax through D5–D6 or more than 10 cm maximum diameter.

Other locations are less frequent.

Pulmonary involvement is often associated with mediastinal lymph node localization, and is best demonstrated by a CT scan, which should always be recommended (if available) to clarify the subsequent radiation fields. This may be through an extension to the adjacent lymph nodes or rarely because of hematogenous dissemination.

Neurological involvement is usually late in the disease progression, and may also be related to a particular compression locoregional if paravertebral lymph nodes are involved. This may then give rise to epidural spinal cord compression, and less frequently involve hematogenous spread.

Intracerebral damage, described in the literature, can be characterized by cerebral seizures or neurological deficits, though this is not a common finding.

Bone involvement is usually demonstrated as bone pain and is rarely isolated.

Involvement of the spleen and/or liver is frequently found. Symptoms of bleeding and jaundice may indicate the presence of immune hemolytic anemia and thrombocytopenia.

Involvement of the bone marrow can be suspected in the clinical signs of the step by bone marrow failure. This disease is often subclinical and affects the blood count.

In exceptional cases, the disease can be revealed and accompanied by autoimmune thrombocytopenic purpura or autoimmune hemolytic anemia.

In Africa

Children present with advanced disease and associated comorbidities. Tuberculosis and HIV may coexist and do not exclude the presence of the lymphoma.

Bulky disease is often encountered and confirmed by chest X-rays (Fig. 14.5). Superior vena cava syndrome if present should be treated immediately.

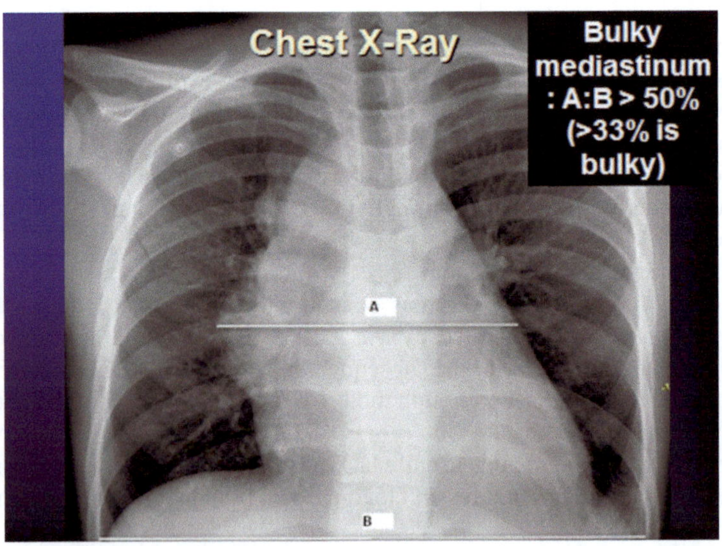

Fig. 14.5 Bulky disease confirmed by chest X-rays

Diagnosis of HL and Histology

The diagnosis of Hodgkin lymphoma is based on the histopathology of a biopsy of a lymph node or default of another organ or tissue.

FNA (fine needle aspiration) can diagnose Classical Hodgkin lymphoma together with immunostains but cannot identify subtypes, which are not needed for treatment.

Description of Pathology

Diagnosis is made by the presence of RS cells in the context of inflammatory granuloma resulting from lymphocytes, granulocytes, and plasma cells and eosinophils. The RS cells are large cells usually having two lobes with prominent nucleoli (Fig. 14.6).

The WHO recognizes two major subtypes of HL: the classical and nodular lymphocyte predominant HL (Fig. 14.7a, b below—pathology classification).

Classical Hodgkin lymphoma has four forms:

- Nodular sclerosis
- Mixed cellularity
- Lymphocyte depleted
- Lymphocyte predominant

Immunophenotyping is recommended as a routine diagnostic tool.

If not available for all patients, it should be done when clinical and/or pathological morphological findings are not clearly consistent with HL.

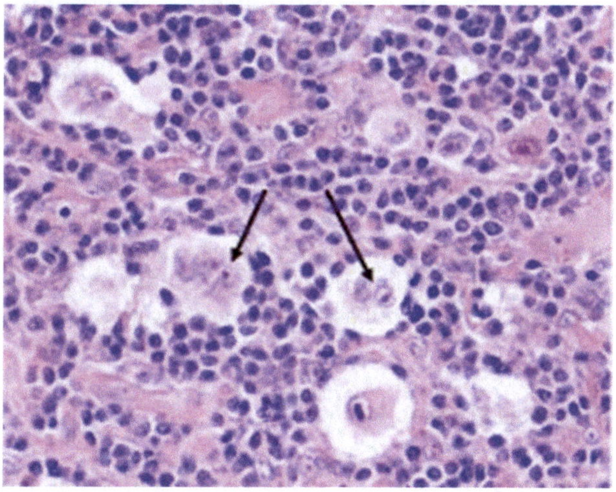

Fig. 14.6 Reed-Sternberg cells

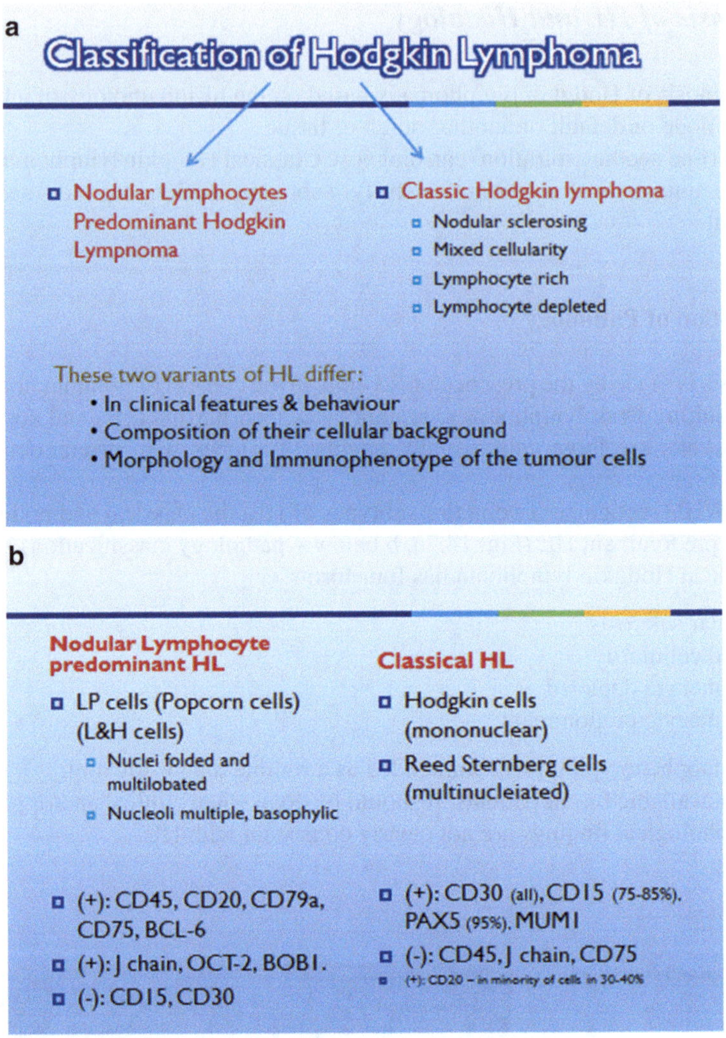

Fig. 14.7 Pathology classification of Hodgkin lymphoma

Immunohistochemistry usually shows in the conventional form of positive markers CD15 and CD30, whereas CD20 is often negative. The LMP antigen, a marker of EBV is present in tumor cells especially in the mixed cellularity type. In the nodular lymphocytic form CD20 and CD45 are positive against CD15 and CD20, while the EBV as well as markers are negative.

Diagnosis Workup

Laboratory tests are usually noncontributory as far as staging is concerned, but are important to monitor progress and FBC, renal and hepatic functions are important.

Laboratory Tests

Hematology Studies

Complete blood count (CBC).
Erythrocyte sedimentation rate (ESR).

The full blood count may show different anomalies, such as frequently observed neutrophilic leukocytosis and hypereosinophilia. Lymphopenia is less common in children. Hypochromic anemia of inflammatory origin reflects the progression of the disease. Autoimmune hemolytic anemia can be observed as well as thrombocytopenia or autoimmune neutropenia. More rarely, pancytopenia can confirm bone marrow involvement.

Bone marrow biopsy allows confirmation of the involvement, but has been replaced by the use of the PET scan in resourced countries.

Under the staging, in Africa in the absence of the PET scan, two bone marrow biopsies looking for Hodgkin location, given the nature of focal bone marrow infiltration, is recommended.

Biochemical Studies

Liver function tests (AST, alkaline phosphatase, total protein/albumin, lactic dehydrogenase, and bilirubin).
Renal function studies (blood urea nitrogen, creatinine, serum electrolytes, and urinalysis).

Other tests described in the literature include the following: Serum copper, fibrinogen, haptoglobin, Immunoglobulins, Serum ferritin and transferrin, Serum $ß_2$ macroglobin, Serum-soluble interleukin-2 receptor (sIL-2R), T_4/TSH, LH/FSH.

On the African continent these tests as well as the *immunologic evaluation of the patient are not recommended* (the absolute lymphocyte count, T- and B-cell counts).

Viral studies: Hepatitis B and C serology, HIV antibody, HSV antibody, CMV antibody, varicella antibody.

Radiologic studies include the following investigations:

- Chest radiograph (posterior, anterior, and lateral).
- Ultrasound examination of abdomen (special attention to liver and spleen).
- CT scan of the chest and abdomen.

Other investigations used for the diagnostic workup of the disease include MRI or/and PET scans which are expensive and in most cases not available.

The bone scan and Gallium scan used in the past are not recommended anymore.

Radiological signs are variable but predominantly lytic. Vertebral fractures can occur with the risk of spinal cord compression (Table 14.1).

Table 14.1 Initial assessment of Hodgkin lymphoma and minimal investigations required for the diagnosis

History	Fever, night sweats, loss of weight, pruritus, enlargement of lymph nodes
Clinical examination	Lymphadenopathy, hepatosplenomegaly
Hematology and biochemistry	CBC, ESR, UKE, LFT
Viral studies	HIV, EBV, CMV, hepatitis
Radiological investigations	Chest X-ray, abdominal ultrasound (preferably CT scan of chest and abdomen)
Exclude tuberculosis if in high prevalence area	

Table 14.2 Ann-Arbor classification

Stage	Description
I	Involvement of a single lymph node site or lymphoid structure
II	Involvement of at least two nodal areas on the same side of the diaphragm
III	Involvement of lymph nodes both in the chest and the abdomen
IV	Extranodal involvement present

Note: Splenic involvement is considered an infringement of a lymph node area

E Subscript of the stage: extranodal involvement by contiguity

Prognosis

The prognosis is closely related to the expansion stage of the disease according to the Ann-Arbor (Table 14.2) classification (Fig. 14.8).

Classification A or B is considered according to the presence or absence of clinical signs (Fever: >38 °C for >1 week, Weight loss >10 % within 6 months, heavy night sweats).

Another classification that is used is divided into three groups depending on the disease involvement and the presence of A or B symptoms (Table 14.3).

A simplified risk classification used includes only two groups (Table 14.4).

Approach to Therapy

The choice of treatment is based on the stage, associated comorbidities, and availability and affordability of therapy.

Each patient should receive the treatment which optimizes his/her chance to be cured based on risk assessment, response adapted, and the availability of drugs and treatment.

One of the most common used protocols in the treatment of HL is the ABVD (Adriamycin, Bleomycin, Vinblastine, Dacarbazine).

This regimen comprises the administration of Adriamycin, Bleomycin, Vinblastine and Dacarbazine, and is usually given for 6 cycles at 2-week intervals and can be given as an outpatient therapy.

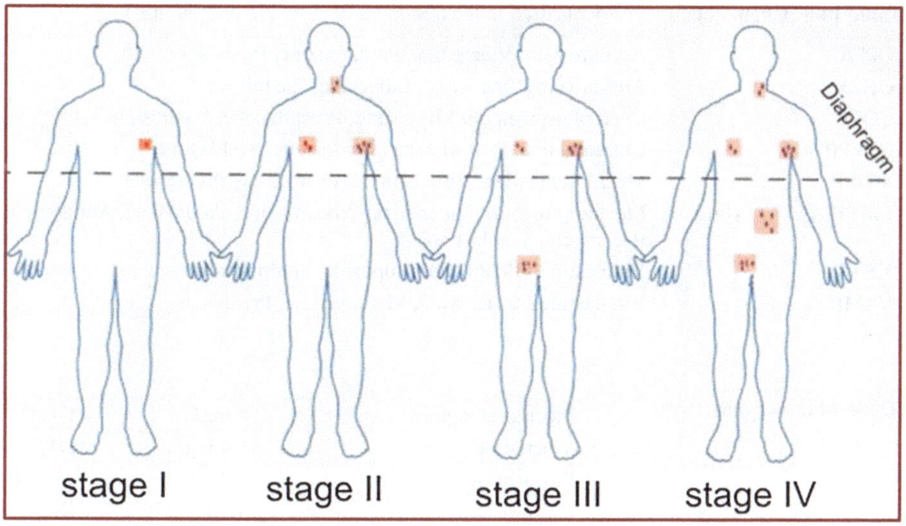

Fig. 14.8 Staging classification

Table 14.3 Risk classification (St. Jude)

Risk	Description
Favorable	Stage I and II A Nonbulky mediastinal disease <3 involved nodal regions
Intermediate	Stage I and II A with bulky mediastinal disease or ≥ nodal regions Stage IIIA
Unfavorable	Stages IIB, IIIB, IVA, and IVB

Table 14.4 Simplified risk classification

Risk	Description
Favorable	Stage I and II A No bulky mediastinal disease <3 involved nodal regions
Less favorable	All other cases

Other regimens used in the treatment of the disease are presented in Tables 14.5 and 14.6.

The choice of treatment is dependent on the availability of the drugs avoiding delays in administration of the chemotherapy.

Substitution when no controlled study is available

A missing drug should be replaced with something else (Table 14.7).

Cure requires remission and consolidation. Current treatment aims to minimize the apparition of late effect and increased risk of toxicity without losing or improve survival rates and by successive refinements of treatment based on prognosis and the search for alternatives to treatment with potential toxicity.

Table 14.5 Chemotherapy protocols used in the treatment of Hodgkin lymphoma

OPPA	Adriamycyin, Vincristine, Procarbazine, Prednisone
OEPA	Adriamycin, Vincristine, Etoposide, Prednisone
COPP	Cyclophosphamide, Vincristine, Procarbazine, Prednisone
CLVPP	Chlorambucil, Procarbazine, Prednisone, Vinblastine
MOPP	Mechlorethamine, Vincristine, Procarbazine, Prednisone
MOPP/ABVD hybrid	Mechlorethamine, Vincristine, Procarbazine, Prednisone, Adriamycin, Bleomycin, Vinblastine
VBVP	Vinblastine, Bleomycin, Etoposide, Prednisone
VAMP	Vinblastine, Adriamycin, Methotrexate, Prednisone

Table 14.6 Staging

Mechlorethamine	6 mg/m^2	D1,8
Vincristine	1.4 mg/m^2	D1,8
Procarbazine	100 mg/m^2	D1–14
Prednisone	40 mg/m^2	D1–14
ABVD (/28 days)		
Adriamycin	25 mg/m^2	D1,15
Bléomycine	10 mg/m^2	D1,15
Vinblastine	6 mg/m^2	D1,15
Dacarbazine (DTIC)	375 mg/m^2	D1,15
MOPP/ABVD hybrid (/28 days)		
Mechlorethamine	6 mg/m^2	D1
Vincristine	1.4 mg/m^2	D1
Procarbazine	100 mg/m^2	D1–7
Prednisone	40 mg/m^2	D1–14
Adriamycin	35 mg/m^2	D8
Bléomycine	10 mg/m^2	D8
Vinblastine	6 mg/m^2	D8
COPP (/28 days)		
Cyclophosphamide	500–600 mg/m^2	D1,8
Vincristine	1.5 mg/m^2	D1,8
Procarbazine	100 mg/m^2	D1–14
Prednisone	40 mg/m^2	D1–14
OPPA (/28 days)		
Vincristine	1.5 mg/m^2	D1,8,15
Procarbazine	100 mg/m^2	D1–15
Prednisone	60 mg/m^2	D1–15

Radiotherapy has been historically part of the treatment, but this use is now decreasing given the concern about its long-term effects.

Favorable risk lymphoma will require one consolidation:

- If CR (complete remission) after 2 cycles—consolidate with another 2 cycles or RT
- If no CR—4 more cycles or 2 cycles + RT

Table 14.7 Replacement drugs

COPP = MOPP (mustard vs. cyclophosphamide)
COPP = cyclophosphamide, oncovin, procarbazine, prednisone
ChIVPP cyclophosphamide, oncovin, procarbazine, prednisone
CVPP = CCNU, Vinblastine, Procarbazine, Prednisone
OPPA = COPP (cyclophosphamide vs. doxorubicin)
Oncovin Procarbazine, Prednisone, Adriamycin

Unfavorable risk consolidation will require two consolidations:

- If CR after 2 cycles—2 more cycles or RT
- If no CR—4 more cycles or 2 more cycles + RT

Radiotherapy is added as treatment in advanced disease or nonresponders. The radiotherapy fields have evolved and become increasingly restricted as radiotherapy is no longer needed to sterilize the disease in all patients.

Total regional and nodal fields have been replaced by involved-field radiation therapy (IFRT) and the total contemporary treatment, in most cases, includes regimens of 15–21 Gy.

The therapeutic results of Hodgkin lymphoma are a real victory of modern oncology so that in most reported series, the 5-year survival exceeds 90 %. The treatment program varies with the stage, the tumor mass, and age. In most cases chemotherapy and radiotherapy are combined.

Follow-Up During Treatment

Throughout the treatment, assessment of the response is of great importance to assess the effectiveness of treatment. Monitoring the size of lymph nodes is valuable, as the reduction in size is a clinical response to the therapy. This should be associated with the disappearance of B symptoms.

Before each cycle of chemotherapy, a CBC is recommended. The international guidelines and the advances in oncology recommend the use of the PET scan after 2–3 cycles of chemotherapy.

In Africa, the radiological evaluation during therapy might be difficult and remains controversial. If the clinical response is adequate a sonar or CT scan depending on the initial site should be performed at the end of the therapy.

Follow-Up After Treatment

One month posttreatment, the response is documented by taking history, a physical examination, CBC, ESR, and biochemistry.

The history should underline the absence of B symptoms and the physical examination to note the disappearance of the enlargement of the lymph nodes.

A raised ESR is an indication for close surveillance.

Table 14.8 presents the recommended follow-up for HL. Figure 14.9 shows the evolution of clinical signs before and after treatment.

Table 14.8 Recommended follow-up for Hodgkin lymphoma

Repeat all relevant investigations after 2 courses
At the completion of treatment
Every 3 months ×2
Every 6 months for 4 years
Once a year for 5 years

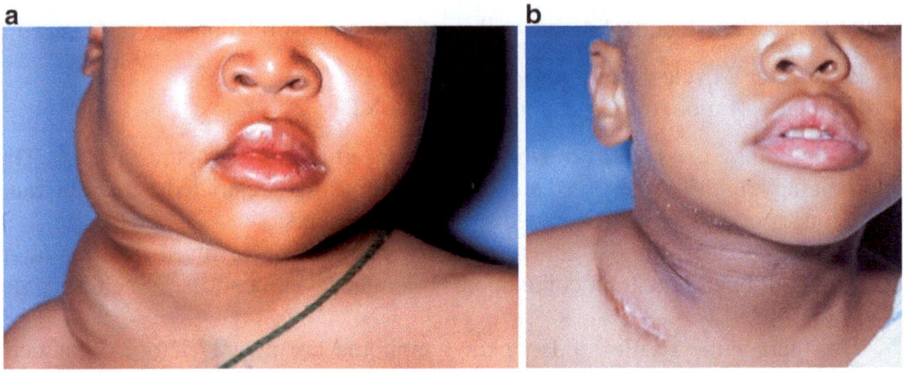

Fig. 14.9 Clinical signs (**a**) Before treatment, (**b**) follow-up after treatment

Complications Related to Therapy

Complications related to therapy can be divided into two groups: acute and late/delayed.

The acute side effects are mainly the consequence of administration of chemotherapy: bone marrow suppression, infection, nausea, susceptibility to infection, decreased lung function (bleomycin use).

The delayed complications are apparition of secondary cancers, following the use of chemotherapy and radiation: breast cancers, thyroid cancers, lung cancers, soft tissue sarcomas, cardiac diseases, acute myeloid leukemia. The risk for secondary cancers is increased 20 fold in children treated for HL.

Late complications that are noted, is the toxicity from anthracycline use with cardiac dysfunction and hypothyroidism from radiation.

Relapse of Hodgkin Lymphoma

Hodgkin lymphoma is a malignancy characterized by the possibility of late relapse up to 10 years posttreatment and apparition of late effects and secondary malignancies.

Rescue therapies described in the literature include second-line chemotherapy protocols, such as ICE, CCNU (Lamustin, VP16, Chlorambucil, and Prednisone), Gemcitabine, Vinorelbine, and the use of radiotherapy.

Supportive care measures are essential in the management of these patients because of an increase in the toxicity of the drugs. Blood and platelet transfusions as well as granulocyte stimulating factor are often included in the therapy.

In Africa

Certain investigations can be omitted to reduce costs, as there are no major advantages in assessing the level of copper, ferritin, and immunoglobulin.

It is important to screen for HIV and tuberculosis (EBV if affordable).

Treatment should be administered as outpatient, on established protocols, giving all drugs with no omissions or delays.

If something is missing (drug, RT) replace this with something else (different drug or additional chemotherapy cycles).

Summary

Hodgkin lymphoma is a relatively common cancer and usually presents with lymphadenopathy with or without systemic symptoms.

Suspect Hodgkin lymphoma in well-appearing older children and adolescents with slowly growing, firm, non-tender lymph nodes.

Perform chest X-rays, hemogram, chemistry panel immediately (in case of NHL or ALL with mediastinal mass).

Accurate tissue diagnosis and staging is essential. Confirm the diagnosis by biopsy and not aspiration.

Carefully document the sites of disease, stage, and risk group.

Many patients can be cured with outpatient chemotherapy. Patients must be followed closely, as many complications of therapy can arise and relapse can occur many years after the initial diagnosis.

A multidisciplinary approach, uniform protocol-based therapy, and abandonment prevention contribute to an increase in survival of the patients diagnosed with Hodgkin disease in Africa.

Suggested Reading

Cartwright RA, Watkins G (2004) Epidemiology of Hodgkin's disease. Hematol Oncol 22:11–26

Freed J, Kelly KM (2010) Current approaches to the management of pediatric Hodgkin lymphoma. Paediatr Drugs 12(2):85–98

Harif M, Madani A, Hessissen L, Zafad S, Khattab M, Quessar A, Benchekroun S (2009) Maladie de Hodgkin de l'enfant: Expérience marocaine. Arch Pediatr 16(6):675–677

Hodgson DC, Hudson MM, Constine LS (2007) Pediatric Hodgkin lymphoma: maximizing efficacy minimizing toxicity. Semin Radiat Oncol 17:230–242

Stefan DC (2013) Hodgkin lymphoma in Africa: present and future. Transfus Apher Sci 49(2):144–146. doi:10.1016/j.transci.2013.07.016, Epub Aug 13 2013 review

Chapter 15
Non-Hodgkin Lymphoma

Case Presentation 1

A 13-year-old boy, previously healthy, presented with a 1-month history of cervical and bilateral axillary lymphadenopathy. Two weeks prior to his presentation, he also started developing respiratory distress which was worsening (Fig. 15.1).

Findings on examination:

The boy appeared acutely ill.

Weight: 45 kg; Height: 148 cm.

Observations: Pulse rate 123/min, respiratory rate 38/min, oxygen saturation 92 %, blood pressure 118/65 mmHg.

Cervical, submandibular and bilateral axillary lymphadenopathy with a diameter of 1.5–2 cm was present. Mild pallor and facial edema were also noted.

On respiratory examination, signs of respiratory distress were found: tachypnea, orthopnea, intercostal recession, and alar flaring. The left side of the thorax was more prominent than the right. The trachea was central. There was good air entry on both sides of the chest with no adventitious sounds heard.

On cardiovascular examination, the boy was tachycardic and had a raised jugular venous pressure. The area of cardiac dullness appeared increased. The heart sounds were normal, there were no murmurs, and no signs of cardiac failure were noted.

On examination of the abdomen, the liver was palpated 5 cm below the costal margin and the spleen 4 cm below the costal margin.

The neurological system was normal.

D.C. Stefan, M. Harif, *Pediatric Cancer in Africa*,
DOI 10.1007/978-3-319-17936-0_15

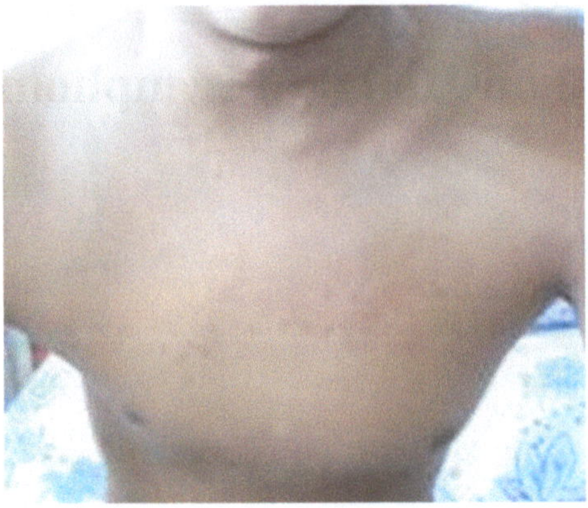

Fig. 15.1 Prominent left hemithorax

What Is Differential Diagnosis?

Infections: tuberculosis, human immunodeficiency virus (with a superimposed infection), Cytomegalovirus, Ebstein Barr virus, etc.

Neoplasms: Hodgkin lymphoma, NHL (Burkitt lymphoma (BL)), diffuse large B-cell lymphoma, anaplastic large cell lymphoma, T- or B-cell lymphoblastic lymphoma, acute lymphoblastic or myeloid leukemia, chronic myeloid leukemia.

Other, e.g., autoimmune lymphoproliferative disorder, Rosai-Dorfmann disease.

What Investigations Would You Like to Request?

- Full blood and differential count, reticulocyte count, peripheral blood smear
- Biochemistry: electrolytes (including calcium, magnesium, and phosphate), renal function, uric acid
- LDH
- Chest X-ray (PA and lateral)
- Abdominal sonar
- Then lymph node biopsy or fine needle aspiration of a lymph node with flow cytometry

Herein listed are available results for this case scenario:

Wcc	Hb	MCV	Pl	Neutro	Mono	Lymph	Eosino	Baso	Retic
9.5	11	80	368	5.5	0.5	3	0.3	0.2	1.1 %

Na	K	Urea	Creat	Calcium	Magnesium	Phosphate	Uric acid	LDH
136	4.2	5.7	53	2.1	0.78	1.2	0.53	798

Abdominal ultrasound: multiple enlarged lymph nodes present with an enlarged liver and spleen. No other abnormalities were seen (Fig. 15.2).

FNA of lymph node with flow cytometry: T-cell lymphoblastic lymphoma

What other important staging investigation needs to be performed now and why?

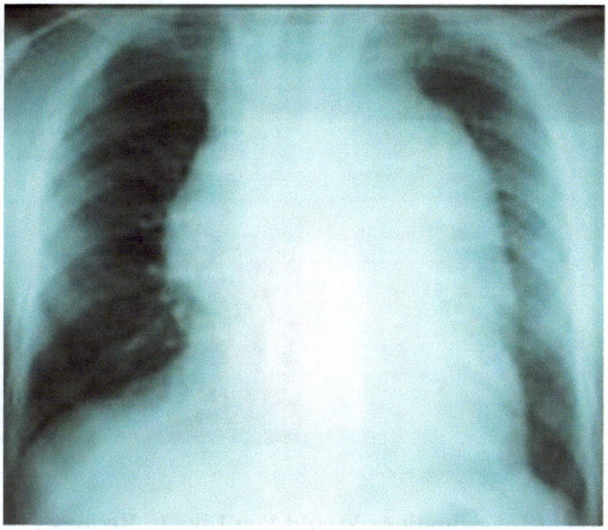

Fig. 15.2 Mediastinal mass

Bone marrow aspiration and trephine biopsy: to assess the number of blasts in the bone marrow to diagnose either T-cell lymphoblastic lymphoma (<20 % blasts) or T-cell acute lymphoblastic leukemia (>20 % blasts).

Case Presentation 2

A 4-year-old boy was admitted to hospital after presenting with a 1-week history of an enlarging left-sided jaw mass as well as progressive swelling of the left eye for 3 days prior to presentation. He also had a reduced appetite.

Findings on examination:

He did not look acutely or chronically ill
Weight: 18 kg; Height: 93 cm

The most obvious finding was a painless left-sided jaw mass, which displaced the left-sided molars as well as left-sided periorbital swelling and proptosis. There was also associated left cervical and submandibular lymphadenopathy. On further examination, the only other significant finding was hepatosplenomegaly (Fig. 15.3).

What Is Differential Diagnosis?

Infections: cellulitis of the involved areas, dental abscess
Neoplasms: BL, diffuse large B-cell lymphoma, rhabdomyosarcoma, acute myeloid leukemia, myeloid sarcoma.

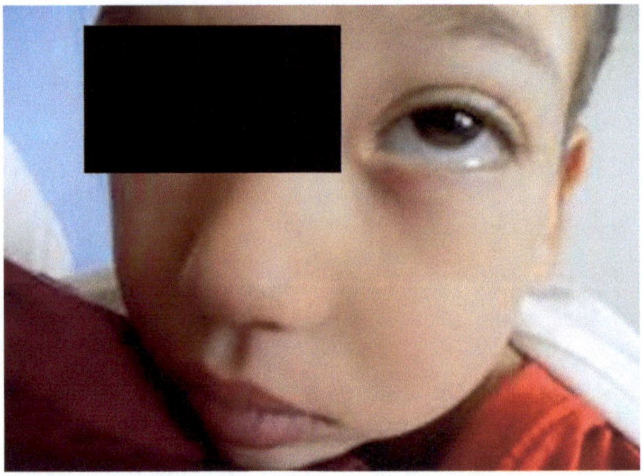

Fig. 15.3 Left-sided periorbital swelling and jaw mass

What Investigations Would You Like to Request?

- Full blood and differential count, reticulocyte count, peripheral blood smear
- Biochemistry: electrolytes (including calcium, magnesium, and phosphate), renal function, uric acid
- LDH
- Chest X-ray (PA and lateral)
- Abdominal sonar
- CT or MRI of head, if available
- Biopsy or fine needle aspiration of the jaw mass with flow cytometry

Herein listed are available results for this case scenario:

Wcc	Hb	MCV	Pl	Neutro	Mono	Lymph	Eosino	Baso	Retic
7.6	9.9	78	265	2.4	0.4	3.3	0.28	0.2	1.5 %

Na	K	Urea	Creat	Calcium	Magnesium	Phosphate	Uric acid	LDH
138	4.8	7.8	66	2.3	0.86	1.15	0.61	1198

Abdominal ultrasound: multiple enlarged lymph nodes were seen throughout the abdomen; hepatosplenomegaly was noted; no other abnormal findings.

Fine needle aspiration of the jaw mass: Burkitt lymphoma.

Non-Hodgkin Lymphoma

The NHLs constitute a mixed group of malignancies with a lymphoid clonality of either B- or T-cells in common. Childhood NHLs differ substantially from those seen in adults according to histology, aggressiveness, their primary extra-nodal localization

Table 15.1 Classification of the NHLs of childhood

B-cell origin	T-cell origin	Uncommon
BL and Burkitt-like lymphoma	Anaplastic large cell lymphoma – Systemic – Cutaneous	Lymphoproliferative disease associated with immunodeficiency
Diffuse large B-cell lymphoma	Precursor T-cell lymphoblastic lymphoma	Pediatric follicular lymphoma
Precursor B-cell lymphoblastic lymphoma		Primary CNS lymphoma
		Peripheral T-cell lymphoma

as well as the fact that they often have medullary and central nervous system (CNS) involvement. Nowadays, more than 90 % of children with early stage disease can be cured by modern treatment protocols and good supportive care.

In the classification of lymphoma, those of B-cell origin are distinguished from those with a T-cell origin. Thus, the NHLs of B-cell origin are: BL and Burkitt-like lymphoma, diffuse large B-cell lymphoma and precursor B-cell lymphoblastic lymphoma, while the T-cell lymphomas are anaplastic large cell lymphomas (systemic and cutaneous) and precursor T-cell lymphoblastic lymphomas (Table 15.1). Other rare types include lymphoproliferative disease associated with immunodeficiency, pediatric follicular lymphoma, primary CNS lymphoma, and peripheral T-cell lymphoma.

Epidemiology

Non-Hodgkin lymphoma is one of the most frequent childhood cancers (about 7 % of all childhood cancers). Factors influencing the incidence are age, gender, ethnicity, and histology. In most Western country registries, NHL is the third most common cancer, after acute leukemia and brain tumors. Children affected are mostly 3 years and older. NHL rarely occurs in infants and a male predominance is seen in most studies.

The geographical distribution of NHL is heterogeneous and reflects the impact of environmental factors. BL is particularly frequent in sub-Saharan Africa, where it is the common childhood cancer, is endemic to the region, and therefore termed "endemic Burkitt lymphoma." In the rest of the world, the term "sporadic Burkitt lymphoma" is used. HIV-associated BL occurs in patients with the HIV disease. Almost 85 % of endemic cases are associated with Ebstein Barr virus (EBV) infection, compared to 15 % of sporadic cases. The role of EBV in carcinogenesis, however, is not elucidated. Children with acquired or inherited immunodeficiency have an increased risk of developing NHL, usually of B-cell origin (Table 15.2).

Table 15.2 Conditions with an increased risk for NHL

Inherited immunodeficiency (primary immune deficiency)
Ataxia telangiectasia
Wiskott Aldrich syndrome
X-linked lymphoproliferative disorder
Acquired immune suppression, e.g., HIV disease, following cancer treatment

Clinical Presentation

The most common clinical presentation is that of lymphadenopathy and/or a painless abdominal mass (40 %) or mediastinal mass (30 %). This can cause symptoms caused by compression, particularly mediastinal compression. Symptoms and signs of bone marrow failure as a result of infiltration may be present. CNS complaints and signs may also occur, indicating advanced disease. The history of complaints is usually short, because of the highly aggressive nature of NHLs, especially BL, which has a doubling time of 18–24 h.

Burkitt- and Burkitt-Like Lymphoma

These types of lymphoma are usually seen in children between ages 3 and 15 years. The clinical presentation of BL and Burkitt-like lymphoma is very similar and can only be distinguished by pathology. A patient with an abdominal mass may present with nausea, vomiting, constipation, or a mass noted by the patient or caregiver. BL may also present with an acute abdomen, caused by bowel perforation or intussusception. Bowel perforation occurs when the lymphoma which originates in the gut-associated lymphoid tissue (GALT), ruptures the bowel wall as a result of growth. Intussusception occurs because of a lymph node mass being the lead point.

A periorbital or facial mass is often seen in BL, involving the maxilla, mandible, or orbit. The facial mass is typical of endemic BL. Usually the maxilla is infiltrated, leading to loose teeth and contiguous extension to the orbit is seen, causing proptosis. A jaw mass is usually painless, but may interfere with the ability to eat and drink. Clinically, these tumors may be misdiagnosed as dental abscesses and therefore may be treated as such with antibiotics and anti-inflammatory drugs, delaying the cancer diagnosis.

Other areas of involvement include the CNS, skin, bone marrow, bone, testes, ovaries, kidneys, liver, spleen, brain, and a paraspinal mass may also occur.

Precursor B- or T-Cell Lymphoblastic Lymphoma

The clinical presentation of these two types of lymphoma is similar: generalized lymphadenopathy and hepatosplenomegaly. A mediastinal mass is commonly seen in T-cell lymphoblastic lymphoma and may lead to coughing, dyspnea, ortopnea, wheezing, and eventually superior vena cava syndrome in advanced cases. Prominence of the one side of the chest may be observed. Other possible sites of disease include: skin, bone, bone marrow, CNS, testes, and the ring of Waldeyer. Rarely, abdominal involvement is seen. If more than 25 % blasts are seen in the bone marrow, the diagnosis is acute lymphoblastic leukemia.

Large Cell Anaplastic Lymphoma

Lymphadenopathy is the usual clinical abnormality and various other sites may be involved including skin, bone, lung, pleura, muscles, and the gastrointestinal tract. Patients may complain of systemic symptoms, such as fever and weight loss.

Diagnosis of NHL

Because of the rapid rate of proliferation, if a NHL is suspected, the diagnosis should be made urgently in the fastest way possible. In areas where the Burkitt tumor is endemic, a clinical diagnosis may be made if there is no time for special investigations or where radiological/pathological investigations are not available.

Laboratory Tests

Hematological Investigations

A full blood and differential count, reticulocyte count, and peripheral blood smear should be performed. Cytopenias may be present, but is expected to be mild to moderate if the bone marrow infiltration is <25 %.

Biochemistry

Non-Hodgkin lymphoma can lead to tumor lysis syndrome (TLS); BL is most often the cause. Features of TLS including abnormal renal function, hyperkalemia, hyperphosphatemia, hypocalcemia, and raised uric acid should be sought. As soon as a clinical diagnosis of NHL is being considered and bulky disease is present, hyperhydration and allopurinol should be started and intake and urinary output carefully monitored. Lactate dehydrogenase (LDH) is usually elevated in NHL. Liver function should be tested before starting chemotherapy to ensure that it is normal.

Radiological Investigations

A chest X-ray should be performed to look for hilar and mediastinal lymphadenopathy (mediastinal mass) as well as pulmonary involvement. In areas with a high incidence of tuberculosis, the X-ray should be scrutinized for signs consistent with tuberculosis.

When a patient presents with an acute abdomen, an abdominal X-ray and lateral shoot-through is valuable to confirm free air. Otherwise, an abdominal ultrasound is the investigation of choice for a patient presenting with an abdominal mass. A mass, closely associated with the bowel or one or more nodal masses or lesions in the kidneys, spleen or/and liver, may be demonstrated. Intussusception may also be suggested.

If available, a CT- or MRI scan of the mass may be performed to allow better anatomical delineation. Patients with airway compression should be scanned in a lateral or prone position and sedation should be avoided if at all possible.

If bony involvement is suspected, a bone scan may be performed. PET CT is used more and more nowadays, but is still not considered a standard investigation in NHL.

Confirming the Diagnosis

Ideally, the diagnosis should be confirmed histologically. The exception is where BL is strongly suspected, and there is insufficient time to make a diagnosis or special investigations are not available. WHAT is extremely important is to confirm the diagnosis of NHL in the quickest, least invasive way, since the tumor is so aggressive and the patients may be gravely ill with TLS, renal failure, bowel perforation, superior vena cava syndrome, etc.

If a pathologist skilled in the interpretation of cytology is available, a fine needle aspiration may be performed for cytological interpretation as well as flow cytometry. Otherwise, an urgent biopsy may be performed, if the patient is stable enough to tolerate anesthesia. Alternatively, ascites fluid or a pleural effusion sample may be sent for cytology and flow cytometry.

Pathology

The three most frequent histopathological types are BL (30 % of NHL) and Burkitt-like lymphoma (10–20 %), precursor T- or B-cell lymphoblastic lymphoma (20 %), and large cell anaplastic lymphoma (10 %). In Table 15.4 the immunohistochemistry of these types are compared.

Burkitt- and Burkitt-Like Lymphoma

Burkitt- and Burkitt-like lymphoma originate from mature cells B and is characterized by specific chromosomal anomalies, i.e., t(8,14), t(8,22), or t(2,8) in order of occurrence. These translocations cause inappropriate expression of c-myc, the presence of which is the gold standard for diagnosing BL. They are not specific to BL, however, and may also be found in diffuse large B-cell or follicular lymphoma.

Burkitt acute lymphoblastic leukemia has the same cytological, immunological, and cytogenetic characteristics and is diagnosed when the percentage of blasts in the bone marrow is >25 %. A diffuse infiltration of small cells is seen in BL, often with vacuolated basophilic cytoplasm and dense chromatin, creating the "starry sky" appearance. Figures of mitoses and apoptosis are frequent and reflect the high proliferative potential of BL.

The diagnosis of diffuse large B-cell lymphoma is made when c-myc cannot be proven, the evidence points towards BL, but the cells are large and the Ki-67 is ≥99 %.

Burkitt lymphoma is characterized by the following immunohistological positive findings: CD19, CD20, CD22, and CD79a as well as the expression of surface immunoglobulin (mostly IgM), with kappa or lambda light chains. CD10 is expressed in almost all cases. In endemic cases, EBV may be demonstrated more frequently.

Diffuse large B-cell lymphoma also expresses the B-cell markers, i.e., CD19, CD20, CD22, and CD79a. Surface immunoglobulins are expressed in more than half of the cases. More rarely, they may express CD5, CD10, BCL2, or BCL6. Ki-67 usually has weaker expression than in BL. The molecular studies frequently show expression of BCL6, BCL2, and c-myc.

Lymphoblastic Lymphoma

Lymphoblastic lymphoma comprises two immunological phenotypes: T-cell, seen in most of the cases and B-cell (Tables 15.3 and 15.4). Lymphoblastic lymphoma is cytologically identical to lymphoblastic leukemia; the percentage of blasts in the bone marrow will determine whether the diagnosis is lymphoma or leukemia. The lymphoblast is characterized by a small amount of cytoplasm which is basophilic and fine chromatin as well as a convoluted appearance at times. Various cytogenetic anomalies have been described in lymphoblastic lymphoma. Primarily translocations t(9,17) and more rarely t(8,13) are seen. These anomalies do not have prognostic significance.

Large Cell Anaplastic Lymphoma

Large cell anaplastic lymphoma more often occurs in the older child and adolescent. The tumor cells are often broad, pleomorphic and express CD30 and ALK (anaplastic lymphoma kinase). Translocation t(2;5)(p23;q35) is frequently found.

Staging and Prognosis

The prognosis is closely related to the tumor burden and the extent of disease. Other important prognostic factors are age, site of disease, response to therapy, and the presence of chromosomal abnormalities: poor outcome in BL for chromosomal

Table 15.3 Diagnostic work-up

Medical history and clinical examination
Blood investigations
Full blood and differential count
Reticulocyte count
Peripheral blood smear
Biochemistry
Electrolytes, including calcium, magnesium and phosphate, renal function
Uric acid
Liver function (bilirubin, AST, ALT)
Radiology
Chest X-ray
Abdominal ultrasound
CT or MRI of the mass, if available
Aspiration of ascites fluid or pleural effusion (flow cytometry)
Fine needle aspiration/biopsy of a lymph node or other mass
Bone marrow aspirate and trephine biopsy

Table 15.4 Immunological phenotype of lymphoblastic lymphomas and Burkitt lymphoma

Subtype	CD45	CD34	TDT	CD3	CD5	CD7	CD19	CD20	CD22	CD79α	CD10	Immuno globulins
Precursor B	+	±	+	−	−	−	+	±	+	+	+	Negative for IgM, sIgM, kappa, and lambda
B	+	±	±	−	−	−	+	±	+	+	+	Positive for IgM, sIgM, and kappa or lambda
T	+	±	±	+	±	+	−	−	−	±	−	

Ig Cytoplasmic Immunoglobulin, sIg surface Immunoglobulin

abnormalities other than c-myc, MYC (8q24) in diffuse large B-cell and loss of heterozygosity at chromosome 6q in T-cell lymphoblastic lymphoma. Infants and adolescents (except in adolescents with BL and Burkitt-like lymphoma) have a poorer outcome. Early stage disease has an excellent prognosis with a 5-year survival rate of more than 90 %. Mediastinal involvement usually predicts a poor outcome. Involvement of the bone marrow or CNS also indicates an inferior outcome.

Early stage B-cell lymphoma has an excellent outcome of >90 % and even patients with stage III and IV disease have a very good outcome (80–90 %). The survival rate of patients with advanced anaplastic large cell lymphoma is 60–75 %.

Relapsed Disease

Recurrent B-cell lymphoma has a poor outcome of 10–20 % and resistance to chemotherapy is a problem. There is no standard salvage regimen available but the use of new protocols (RICE) or drugs such as Rituximab show promising results. Patients with relapsed lymphoblastic lymphoma also fare poorly (10–40 %), while in relapsed anaplastic large cell lymphoma, 40–60 % of patients may be cured.

Table 15.5 The St Jude (Murphy) lymphoma staging system

Stage	Extension of the malignancy
Stage I	Involvement of a single group of lymph nodes (other than mediastinal or abdominal) or a single extra-nodal mass
Stage II	Single nodal mass with the regional lymph node involved, two or more tumors or nodal masses on one side of the diaphragm, gastrointestinal tract tumor (completely resected) with or without regional lymph node involvement
Stage III	Lymph node involvement or extra-nodal involvement on both sides of the diaphragm, as well as any primary intrathoracic disease, extensive abdominal disease, and any paraspinal or epidural masses
Stage IV	Bone marrow (at least 5 % blasts) or CNS involvement (presence of malignant cells in the cerebrospinal fluid)

Table 15.6 The French LMB staging system

Group	Details
A	Completely resected stage I or abdominal stage II
B	Multiple extra-abdominal sites of disease, non-resected stage I, II, III, and IV (bone marrow <25 % and no involvement of the central nervous system)
C	Bone marrow infiltration ≥25 % and/or central nervous system involvement

Two major staging systems are used, i.e., the Murphy staging system (Table 15.5) and the French LMB staging system (Table 15.6). In the event of bone marrow involvement of more than 25 %, the diagnosis is that of acute leukemia.

Treatment

The type of treatment protocol is determined by the histological subtype as well as the stage of disease. Before treatment is started, measures to prevent TLS should be taken, e.g., allopurinol, hyperhydration, and frequent monitoring. Rasburicase may also be used, if available. In some cases, because of critical illness, airway compression or TLS, treatment should be initiated even without confirming the diagnosis first.

Surgery is only indicated to perform a minimally invasive biopsy or in the case of intussusception or bowel perforation. Tumor debulking should not be performed empirically, since the lymphoma responds very well to chemotherapy only. Radiotherapy is rarely indicated.

Good supportive care must be provided when NHL is treated, since significant treatment-related toxicity is expected.

B-Cell Lymphomas (Burkitt, Diffuse Large B-Cell)

Several chemotherapy regimens are available for the treatment of B-cell lymphomas, of which the French LMB regimen is used most commonly. Patients are stratified as group A (resected stage I or abdominal stage II disease), group B (unresected stage I/II disease), or group C (with CNS or bone marrow involvement) (Table 15.6). The German BFM (Berlin-Frankfurt-Munster) protocol is also often used and the outcomes of both regimens are comparable. Very good outcomes are obtained for early stage disease and moderate outcomes for more advanced disease.

The LMB treatment comprises a less intensive prephase of 1 or 2 weeks, with the aim of minimizing the risk of TLS, while reducing tumor volume. Thereafter, an intensive phase of about 5–6 months duration is divided into courses of 6–7 days, every 2–3 weeks.

In Africa

In some African countries, endemic BL is treated with modified, less intense chemotherapy protocols, because of a lack of drugs and supportive care. The Groupe Franco-Africain d'Oncologie Pédiatrique (GFAOP) modified the LMB89 protocol (Table 15.7 and Fig. 15.4) and achieved a 3-year overall survival rate of 61 %. Limited treatment with cyclophosphamide and intrathecal methotrexate with every course seemed sufficient for most of the cases with stage I and II disease in a study performed in Malawi (Table 15.7 and Fig. 15.5). Relapsed disease has been treated with a higher dose of cyclophosphamide, intrathecal methotrexate, and vincristine and 35 % of patients survived.

In BL, relapses are almost limited to the first year of follow-up. Beyond 1 year off treatment, children are regarded as cured with a minimal risk of relapse.

Lymphoblastic Lymphoma

Lymphoblastic lymphoma is treated using protocols very similar or identical to that of high-risk acute lymphoblastic leukemia (Tables 15.8 and 15.9). In the case of a mediastinal mass, admission to an intensive care unit may be required due to airway compression. Sedation should only be undertaken when absolutely necessary, with supportive staff available. A pleural or pericardial therapeutic tap may be necessary to relieve symptoms. The duration of treatment is usually 2 years. The event-free survival can reach 70–80 %.

Large Cell Anaplastic Lymphoma

The treatment and prognosis vary according to the site of the disease. The protocols are similar to those for B-cell lymphoma and leukemia (Tables 15.7 and 15.9). Vinblastine monotherapy has been used very successfully in patients with relapsed disease (Table 15.10).

In the event of a poor response on day 15, continue with COPM1and2 and CYM1and2 with 2–3 week intervals between courses:

Table 15.7 B-cell lymphoma: Protocol LMB89 adapted by the GFAOP

GROUP A: COPAD 1 and 2 with a 3-week interval		
COPAD		
Drug	Dose	Day
Vincristine	2 mg/m² IV bolus (max 2 mg)	Day 1, 6
Predniso(lo)ne	60 mg/m² po	Days 1–5, then wean over 3 days
Cyclophosphamide	250 mg/m²/12 h IV	Days 1–3
Adriamycin	60 mg/m² IV	Day 1
NB Courses are started when the neutrophil count is ≥1000/mm³ and the platelets ≥100,000/mm		

GROUP B: Prephase, COPADM 1 and 2, followed by CYM1 and 2 (2–3-week intervals between courses)		
Prephase (may repeat if necessary)		
Cyclophosphamide 300 mg/m² IV	Day 1 (+intrathecal chemo(IT))—see below for doses of IT according to age	
Induction COPADM1 and 2 (1 week after the prephase)		
COPADM 1		
Vincristine	2 mg/m² IV bolus (max 2 mg)	Day 1
Predniso(lo)ne	60 mg/m² po	Days 1–5, then wean over 3 days
Methotrexate (MTX)	3 g/m² over 3 h IV	Day 1(+IT day 2 and 6)
Folinic acid (Leukovorin)	15 mg/m²/dose po/IV 6 hourly	Begin 24 h after commencing MTX infusion (total of 12 doses)
Cyclophosphamide	250 mg/m² 12 hourly IV	Days 2, 3, and 4
Adriamycin	60 mg/m² IV over 6 h	Day 2
COPADM 2 identical to COPADM1		

Consolidation CYM1 and 2		
CYM 1		
Methotrexate	3 g/m² over 3 h IV	Day 1 (+IT days 2 and 6)
Folinic acid	15 mg/m²/dose 12 hourly po/IV	Day 2 and 4
Cytarabine	100 mg/m²/day IV	Day 2–6
CYM 2 identical to CYM 1		

GROUP C: COPADM(8)1 and 2 followed by CYVE1 and 2, followed by Seq1–4 (2–3-week intervals between courses)		
Prephase: may repeat if necessary		
Cyclophosphamide	500 mg/m² IV	Day 1 (+IT days 1, 3, and 5)
Folinic acid	15 mg/m²/dose 12 hourly po/IV	Day 2 and 4
Induction COPADM(8) 1 and 2		
COPADM(8) 1		
Vincristine	2 mg/m² IV	Day 1
Predniso(lo)ne	60 mg/m² po divided in 2 doses	Day 1–5, then wean over 3 days
Methotrexate	8 g/m² over 4 h IV	Day 1 (+IT days 2, 4, and 6)
Folinic acid	15 mg/m²/dose po/IV 6 hourly	Begin 24 h after commencing MTX infusion (total of 12 doses)
Cyclophosphamide	250 mg/m²/dose 12 hourly IV	Days 2, 3, and 4

(continued)

Table 15.7 (continued)

GROUP C: COPADM(8)1 and 2 followed by CYVE1 and 2, followed by Seq1–4 (2–3-week intervals between courses)		
Prephase: may repeat if necessary		
Adriamycin	60 mg/m^2 IV over 6 h	Day 2
COPADM(8) 2 identical to CPADM(8) 1		

Consolidation CYVE1 and 2		
CYVE1		
Cytarabine	50 mg/m^2 IV over 12 h (infuse from 20h00 to 08h00)	Days 1–5
Cytarabine	3 g/m^2 over 3 h IV (infuse from 08h00 to 11h00)	Days 2–5
VP16	200 mg/m^2 IV over 2 h (infuse from 14h00 to 16h00)	Days 2–5
CYVE 2 identical to CYVE1		

Maintenance		
Sequence 1		
Vincristine	2 mg/m^2 IV bolus (max 2 mg)	Day 1
Predniso(lo)ne	60 mg/m^2 (in 2 divided doses) IV/po	Day 1–5, then wean over 3 days
Cyclophosphamide	500 mg/m^2 IV over 30 min	Day 2 and 3
Methotrexate	8 g/m^2 over 4 h IV	Day 1 (+IT day 2)
Folinic acid	15 mg/m^2/dose po/IV 6 hourly	Begin 24 h after commencing MTX infusion (total of 12 doses)
Adriamycin	60 mg/m^2 over 6 h	Day 2 after 1st dose of cyclophosphamide
Sequence 2		
Cytarabine	50 mg/m^2 subcutaneous every 12 h	Days 1–5
VP16	150 mg/m^2 over 90 min IV	Day 1–3
Sequence 3		
Vincristine	2 mg/m^2 IV bolus (max 2 mg)	Day 1
Predniso(lo)ne	60 mg/m^2/day	Day 1–5, then wean over 3 days
Cyclophosphamide	500 mg/m^2/day over 30 min	Day 1 and 2
Adriamycin	60 mg/m^2 IV over 6 h	Day 1 after 1st dose of cyclophosphamide
Sequence 4		
Cytarabine	50 mg/m^2 subcutaneous every 12 h	Day 1–5
VP16	150 mg/m^2 over 90 min IV	Day 1–3

Doses for intrathecal chemotherapy according to age		
Age (year)	Methotrexate and hydrocortisone (mg)	Cytarabine (mg)
<1	8	15
1–2	10	20
2–3	12	25
>3	15	30

Fig. 15.4 Chest X-ray: normal

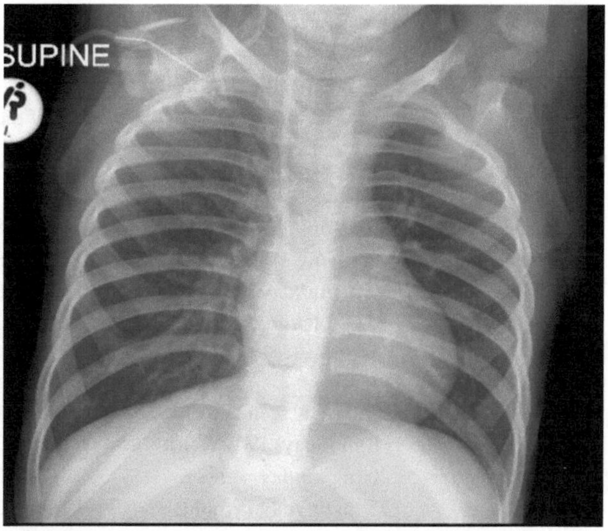

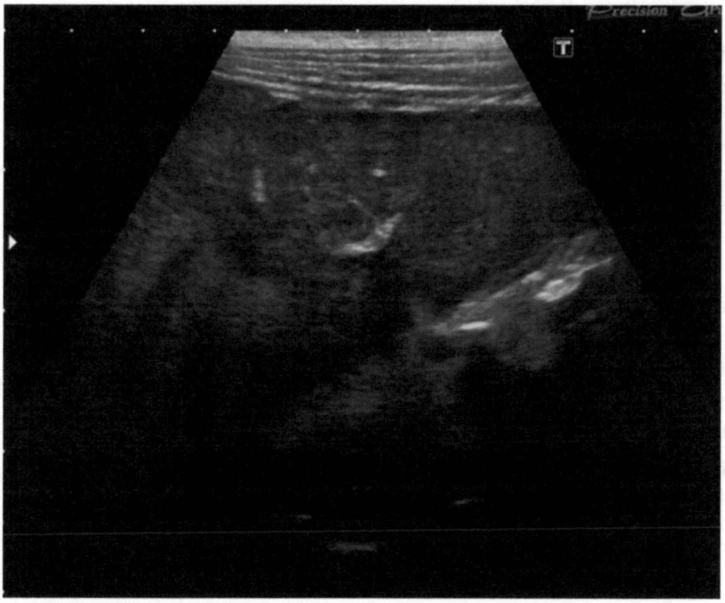

Fig. 15.5 Abdominal ultrasound

Table 15.8 Euro-lb02 protocol for lymphoblastic lymphoma

Prephase		
Prednisone	60 mg/m²/day in 3 divided doses	Days 1–7
IT		Day 1 (if the clinical condition allows an IT)
Induction		
Protocol Ia		
Prednisone	60 mg/m²/day in 3 divided doses	Days 8–28, then wean over 1 week
Vincristine	1.5 mg/m² IV bolus (max 2 mg)	Days 8, 15, 22, and 29
Daunorubicin	30 mg/m²/day IV over 1 h	Days 8, 15, 22, and 29
Asparaginase	10,000 IU/m²/day	Days 12, 15, 18, 21, 24, 27, 30, and 33
IT		Days 12 and 33 (if CNS involvement at diagnosis, also on days 18 and 27)
Protocol Ib if a good response is seen and blood counts have recovered		
Cyclophosphamide	(1 g/m²/day) IV over 1 h	Days 36 and 64
6-Mercaptopurine	60 mg/m²/day po nocte	Days 36–63
Cytarabine	75 mg/m²/day IV bolus	Days 38–41, 45–48, 52–55, 59–62
IT		Days 45 and 59
Protocol M: to start 2 weeks after the end of protocol I		
6-Mercaptopurine	25 mg/m²/day po nocte	Days 1–56
Methotrexate	5 g/m²/day IV over 3 h	Days 8, 22, 36, and 50
Folinic acid	15 mg/m²/dose po/IV 6 hourly	Begin 24 h after commencing MTX infusion (total of 12 doses)
IT		Give 2 h after commencing methotrexate infusion
Protocol IIa and b: intensification (Stages III and IV only)		
Protocol IIa (to start 2 weeks after the end of protocol M)		
Dexamethasone	10 mg/m²/day in 3 divided doses po	Days 1–21, then wean over 1 week
Vincristine	1.5 mg/m² IV bolus (max 2 mg)	Days 8, 15, 22, and 29
Doxorubicin	30 mg/m²/day over 1 h	Days 8, 15, 22, and 29
Asparaginase	10,000 IU/m²/day IM	Days 8, 11, 15, and 18
Phase IIb		
6 Mercaptopurine	60 mg/m²/day po nocte	Days 36–49
Cyclophosphamide	1 g/m²/day IV over 1 h	Day 36
Cytarabine	75 mg/m²/day IV	Days 38–41 and 45–48
IT		Days 38 and 45

Table 15.9 Large cell anaplastic lymphoma: Protocol ALCL99

Prephase		
Dexamethasone	5 mg/m²/day on days 1 and 2, followed by 10 mg/m²/day in 2 divided doses days 3–5 (IV or po)	
Cyclophosphamide	200 mg/m² over 1 h	Days 1 and 2
IT		Day 1

AM (AM1, AM2 and AM3)		
Dexamethasone	10 mg/m²/day po in 2 divided doses	Days 1–5
Methotrexate	3 g/m² IV over 3 h	Day 1
Folinic acid	15 mg/m²/dose po/IV 6 hourly	Begin 24 h after commencing MTX infusion (total of 12 doses)
Ifosfamide	800 mg/m²/day over 1 h	Days 1–5
Mesna	330 mg/m²/dose IV	At hours 0, 4, and 8 after commencing ifosfamide infusion
Cytarabine	150 mg/m²/dose 12 hourly	Days 4 and 5
VP16	100 mg/m²/day over 2 h	Days 4 and 5

BM (BM1, BM2, and BM3)		
Dexamethasone	10 mg/m²/day in 2 divided doses	Days 1–5
Methotrexate	3 g/m² over 3 h	Day 1
Folinic acid	15 mg/m²/dose po/IV 6 hourly	Begin 24 h after commencing MTX infusion (total of 12 doses)
Cyclophosphamide	200 mg/m²/day IV	Days 1–5
Doxorubicin	25 mg/m²/day IV over 1 h	Days 4 and 5

COPM1		
Vincristine	2 mg/m² IV bolus (max 2 mg)	Day 1
Predniso(lo)ne	60 mg/m²/day po	Days 1–5, then wean over 3 days
Cyclophosphamide	500 mg/m² IV over 30 min	Days 2–4
Methotrexate	3 g/m² IV over 4 h	Day 1 (+IT days 2 and 6)
Folinic acid	15 mg/m²/dose po/IV 6 hourly	Begin 24 h after commencing MTX infusion (total of 12 doses)
COPM2 identical to COPM1		
CYM 1		
Methotrexate	3 g/m² IV over 3 h	Day 1 (+IT days 2 and 6)
Folinic acid	15 mg/m²/dose po/IV 6 hourly	Begin 24 h after commencing MTX infusion (total of 12 doses)
Cytarabine	100 mg/m²/day continuous infusion over 24 h	Days 2–6
CYM 2 identical to CYM1		

Table 15.10 Cyclophosphamide treatment protocol for Burkitt lymphoma—GFAOP

Stages 1 and 2	
Cyclophosphamide 40 mg/kg (1.2 mg/m^2)	Days 1, 8, 15 (+IT Days 1, 8, and 15)
Stages 3 and 4	
Cyclophosphamide 40 mg/kg (1.2 mg/m^2)	Days 1, 8, 15, 29, 43, 57 (+IT Days 1, 8, 15, 29, 43, and 57)

Maintenance Treatment

The maintenance phase should start 2 weeks after protocol M for stages I and II or after protocol II for stages III and IV and should continue for a total of 24 months, starting from the prephase:

6-Mercaptopurine 50 mg/m^2/day po nocte
Methotrexate 20 mg/m^2 weekly po or IM

Risk Stratification

Isolated cutaneous lesions: careful monitoring of disease; no chemotherapy initially
Low-risk group: Stage 1 complete resection
Prephase, then 3 courses: P—AM1—BM1—AM2
Total duration of treatment: 10 weeks
Standard risk group: No proven cutaneous, mediastinal, hepatic, splenic, or pulmonary involvement
Prephase, then 6 courses: P—AM1—BM1—AM2—BM2—AM3—BM3
All patients to receive methotrexate 3 g/m^2 without intrathecal chemotherapy
Total duration of treatment: 19 weeks
High-risk group: histologically proven cutaneous lesion (not isolated skin lesions <5 lesions) as well as mediastinal, hepatic, splenic, or pulmonary involvement
Prephase then 6 courses: P—AM1—BM1—AM2—BM2—AM3—BM3
All patients to receive methotrexate 3 g/m^2 without intrathecal chemotherapy
Total duration of treatment: 19 weeks
Group Nm (CNS involvement)
Patients will be treated according to the LMB89 protocol group C (including cranial radiotherapy)

Summary

- NHL is one of the most frequent childhood cancers.
- The most frequent subtypes are Burkitt- and Burkitt-like lymphoma, lymphoblastic leukemia, and anaplastic large cell lymphoma.

- Endemic BL occurs in sub-Saharan Africa and is strongly associated with EBV infection; sporadic BL occurs in the rest of the world. A third subtype is associated with HIV infection.
- Patients with NHL are at risk for airway compression and tumor lysis syndrome.
- The diagnosis of NHL is confirmed by cytological and/or histological evaluation.
- An abdominal or maxillofacial mass points towards a B-cell lymphoma, whereas a mediastinal mass supports the diagnosis of a T-cell lymphoma.
- The prognosis varies according to the age of the patient, histological type, tumor burden, site of disease, response to therapy, as well as the presence of metastatic lesions/involvement.
- Patients with early stage disease have an excellent outcome.

Suggested Reading

Harif M, Barsaoui S, Benchekroun S, Bouhas R, Doumbe P, Khattab M, Ladjaj Y, Moreira C, Msefer-Aloui F, Patte C, Rakotonirina G, Raphael M, Raquin M, Lemerle J (2008) Treatment of B-cell lymphoma with LMB modified protocols in Africa—report of the French-African Pediatric Oncology Group (GFAOP). Pediatr Blood Cancer 50:1138–1142

Hesseling PB, Israels T, Harif M, Chantada G, Molyneux E (2013) Practical recommendations for the management of children with endemic Burkitt lymphoma (BL) in a resource limited setting. Pediatr Blood Cancer 60(3):357–362

Le Deley M, Reiter A, Williams D, Delsol G, Oschlies I, McCarthy K, Zimmermann M, Brugieres L (2008) Prognostic factors in childhood anaplastic lymphoma. Blood 111(3):1560

Molyneux E, Rotchford R, Griffin B, Newton R, Jackson G, Menon G, Harrison CJ, Israels T, Bailey S (2012) Burkitt's lymphoma. Lancet 379:1234–1244

www.cancer.gov/cancertopics/pdq/treatment/child-non-hodgkind/HealthProfessional/page1. Accessed 19 April.

Chapter 16
Acute Leukemia

Case Presentation

A 14-year-old boy was admitted for fever, gingival hemorrhage, and pallor for 10 days. Examination found bruises on the lower limbs, with gingival hypertrophy (Fig. 16.1). The CBC showed 70,000 WBC/mm^3 made of 90 % of blasts, a hemoglobin 6.1 g/100 mL and 17,000/mm^3 of platelets.

1. How would you proceed with the diagnostic confirmation?
2. What are the symptomatic measures?
3. What are the principles of the specific treatment?

Acute leukemia is the most common cancer in childhood. This is a heterogeneous group of clinical–biological entities as a result of monoclonal proliferation of the progenitor hematopoietic stem cell. The development of immunological studies and genetics has allowed better characterization of various entities and also generated new approaches for understanding and care of acute types of leukemia. Improved refinement of prognostic factors and in the supportive care allows long-term survival rates of 70–80 % of acute lymphoblastic leukemia (ALL) and 50–60 % of acute myeloblastic leukemia (AML). In Africa, acute types of leukemia seem to present less frequent. However, because of the high incidence of HIV infection, malaria, and other more frequent hematologic diseases, i.e., sickle cell anemia, as well as insufficient laboratory infrastructure, leukemia may not be diagnosed because of unspecified clinical expression.

D.C. Stefan, M. Harif, *Pediatric Cancer in Africa*,
DOI 10.1007/978-3-319-17936-0_16

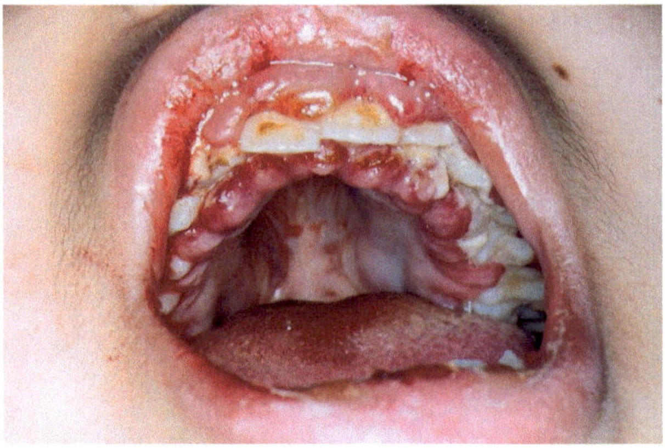

Fig. 16.1 Ginigival hypertrophy

Epidemiology and Etiology

Acute leukemia represents 30–40 % of childhood cancers in the western population. Of leukemia, 75–80 % are of lymphoid types. ALL occurs with high frequency in the 2–5-year age group, while AML occurs more frequently in infants and adolescents. Undifferentiated or bilinear forms are seen in about 5 % of cases.

Hereditary predisposing factors to the types of leukemia are rarely found. However, a higher incidence of leukemia has been reported in patients with congenital agammaglobulinemia, Bloom syndrome, Shwachman syndrome, ataxia-telangiectasia, Li–Fraumeni syndrome, neurofibromatosis, Blackfan-Diamond syndrome, and Kostmann disease. The risk of developing leukemia is 10–20 times higher in children with Down syndrome compared to the general childhood population.

Among the environmental predisposing factors, exposure to in-utero ionizing radiation or treatment of primary cancer with radiotherapy and/or chemotherapy, particularly alkylating (cyclophosphamide) agents and inhibitors of topoisomerases II (VP16), are the most reported ones. Other factors such as exposure to electric or magnetic fields, the consumption of alcohol, marijuana, or tobacco during pregnancy, and exposure to pesticides have not been confirmed.

Clinical Presentation

Symptoms and signs of acute types of leukemia are related to bone-marrow failure caused by replacement of normal bone marrow by leukemia cells and by blast infiltration of lymphoid and non-lymphoid organs and tissues.

Pallor, fatigue, lethargy (sometimes), and headaches are manifestations of anemia; and a fever with or without chills and sometimes mouth ulcers are related to neutropenia. While severe hemorrhagic syndrome with petechiae, bruising, and epistaxis, gingival bleeding and sometimes visceral or cerebro-subarachnoid hemorrhage are more or less attributable to thrombocytopenia. Thrombocytopenia may be the result of bone marrow failure, but also of consumptive coagulopathy, better known as disseminated intravascular coagulation (DIC). Infiltration of lymphoid organs is inconstant (not always present) and peripheral, non-inflammatory lymph nodes located deep in subcutaneous tissue can be enlarged on palpation. Abdominal or mediastinal lymphadenopathies may also be observed, however they rarely cause compression of the regional organs or vessels. Splenomegaly and hepatomegaly are very frequently associated with lymph node infiltration.

Bone pains have been reported in 20–25 % of patients. They reflect leukemic bone infiltration and can be mistaken for rheumatoid- or sickle cell disease.

Involvement of other tissue or organs is less frequent, though seen in some leukemia subtypes. Testicular (Fig. 16.2) or central nervous system (CNS) infiltration (Fig. 16.3) is more frequently seen in ALL, whereas gingival infiltration is seen in myeloblastic leukemia. A malignant tumor, chloroma, usually found in the orbital part of the brain can reveal or accompany an acute myelogenous leukemia.

A high leukocyte count can induce a leukostasis secondary to abnormal aggregation and clumping and occluded microcirculation, particularly in the lungs and the brain. Clinical expression is usually dyspnea with or without neurological symptoms that may be life-threatening in severe cases.

Diagnosis

The diagnosis of acute leukemia is based on the characterization of leukemic cells in the blood, and in the bone marrow.

In most cases complete blood count usually shows normochromic normocytic anemia, leukocytosis mainly consisting of blast cells with neutropenia and

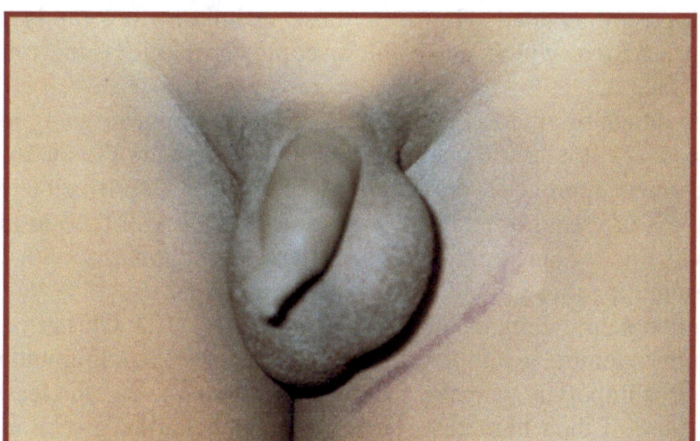

Fig. 16.2 Testicular involvement in ALL

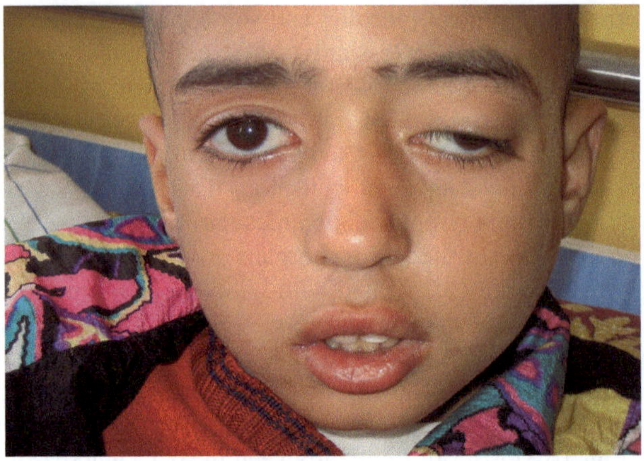

Fig. 16.3 CNS involvement in ALL

thrombocytopenia. The bone marrow aspiration shows a rich smear and blast cell infiltration. The diagnosis of acute leukemia is made when blast cells exceed 20 % of the bone marrow cellularity. When specific cytogenetic abnormality is found the diagnosis of acute leukemia can be accepted even at a reduced percentage of blast cells in the bone marrow. This diagnosis requires additional cytochemistry, and mostly in immunology and cytogenetic studies.

Analysis of bone marrow smears after May-Grunwald-Giemsa and myeloperoxidase (MPO) staining is mandatory for initial diagnosis evaluation. Lymphoblasts are often small-sized and characterized by dense chromatin, little or no nucleolus and sparse and non-granular cytoplasm. The myeloblasts are typically larger in size, have a loose chromatin nucleus with several nucleoli and relatively abundant cytoplasm-containing MPO positive granules. Auer rods, representing abnormal condensation of cytoplasmic granules, may be observed in myeloblasts. Additional characterization of leukemia using immunophenotyping assays and genetic analysis is highly recommended. However, these techniques are rarely available in most parts of Africa, which make microscopic morphology the only available diagnostic tool.

WHO classification of ALL is based on the immunophenotyping identification of membrane and cytoplasmic markers using flow cytometry (Table 16.1). Because different treatment approaches are proposed for children with B-cell leukemia, their identification is of great importance. The mature B-cell ALL (L3) in most cases is identified via microscopic morphology as large lymphoblasts with cytoplasmic vacuoles resembling those found in Burkitt's lymphoma.

The immunophenotyping techniques use antibodies (CD: Cluster of differentiation) to identify membrane antigens by flow cytometry. When immunophenotyping is available it is important to make a stepwise approach to use the least number of markers because of their high cost. Three immunophenotype groups are identified in ALL: the pre-B phenotype constituting 70–80 %, the T phenotype (15 %), and mature B-cell phenotype corresponding to the type Burkitt leukemia (2–5 %).

Table 16.1 Acute lymphoblastic leukemia (ALL) phenotype classification

	Phenotype				Comment
ALL subtype	CD19	CD10	clg	slg	
Pre-pre-B	+	–	–	–	Mostly infants, poor prognosis, frequent MLL/11q23 rearrangements
Early Pre-B	+	+	–	–	Common ALL, young children, good prognosis
Pre-B	+	+	+	–	Older children, good prognosis with intense therapy
B-cell	+	+	+	+	Burkitt leukemia, MYC/lg fusion genes, good prognosis with B-cell lymphoma-type therapy
T-cell	–	–	–	–	Adolescents, anterior mediastinal mass, CNS involvement, good prognosis with intense therapy

The phenotype T seems more common in developing countries. Usually blast cells in AML express CD11, CD13, CD15, CD33, and CD34 antigens. In some cases, the distinction between LAL and LAM may be difficult. The immunophenotype profile may help in distinguishing these leukemia groups. In rare cases, aberrant expression of markers of two lineages, identifying the so-called biphenotypic leukemia is found. In western populations, early pre-B and pre-B subtypes are predominant.

According to the WHO, the diagnostic and prognostic classification of AML should take into account morphological analysis according to the French–American–British (FAB) criteria as well as genetic studies (Table 16.2).

Genetic studies of blast cells, when evaluated, should be routinely performed in acute types of leukemia. Karyotype analysis shows abnormalities in the number and structures of chromosomes. Molecular biology techniques are useful for evaluation of possible fusion genes.

In the ALL, hyperdiploidy (>50 chromosomes or DNA index >1.16) is found in 25 % of cases of pre-B phenotype. This is associated with a good prognosis. The fusion gene TEL/AML1 t(12;21) is also found in 25 % of patients and is also associated with a good response to treatment. The MLL gene abnormalities are mainly found in infants with ALL (80 %) and carry a poor prognosis. Translocation t(9;22) inducing BCR/ABL fusion gene is found in 3 % of childhood ALL. This is much more common in adults and is similarly associated with a poor response to treatment. In ALL3, translocations involving the immunoglobulin gene are found, as in Burkitt's lymphoma. FLT3 mutations are the most common AML genetic abnormalities (20–35 %) and are associated with a poor prognosis in the FLT3/ITD association. Chromosomal abnormalities involving the MLL/11q23 gene, found in 15–20 % of patients, are often associated with M4 or M5 phenotype and also have a poor prognosis.

The rare monosomy 7 and del 5q also have a poor prognosis. Trisomy 21, translocations t(8;21) and t(15;17) found in AML3, and inv(16) found in eosinophilic AML4 are considered good prognostic factors. Translocation t(8;21) is frequently associated with chloroma and seems more common in Morocco.

Table 16.2 Classification of acute myeloid leukemia according to French–American–British classification (FAB)

Subtype	Features	Cytogenetic abnormalities	Comment
M0	Acute myeloblastic leukemia (AML), minimally differentiated		
M1	AML, without maturation		
M2	AML, with granulocytic maturation	t(8;21) (q22;q22), t(6;9)	Frequent association with chloroma
M3	Acute promyelocytic leukemia	t(15;17)	Association with consumptive coagulopathy
M4	AML	inv(16) (p13q22), del(16q)	Frequent association with gingival Infiltration
M4eo	Myelomonocytic together with bone marrow eosinophilia	inv(16), t(16;16)	Frequent association with gingival Infiltration
M5	Acute monocytic leukemia • Acute monoblastic (M5a) or • Acute_monocytic_leukemia (M5b)	del(11q), t(9;11), t(11;19)	Frequent association with gingival Infiltration
M6	Acute erythroid leukemia		
M7	Acute megakaryoblastic leukemia	t(1;22)	Myelofibrosis

Work-Up

The patient assessment must include a chest X-ray searching for possible mediastinal mass (Fig. 16.4), seen particularly in T-ALL. Also look for a pulmonary infectious process that may complicate the disease. Abdominal ultrasound is also recommended to evaluate the possible abdominal organ involvement. CSF is also evaluated for blast cells.

Blood electrolyte, serum urea, and creatinine are important to evaluate tumor lysis syndrome especially in high leukocyte-count types of leukemia. Hemostasis should also be evaluated for possible DIC. Hepatic evaluation, EKG, and echocardiography with measurement of systolic ejection fraction are recommended before chemotherapy.

Prognosis

Identifying factors leading to the prognosis is essential for the adaptation of treatment. These factors can be classified according to whether they are related to the host, to the disease or to the initial response to the treatment.

The main prognostic factors in ALL are age, CNS involvement, white blood cell count, immunological phenotype, genetic abnormalities, and response to steroid therapy or induction chemotherapy (Table 16.3).

In AML, risk factors are related mainly to genetic anomalies (Table 16.4).

Fig. 16.4 Mediastinal involvement in T-ALL patients

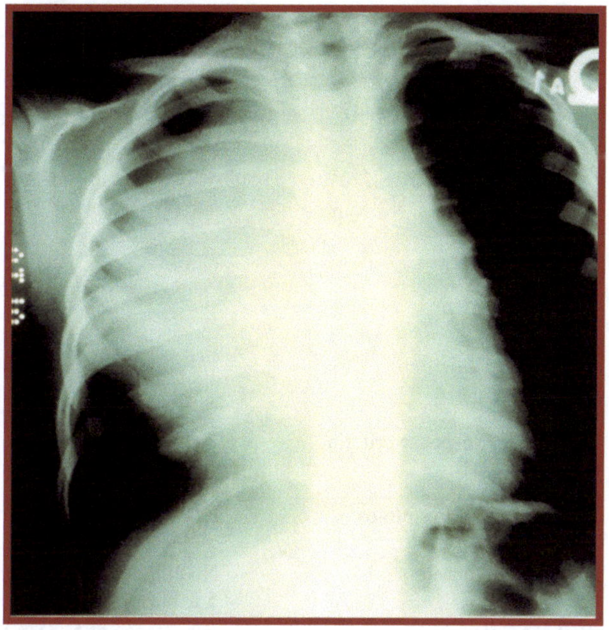

Table 16.3 ALL prognosis factors

Risk factor	Standard risk	High risk
Age	1–9 years	<1 or >9 years
Sex	Female	Male
White blood count	<50,000/mm^3	>50,000/mm^3
Immunophenotype	Pre-B CD10+	Pre-B CD–, T
Genetic abnormalities	Hyperdiploïdy (>50 chromosomes); Tel/AML1 or t(12;21)	Hypodoploïdy (>45 chromosomes); t(9;22) or BCR/ABL; t(4;11) or MLL/AF4
Response to steroids	<1000 blasts at D8	>1000 blasts at D8
Response to chemotherapy	<5 % bone marrow blasts at D15	>25 % bone marrow blasts at D15
Minimal residual disease	<10–4 bone marrow blasts at week 5	<10–3 bone marrow blasts at week 5

Treatment

Treatment is adapted to prognostic factors. Special attention should be given to prevention and treatment of infections, hemorrhage, and tumor lysis syndrome. These patients are best treated in specialized units of pediatric oncology, while high-risk patients should be treated in an intensive care unit. An accurate vascular assessment should be secured. In infants and small children it is recommended to insert a central venous catheter.

Table 16.4 AML prognostic factors

Low risk	Standard risk	High risk
Inv(16) or t(16;16)		FLT3-ITD
T(8;21)		M6
T(15;17)	No low- or high-risk criteria	M7
Trisomy 21		T(6;9)
		Monosomy 7
		Del 5q
		Secondary AML
		Induction failure

Table 16.5 Response criteria

Response	Criteria
Good response to steroids	Less than 1000 blasts/mm^3 at day 8
Complete remission	No clinical or biologic sign of the disease with less than 5 % blast in bone marrow smear
Partial response	Persistence of 5–25 % blast in bone marrow
Failure	More than 25 % blasts in bone marrow

Principles of Treatment of ALL

Multidrug chemotherapy is the backbone of ALL treatment. The induction phase to achieve complete remission is followed by consolidation, late intensification, and maintenance. The total duration of treatment varies from 2–3 years.

The induction phase, which lasts 4–6 weeks, uses steroids (prednisone or dexamethasone), vincristine, L-asparaginase, and where appropriate an anthracycline (daunorubicin or doxorubicin). Evaluation of the response to treatment during this phase is of great importance for further treatment options (Table 16.5).

Complete remission is achieved in 98 % of cases after the induction phase. In Africa, this period is associated with high mortality because of tumor lysis syndrome, infection, and hemorrhage. Special attention should be given to these children and if possible they should be kept in the hospital.

The intensity and duration of post-induction treatment are adapted according to the prognostic group. The consolidation phase goal is to overcome resistance of residual leukemic cells. Maintenance treatment includes daily 6-mercaptopurine associated with methotrexate at low doses and monthly injections of vincristine associated with steroids.

CNS intrathecal (IT) treatment is recommended in all phases of the treatment. The central nervous system is considered a sanctuary for blast cells because of the physiological blood–brain barrier for intravenous chemotherapy. This treatment combines methotrexate, cytarabine, and hydrocortisone. The use of high-dose methotrexate contributes to the treatment of CNS disease. Prophylactic irradiation has been abandoned in most of the protocols because of the neurocognitive sequelae and the risk of secondary cancer.

In high-risk groups and in relapses, allogeneic hematopoietic stem cell transplantation is recommended. In patients with a translocation t(9;22), treatment with imatinib, inhibitor tyrosine kinase is recommended. In most of these patients, palliative care would be the best option in limited resource settings.

Principles of Treatment of the AML

The treatment approach of AML is based on intensive chemotherapy to achieve complete remission followed by a consolidation. In a good prognostic group no further treatment is added. In other patients, allogeneic hematopoietic stem cells transplantation should be considered.

The initial treatment consists of the association anthracyclin (daunorubicin, doxorubicin, or idarubicin) and cytarabine. After two cures, a complete remission is achieved in 80–90 % of cases.

After complete remission, consolidation with 2–3 courses of high-dose aracytine combined with anthracycline or L-Asparaginase and for some cases vepeside should be added.

In AML3 acid, all-trans retinoic (ATRA) and, more recently, arsenic acid should be used in conjunction with chemotherapy. These medications induce maturation of blast cells unlike chemotherapy which induces a cell lysis. This approach prevents coagulopathy, one of the leading causes of mortality and morbidity in this disease.

Allogeneic hematopoietic stem cell transplantation significantly improves the survival in AML and particularly in high-risk forms. This approach is recommended for high-risk AML or intermediate-risk AML with compatible donors. This procedure is not indicated for good prognosis AML such as AMLwith the translocations t(8; 21), t(15;17), or inv(16).

Practical Recommendations in Africa

Diagnostic Approach

- Good CBC and bone marrow smears with MGG and MPO staining determine the diagnosis in most cases;
- Immunophenotyping and genetic studies may be helpful

Prognosis

- ALL:
  - Standard risk: Age 1–9 years; WBC less than 50,000, Good response to steroids
  - High risk: Age less than 1 year or more than 9 years; WBC more than 50,000/ mm^3; bad response to steroids
- AML: Mainly karyotype when available

Treatment

Patients with leukemia are at high risk of life-threatening complications including tumor lysis syndrome, infection, and hemorrhage caused by high leukocyte-count and bone-marrow failures.

- ALL:
  - Standard risk:
    - (a) Induction: steroids, vincristine, asparaginase, IT
    - (b) Consolidation: steroids, vincristine, 6-mercaptopurine, methotrexate, IT
    - (c) Intensification: Steroids, anthracyclin, vincristine, 6-mercaptopurine, cytarabine IT
    - (d) Maintenance 18 months: 6-mercaptopurine; methotrexate, IT
  - High risk:
    - (a) Induction: steroids, vincristine, anthracyclin, asparaginase, IT
    - (b) Consolidation: steroids, vincristine, 6-mercaptopurine, high-dose methotrexate, IT
    - (c) Intensification: Steroids, anthracyclin, vincristine, 6-mercaptopurine, cytarabin IT
    - (d) Induction 2: steroids, vincristine, anthracyclin, 6-mercaptopurine, IT
    - (e) Intensification 2: steroids, vincristine, anthracyclin, asparaginase, 6-mercaptopurine, IT
    - (f) Maintenance 24 months: 6-mercaptopurine; methotrexate, IT
- AML:
  - Induction 1 and 2 with anthracyclin and cytarabine
  - Intensification 1 and 2 with high-dose cytarabine, anthracyclin, or VP16

In case of AML3 treatment with ATRA with or without arsenic acid is necessary.

If complete remission is not achieved after induction, the prognosis is very bad if bone marrow transplantation is not available. Palliative care is the best option.

Suggested Reading

Bachir F, Bennani S, Lahjouji A et al (2009) Characterization of acute lymphoblastic leukemia subtypes in Moroccan children. Int J Pediatr 1–7. doi:10.1155/2009/674801
Bachir F, Bennani S, Lahjouji A (2009b) Characterization of acute lymphoblastic leukemia subtypes in Moroccan children. Int J Pediatr. doi:10.1155/2009/674801
Ekouya Bowassa G, Okouango Ova J-D, Ngolet L, Okoko A-R, Elira-Dokekias A (2012) Leucémies aigues de l'enfant à Brazzaville. Arch Pediatr 19:1123–1124
Had N, Chadli B, Bousfiha A, Trachli A, Harif M, Benslimane A (1996) Cytogenetic survey of 53 Moroccan patients with acute myeloblastic leukemia. Cancer Genet Cytogenet 86(2):124–128
Kaspers GJL, Zwaan CM (2007) Pediatric acute myeloid leukemia: towards high-quality treatment of all patients. Haematologica 92:1519–1532
Pieters R, Carroll WL (2008) Biology and treatment of acute lymphoblastic leukemia. Pediatr Clin N Am 55:1–20
Togo B, Traoré F, Diakité AA et al (2011) Leucémie aigue lymphoblastique de l'enfant: 12 observations au Mali. Med Trop 71:629–631

Chapter 17
Chronic Leukemias

Chronic Myeloid Leukemia

This disease occurs more commonly in young adults. It is rare in children and is seen especially in older children and adolescents. It is a myeloproliferative disorder characterized by the presence of translocation t (9;22) commonly referred to as the Philadelphia (Ph1) chromosome.

The disease has three phases: the chronic, accelerated, and acute. The If CML is not adequately treated, the transition from chronic to acute phases can occur with disastrous consequences between forms if not treated adequately can occur rapidly with disastrous consequences.

Philadelphia (Ph1) chromosome is the result of a translocation between 2 chromosomes: 9 and 22 (q34q11). This translocation leads to the juxtaposition of proto-oncogene c-ABL (chromosome 9) and BCL gene (chromosome 22). The chimeric gene produces a tyrosine kinase protein which has an anti-apoptotic effect with loss of adhesion to the stromal matrix molecules.

Few symptoms are noticed during the chronic phase. Some CML may be asymptomatic. Nonspecific signs such as fever, night sweats, or a vague pain of the left hypochondria are the most commonly reported symptoms. Clinical examination is in most cases dominated by a grossly enlarged spleen and sometimes moderate anemia. Complete blood count shows a leukocytosis often exceeding 100,000/mm^3 with a left shift extending to blast cells, basophilia, thrombocytosis, and a moderate normochromic anemia. The bone marrow aspirate adds valuable information and is characterized by a hyperplasia of the granulocytic lineage with normal maturation. During accelerated phase, an increased rate of immature blasts is found in bone marrow. Acute transformation can give rise to myeloid or lymphoid leukemia. The disease may rarely lead to thrombotic events and in particular to priapism. The thrombosis is related to the blood hyperviscosity caused by leukocytosis, lower deformability of the blasts, and thrombocytosis.

D.C. Stefan, M. Harif, *Pediatric Cancer in Africa*,
DOI 10.1007/978-3-319-17936-0_17

A complete diagnosis of the disease requires the karyotype or molecular analysis. However, in African setting these analyses may not be available.

A high degree of suspicion is present in an older child or young adult with a chronic anemia, tiredness, and splenomegaly. The suspicion is in most cases confirmed by a high leucocyte count with a left shift.

The initial treatment may be started with Hydroxyurea (10–20 mg/kg/day) and will provide hematologic response but without eradication of the malignant clone.

The drug of choice remains a tyrosine kinase inhibitor and hematopoietic stem cell transplantation for patients who fail to respond to TKI. or allogeneic bone marrow transplantation. In the absence of the ideal therapy, the inevitably progressing to the refractory acute form. Interferon therapy allows in less than 20 % of the cases an eradication of the malignant clone proved by the negativity of the BCR-ABL chimeric protein. The allogeneic hematopoietic stem cells transplant from HLA compatible donor and particularly in the siblings is a treatment that allows the eradication of malignant clone. This approach however has a significant morbidity and mortality.

The use of tyrosine kinase inhibitor (TKI) as therapy has been a successful revolution in curing the disease.

Children receiving a daily dose of 340 mg/m^2 dose of imatinib achieves a complete cytogenetic and molecular remission in more than 90 % of the cases. The very few cases that become resistant to the first class of drugs are now treated with second generation of inhibitors of tyrosine kinase such as dasatinib and nilotinib that are available. However, the best results are obtained in patients at chronic phase.

In Africa, access to cytogenetic analysis and molecular biology is limited. Availability of TKI is also an important issue and is related to cost. The Glivec International Patient Assistance Program (GIPAP) is a mechanism which facilitates access to the drugs. It started in 2001 through the support of Novartis in order to improve the access to imatinib of patients with CML or gastrointestinal stromal tumors. African patients benefit of the medication through GIPAP. However in some circumstances the consumption of some indigenous herbs and traditional medicines increased the risk of toxicity of this medication.

Juvenile Myelomonocytic Leukemia

Juvenile myelomonocytic leukemia (JMML) is more common in patients with type-1 neurofibromatosis, Noonan syndrome (facial dysmorphia, dwarfism, mental retardation, and congenital heart disease) and Trisomy 8 (mental retardation, various dysmorphias, genitourinary malformations). Monosomy 7 may also be found.

The main biologic abnormality is a hypersensitivity of stem cell to cytokines stimulation, in particular, GM-CSF, TNF, and IL-1 b. Autocrine production contributes to spontaneous cell proliferation in vitro. Gene RAS activation seem to be the origin of this anomaly.

This disease is mainly encountered in children younger than 2 years of age. Clinical manifestations include pallor, respiratory signs, hemorrhagic syndrome, skin lesions (rash, eczema, and xanthoma), an enlarged spleen and/or hepatomegaly, lymphadenopathy or diarrhea. The hemogram shows leukocytosis with monocytosis, thrombocytopenia, erythro-myelemia, occasionally blasts. The bone marrow smears consists in hyperplasia of granulocyte lineage with signs of myelodysplasia involving granulocytic and megakaryocytic lineage and often a moderate blasts infiltration. Electrophoresis of hemoglobin is dominated by a high hemoglobin F level. The cytogenetic exploration does not show specific anomaly and in particular absence of translocation t(9, 22).

This disease is usually associated with a poor prognosis. 6-mercaptopurine with or without low-dose aracytine or more intensive regimen, similar to those used in acute myeloblastic leukemia reduce blast cell count and improve the quality of life but have no impact on survival in the JMML. Hematopoietic stem cell transplantation from a compatible family donor allows 50 % long-term survival. The use of 13 cis-retinoic acid inhibit in vitro monocytic proliferation but the response is however transient.

Practical Recommendations in Limited Resource Setting

- The diagnosis of CML should be considered in adolescent presenting with splenomegaly and very high leukocyte count with a left shift and myeloid hyperplasia of bone marrow.
- The finding of t(9, 22) or BCR-ABL molecular abnormalities confirm that the diagnosis is needed only if specific treatment is available.
- Hydroxyurea is a good drug for reducing leukocyte count and splenomegaly but does not improve survival.
- TKI treatment should be considered whenever possible through international support.
- The diagnosis of JMML should be considered in a young child with various nonspecific symptoms and signs including large spleen, skin lesions associated with high leukocyte count with left shift and monocytosis. The probability of JMML is higher in type-1 neurofibromatosis.
- 6-mercaptopurine and good supportive care should be provided for patients with LMMJ when allogeneic bone marrow transplantation is not available.

Suggested Reading

Alkhatib MA (2011) Pattern of pediatric chronic myeloid leukemia in Sudan and hematological response to imatinib. Pediatr Hematol Oncol 28(2):100–105

Babatunde TO, Ogun GO, Brown BJ, Akang EE, Aken'Ova YA (2014) Pattern of childhood leukaemia in University College Hospital Ibadan. Afr J Med Sci 43(2):135–138

Boma PO, Durosinmi MA, Adediran IA, Akinola NO, Salawu L (2006) Clinical and prognostic features of Nigerians with chronic myeloid leukemia. Niger Postgrad Med J 13(1):47–52

Hijiya N, Millot F, Suttorp M (2015) Chronic myeloid leukemia in children. Pediatr Clin North Am 62(1):107–119

Kiarie GW, Othieno-Abinya NA, Riyat MS (2009) The GLIVEC international patient assistance programme: the Nairobi experience. East Afr Med J 86(12 Suppl):S106–S107

Satwani P, Kahn J, Dvorak C (2015) Juvenile myelomonocytic leukemia. Pediatr Clin North Am 62(1):95–106

Segbena AY, Kueviakoe IM, Agbetiafa K et al (2012) Chronic myeloid leukemia and imatinib: experience at the Lome Campus teaching hospital (Togo). Med Sante Trop 22(3):307–311

Chapter 18
Tumors of the Central Nervous System

Case Presentation

A 7-year-old child presents with a 3-week history of morning vomiting and walking disorder. CT scan and MRI (Fig. 18.1) highlight a tumor process occupying the brainstem and compressing the 4th ventricle.

1. What complementary diagnostic approach would you recommend?
2. What is the prognosis of this tumor?
3. What treatment do you suggest?

Tumors of the central nervous system (CNS) are the most common solid tumors in children according to Western cancer registries, and one of the main causes of morbidity and mortality in childhood. Advances in neuroradiology neurosurgery and radiation have significantly improved diagnosis procedures and management. CNS tumors are characterized by a high histopathology variability. Treatment takes into consideration the histopathology, the tumor site and extent, and long-term side effects of treatment, particularly with regard to the intellectual development of children.

In Africa, these tumors are rarely reported mostly because of underdiagnosis. In Uganda, for example until 2007, there were only five neurosurgeons in a country with 36 million inhabitants. With the increasing number of trained caregivers and development of the diagnostic infrastructure, and particularly with access to CT scans, these tumors should be diagnosed more frequently.

D.C. Stefan, M. Harif, *Pediatric Cancer in Africa*,
DOI 10.1007/978-3-319-17936-0_18

Fig. 18.1

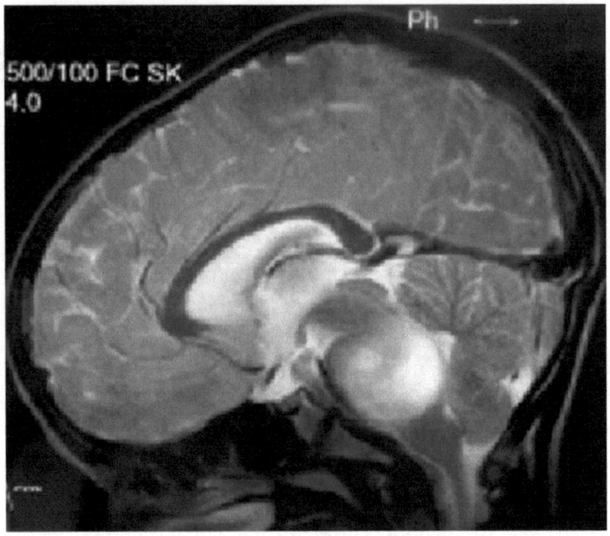

General Consideration

Brain tumors represent almost 20 % of childhood cancers in Western registries. Though the infratentorial location is the most frequent, in infants supratentorial tumors are more frequent.

In only 5–10 %, they are associated to a predisposing syndrome (Table 18.1). Radiotherapy is also a predisposing factor to CNS tumors.

Pathology

In most cases biopsy is necessary to confirm the diagnosis. The stereotactic biopsy technique allows biopsy samples in most locations. In diffuse brain stem tumors, some pineal tumors, and tumors of the optic tract, treatment without histological confirmation can be considered.

CNS tumors are characterized by their great diversity. Immunohistochemistry studies including glial markers (GFAP for glial fibrillary acidic protein) and neural (synaptophysin, the neurofilament protein) ensures a better classification of these tumors.

Types found at infratentorial level, are basically medulloblastoma, cerebellar astrocytoma, brain stem or ependymoma tumors, and in infants rhabdoid tumors. Supratentorial tumors are mostly heterogeneous. Low-grade gliomas represent 75 % of cases in this area. In the suprasellar region, craniopharyngioma or pathway glioma is encountered most frequently. At the pineal region, the germ cell tumor, pineoblastomas and, pineocytoma account for the most of the tumors at this location. Choroid plexus tumors are mostly seen in infants.

Table 18.1 Syndromes predisposing to childhood brain tumors

Genetic syndrome	Brain tumor
Neurofibromatosis type 1	Optic way glioma
Neurofibromatosis type 2	Neuroma (Schwannoma) of the cranial or peripheral nerves
	Meningioma
	Ependymoma
Tuberous sclerosis	Astrocytoma
Li-Fraumeni syndrome	Astrocytoma
	PNET (medulloblastoma)
	Ependymoma
Turcot syndrome	Astrocytoma
	Medulloblastoma
Gorlin syndrome	Medulloblastoma

Clinical Presentation

The clinical presentation of CNS tumors varies according to tumor site, histological nature, and the age of the child. In most cases, the combined symptoms show signs of intracranial hypertension (ICHT) and neurological deficit. The onset of ICHT mainly is related to a deep median tumor or ventricular location causing hydrocephalus rather than to the mass effect of the tumor or peritumoral edema.

Morning headaches, vomiting, and visual disturbances form the classic symptomatic triad of ICHT. Vision disorders may include a decrease in visual acuity, diplopia, or intermittent strabismus. Eye fundoscopy may show papillary edema. Clinical manifestation may be less suggestive and include recurrent or persistent headaches, inappetence with nausea and vomiting, unexplained abdominal pain, a change in behavior, and decrease in performance at school, and rarely torticollis. In infants, the diagnosis is more difficult because of the opening of the cranial sutures and the fontanel and brain plasticity. ICHT induces macrocrania, a bulging of the fontanel and sometimes Parinaud syndrome (paralysis of the verticality of the eye giving it a "sunset" look). Sometimes this is mainly a behavioral change, decrease in playful activity, sleepiness or irritability, and less frequently is expressed by axial hypotonia, apathy, and failure to thrive.

In Africa, patients admitted to neurosurgery are often diagnosed with significant delay and in late stages. Up to 20 % of children with posterior fossa, tumors are blind reflecting long-lasting ICHT.

Other neurologic symptoms may be suggestive of the tumor site (Table 18.2).

Diagnostic Assessment

The development of the neuroimaging techniques have had a major impact on the diagnosis and monitoring of brain tumors. A less invasive diagnosis procedure and better evaluation of locoregional extension and metastatic status are now readily available.

Table 18.2 Clinical presentations directing to tumor localization

Clinical expression	Tumor localization
Convulsions	Cerebral hemisphere
Ataxia	Posterior fossa
Alteration of visual fields	Suprasellar
Paralysis of cranial nerves deficits	Brain stem
Precocious puberty	Pineal or suprasellar
Diencephalic syndrome	Hypothalamus

The *CT scan* (computerized tomography) is a major diagnostic tool that can detect 95 % of tumors particularly with the use of contrast. CT is superior to the MRI in evaluating tumor calcifications. However, it is less accurate in evaluating posterior fossa tumors.

An *MRI* (magnetic resonance imaging) non-irradiating technique is the best choice in the assessment of brain tumors. However, it is more difficult in small children and infants because of the need for prolonged immobilization and most of time general anesthesia. This procedure is more sensitive for the detection of brain tumors, particularly in temporal location and for the evaluation of the perilesionel edema. The classical appearance is in a hyposignal in T1 and hypersignal T2 and T1 after injection of Gadolinium. However MRI characteristics can vary according to the tumor type. Spinal MRI ideally should be done prior to any surgical intervention in case of an aggressive tumor to detect possible spinal metastases. In Africa, where an MRI is not available in most parts, a CT scan with CSF analysis is the best alternative in most cases.

In certain cases, the imaging study can be diagnostic and treatment may be considered without histological confirmation.

- In diffuse pontine tumors, biopsy is not necessary.
- In pineal or suprasellar area tumors, when tumor markers hormonal markers (beta-chorionic gonadotropin (bHCG) and alpha-fetoproteins (aFP) in blood or CSF are positive the diagnosis of malignant germ cell tumors can be made without the need for the histological confirmation.
- In optic pathway glioma, especially in a context of neurofibromatosis type 1, ophthalmologic signs and imaging appearance are often typical allowing treatment to be initiated without tissue biopsy.

The *PET scan* (positron emission tomography) using 2-Deoxyglucose labeled Fluor 18 (FDG) is effective to evaluate the metabolic activity of a tumor. Astrocytomas and oligodendrogliomas are usually hypometabolic, while anaplastic astrocytoma and glioblastoma multiforme are hypermetabolic. The PET scan maybe useful:

- In evaluating the degree of tumor aggressiveness
- To guide the biopsy of the tumor
- To evaluate a residual mass

CSF (cerebrospinal fluid) analysis is an important part of the initial staging, especially in cases of medulloblastoma and other embryonal tumors.

Bone scan, abdominal ultrasound (US), and bone marrow biopsy are indicated in some cases of medulloblastomas and high-grade ependymomas with a high risk of metastases.

Treatment of Brain Tumors

Therapeutic goals are not only to give the child the maximum chance of cure, but also take into account the vulnerability of the developing brain to reduce the risk of long-term sequelae.

Surgery

In most cases surgery is the first and main therapeutic option. Urgent relief of ICHT may be considered as a first option. Biopsy or tumor excision should be performed concomitantly when possible.

Treatment of hydrocephalus using a temporary external ventriculoperitoneal (VP) shunt is the technique of choice in relieving ICHT immediately prior to tumor resection. However in Africa, as in many low and middle income countries most of the patients referred to the neurosurgery department, show an advanced stage of ICHT and undergo aVP shunt insertion. This practice is not optimal as only a minority of patients would require a permanent CSF diversion. Performing an endoscopic ventriculocisternostomy is an alternative. However this technique is not available in most parts of Africa.

The quality of the tumor resection has a major impact on the subsequent survival rate in many pediatric brain tumors. The use of the ultrasonic dissector may be helpful in tumor resection. Progress in techniques of anesthesia and intensive care has significantly reduced surgical mortality of these tumors. However, the complications can be observed: cerebellar mutism and cranial nerves deficits in the context of posterior fossa tumors, endocrinopathies and visual impairments in the surgical management of suprasellar tumors. Perioperative steroids, diuretics, or mannitol treatment is often used to reduce brain edema.

Radiotherapy

Radiotherapy is an effective way to control most childhood brain tumors. However, it is associated with long-term effects particularly in neurocognitive and endocrine alterations. The impact on intellectual development is higher in young children. Endocrine deficits after radiation for brain tumors in children include growth hormone deficits (GHD), thyroid hormone, adrenocorticotropic hormone (ACTH) and

Table 18.3 Examples of chemotherapy protocols

Protocol	Dose	Interval
Vincristine	1.5 mg/m²/s × 8 max	During radiation therapy
CCNU	75 mg/m² PO J1	Every 6 weeks
Vincristine	1.5 mg/m² IV J1, J8, J15	8 cycles
Cisplatin	75 mg/m² PO J1	
Carboplatin	175 mg/m²/week IV × 4 sem	Every 3 weeks
Vincristine	1.5 mg/m²/week IV × 3 sem	12 cycles

sex steroid hormone deficits. In addition craniospinal radiation used largely in medulloblastoma and other tumors with high metastatic potential can also be the cause of stunted growth because of the slow growth of radiated vertebras. This led to the search for dose and field reduction of radiation treatments without jeopardizing the survival. Another option is to consider delaying or avoiding radiation in the very young and rather to use adjuvant chemotherapy or to use conformal radiation to the tumor bed.

The latter has shown benefits in young children with ependymomas and most Western protocols now consider this approach in children with ependymomas over the age of 12 months. Recent developments in equipment and radiation techniques may lead to a reduction of these sequelae. Conformational stereotactic radiotherapy as well as proton-therapy techniques are now available in high income countries. Implementation in low and middle income countries is critical to offer optimal treatment option to this vulnerable population.

Chemotherapy

Chemotherapy plays an important role in the management of a large number of brain tumors. The most effective drugs are vincristine, CCNU, etoposide, cyclophosphamide, ifosfamide cisplatinum, and carboplatin (Table 18.3). Medulloblastoma and malignant germ cell tumors are amongst the most sensitive tumors to chemotherapy. However, no benefit is demonstrated in high-grade glial tumors or high-grade ependymomas. In unresectable glioma, chemotherapy is used to delay or avoid the use of radiotherapy.

Specific Tumors

Medulloblastoma

Medulloblastoma, a primitive neuroectodermal tumor, is the most common malignant brain tumor in children representing 20–30 %, which is usually situated in the 4th ventricle. On histopathology the tumor shows densely cellular

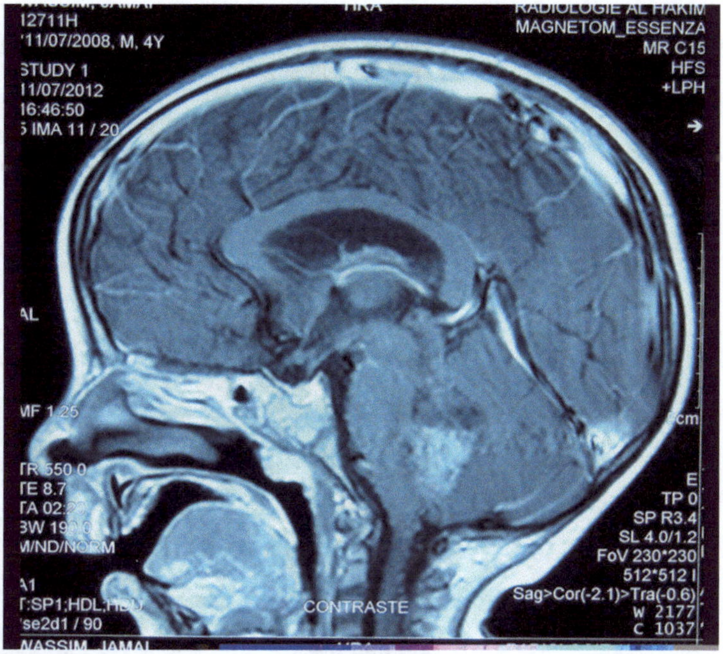

Fig. 18.2 Cerebellar medulloblastoma in a 4-year-old boy

hyperchromatic nuclei, with a high nucleocytoplasmic ratio and numerous mitoses. Immunohistochemistry markers show positivity with vimentin and the synaptophysin. The histopathology classification distinguishes 5 variants: classical, the desmoplastic/nodular medulloblastoma including medulloblastoma with extensive nodularity, anaplastic, and finally, large cell medulloblastoma with a worse prognosis.

When an MRI is available and medulloblastoma is suspected, this should include the brain and the spine prior to surgery if the diagnosis is suspected before proceeding to tumor resection (Fig. 18.2). Otherwise it is recommended to perform the spinal imaging 15 days later to avoid a false positivity associated with postoperative blood and cellular debris. Extraneurologic metastasis work-up (chest and abdomen US or CT scan, bone scan, bone marrow biopsy) is justified only in the presence of suggestive clinical signs or in the presence of metastases to the level of the spinal cord (Fig. 18.3).

The risk category (average risk or high risk) is evaluated according to the Chang classification (Table 18.4) and the quality of resection (Table 18.5).

Several studies have reported that the prognosis of medulloblastoma is closely related to the quality of surgical resection in the absence of metastatic disease. A total or subtotal resection with less than 1.5 cm residual mass is associated with an improved survival. The role of surgery in disseminated disease is less clear.

Radiation therapy is an essential part of medulloblastoma management. Historically patients were treated with craniospinal radiation and boost to posterior fossa.

Fig. 18.3 Leptomeningeal involvements in spinal MRI in a case of medulloblastoma

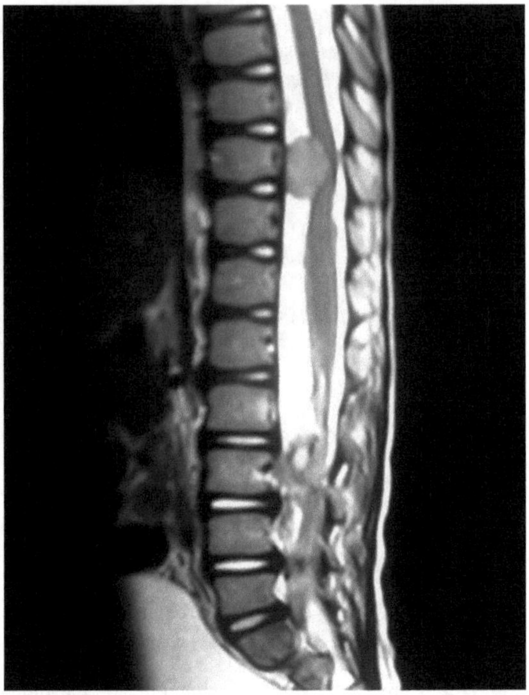

Table 18.4 Modified Chang classification of medulloblastoma

M0	No metastases
M1	Presence of tumor cells in the CSF
M2	Nodules intracranial tumor
M3	Tumor nodules of spaces under arachnoid from the bone marrow
M4	Metastases outside the CNS

Table 18.5 Prognostic groups

	Standard risk	High risk
Tumor extension	M0	M+
Residual mass after surgery	<1.5 cm	>1.5 cm
Age	More than 3 years	Less than 3 years

The dose to the craniospinal axis is determined according to the risk category with 23,4 Gy in 13 fractions for average risk patients and 36 Gy in 20 fractions for high risk patients. A boost was administered to the posterior fossa up to a total of 54Gy. Recent studies have shown that the posterior fossa boost was not necessary and a boost to the total bed was associated with similar outcomes and improved cognitive results. With the combination of craniospinal radiation and chemotherapy the survival rate in average risk patient is between 70-80%. However, these results are obtained with strict conditions and in particular with short interval between surgery and initiation of radiation therapy. In children below the age of 3 years, chemotherapy only strategies have been developed in order to avoid the devastating effects of craniospinal radiation. Results in patients with desmoplastic histological subtpes are encouraging with a 5 year survival rate between 60-80%. However, for patients with non desmoplastic medulloblastoma survival remains low between 30–40%.

Astrocytoma

Cerebellar astrocytomas represent 10–20 % of CNS tumors and usually occur before age 10 years. There are two histological variants:

- The most common is pilocytic astrocytoma occurring in 80–85 %. These tumors are slow growing and benign and cured with resection.
- Diffuse fibrillary astrocytoma (15 %) usually infiltrates adjacent structures and evolves towards the anaplastic form.

Low Grade Cerebral Astrocytoma

The usual clinical manifestation are hydrocephalus, seizures, or neurologic signs or symptoms related to the tumor location. Histologically, these tumors are characterized by the absence of pleomorphism, high cell density or mitotic activity and necrosis.

If surgical resection is complete, no further treatment is necessary. In the case of postsurgical residue, observation, chemotherapy or resection can be discussed.

Cerebellar Astrocytoma

Cerebral Astrocytoma of High Grade

Complete resection is rarely possible because of the invasive nature. In 20–25 % there is an extension to the contra lateral hemisphere through the corpus callosum. Complete resection is associated with improved survival. Postoperative focal radiotherapy with generous margins (2 cm) are recommended. The role of chemotherapy is still unclear in these tumors.

Tumors of the Brain Stem

Gliomas of the brain stem represent 10–20 % of brain tumors. They usually occur between 5 and 9 years of age. Low-grade gliomas have a high survival rate but high-grade gliomas or diffuse pontine gliomas have a 2-year survival rate of less than 10 %.

The diagnosis is made on the clinical and radiological features and a biopsy is not necessary in the context of a diffuse intrinsic pontine glioma (DIPG) involving most of the pons. By contrast resection is recommended for low grade exophytic gliomas.

Treatment of brain stem gliomas and DIPG usually involves focal radiation (50–60 Gy). Given the risk of radiation edema, high-dose steroid therapy should be considered at the same time. Chemotherapy has no role in the treatment of DIPG.

Ependymomas

They represent 5–10 % of tumors of the CNS and are located in the infratentorial compartment, supratentorial region, and more rarely at the spinal cord level.

Surgical excision should be considered. Surgery is the mainstay of treatment and survival in ependymomas is primarely related to the extent of the resection. However, at the level of the 4th ventricle, the morbidity of surgery can be significant and perioperative morbidity is not uncommon.

Radiation therapy increases survival ratesand has become part of the standard treatment whereas the role of chemotherapy remains debatable. However, the benefit of radiotherapy is very limited in the context of an incomplete resection. The recommended dose is 54–59.4 Gy and the technique of choice is a conformal field with 0.5–1 cm margins.

In the case of completely resected ependymomas the survival rate is 70 % at 5 years, while, in incompletely resected tumors this is only 25–35 % at 5 years.

Glioma of the Optic Tract

This type constitutes 5 % of brain tumors. The usual age of onset is 5 years but optic nerve gliomas can be seen in infancy with insiduous presentation such as isolated nystagmus or deincephalic presentation. These tumors are associated with neurofibromatosis in up to 50 % of the cases. Clinical presentation is primarily a decreased visual acuity. At later stages, exophtalmos, optic atrophy, or papilledema can reveal the disease. Histologically, are low-grade astrocytoma (most often grade I: pilocytic astrocytoma).

Clinical and neuroradiology evaluation are the main diagnostic tools. Biopsy may compromise the vision or lead to significant hypothamic or pituitary damage and should only be proposed when the diagnosis is uncertain.

Glioma of the optic pathways can be of low progression. Therapeutic decision must take into account tumor progression evaluated according to radiology and visual alteration.

Prolonged chemotherapy (several months) is efficient and helps eliminate or delay radiation in young children. Radiation therapy can help preserve vision and is indicated especially in the progressive forms in older children who fail the chemotherapy. The recommended dose is 45–50 Gy in the tumor bed. In type-1 neurofibromatosis, radiotherapy is avoided due to increased risk of vasculopathy and stroke.

Craniopharyngioma

Craniopharyngiomas account for 6–9 % of all childhood CNS tumors. They usually occur at ages 5–10. Invasion of the pituitary gland can cause multiple endocrine deficits requiring replacement therapy (hydrocortisone, thyroxine, growth hormone). Craniopharyngiomas are benign tumors with usually slow progressive development.

Complete resection is the treatment of choice, which depends of multiple factors ,such as tumor location (ante or retrochiasmatic), size or consistency. The most significant complication of craniopharyngioma's surgery is hypothalamic damage. For this reason, a number of authors advocate for alternative to aggressive surgery, ie limited surgery followed by radiotherapy. The usual dose is 50–55 or 40–45 Gy in children younger than 5 years. The benefit of chemotherapy has not been demonstrated however for cystic craniophryngiomas, intracystic administration of bleomycin or interferon has shown interesting results.

Five years event free survival survival is around 85 % in the case of complete resection, and 50 % in the case of incomplete resection without radiation therapy, and 60–85 % with radiation.

Intracranial Germ Cell Tumors

These represent 1–3 % of brain tumors and occur usually between ages 10 and 21 years. Different histological types can be found and germ cell tumors are currently divided into 2 main categories: germinomas and non germinomatous germ cell tumors(NGGCT). The latter can contain one or several tissues including, endodermal sinus tumors, embryonal carcinoma, choriocarcinoma, immature or mature teratoma and also some germinoma component. Tumor markers aFP and the bHCG should be measured in the serum and CSF (when safe) as they can be diagnostic if positive. In the initial assessment, craniospinal MRI is recommended. Biopsy is necessary (only) if tumor markers are negative. In the initial assesment of these tumors a craniospinal MRI is recommended.

In benign forms (teratoma), excision surgery is sufficient. Malignant germ cell tumors are chemosensitive. Platinum based chemotherapy is used in both germinomas and nongerminomatous tumors. The role of radiation is critical in these tumors. However the field and teh dose are different between the 2 groups of tumors. These tumors have a very high cure rate, close to 100 % for germinomas and in in the range of 70 % for non germinatomatous tumors.

Intramedullary Tumors

These tumors represent 3–6 % of CNS tumors and can be seen at any age.

Astrocytomas are the most frequent tumors (80 %) followed by ependymomas (10 %). These tumors are usually of low grade, well-differentiated, and sometimes cystic. Tumor growth is usually slow and develops across multiple vertebral segments with spinal cord compression. In high-grade tumors, leptomeningeal dissemination is possible.

Clinical development is usually insidious (several months or years) except in high-grade tumors where growth can be fast. Clinical manifestations vary depending on the level and extension. Motor deficits are variable ranging from monoparesis to quadriplegia. These deficits may be associated with varying degrees of pain or sphincter disorders. Vertebrae pain adjacent to the tumor is sometimes exacerbated by sneezing.

In 15 % of cases, there are signs of ICHT related to an increase of the viscosity of the CSF of the hyperproteinorrachy, arachnoiditis, or obstruction of the 4th ventricle in high cervical tumors.

Various radiological abnormalities are found in spine radiographs. These can be an enlargement of the spinal canal, an erosion of the pedicles or vertebral bodies, posterior scalloping or kyphoscoliosis. The CT scan or MRI with gadolinium injection is necessary for an accurate evaluation of the tumor and its locoregional extension.

Complete surgical excision is rarely possible in astrocytomas. The surgery is often limited to the biopsy. Low grade glioma chemotherapy is often used when resection is incomplete. Complete resection is possible in some ependymomas. This is facilitated by the use of an ultrasonic surgical aspirator. Complete resection, when possible, improves the prognosis.

Radiotherapy has no benefit in completely resected low grade tumors. When radiation is used, a low dose of radiation of 45–50 Gy is recommended.

Five years overall survival rate is 66–70 % in low-grade astrocytomas, and 50–100 % in ependymomas. In high-grade tumors, the the risk of local relapse risk is high and these tumors tend to disseminate. Their prognosis is poor.

Practical Recommendations for Resource-Limited settings

Diagnostic Procedure

- CT scan is good for tumor evaluation and diagnostic.
- CSF analyses should be done in all malignant brain tumors, and in particular in medulloblastoma.
- Biopsy is needed in most cases.

Treatment Approach

- Most of the time, late stage hydrocephaly requires urgent CSF diversion. The use of a shunt should not be systematic as tumor resection can alleviate the hydrocephalus.
- Tumor resection should be performed in all cases where possible.
- In medulloblastoma, the treatment is multidisciplinary and involve surgery, radiotherapy and chemotherapy. Good communication between the treating teams is paramount for optimal management.
- In germ cell tumors, the recommended chemotherapy may involve upfront chemotherapy followed by radiotherapy according to the tumor (germinoma or NGGCT).
- Inpontine tumors, chemotherapy is of no benefit.

Suggested Reading

Stagno V, Mugamba J (2014) Presentation, pathology, and treatment outcome of brain tumors in 172 consecutive children at Cure Children's Hospital of Uganda. The predominance of the visible diagnosis and the uncertainties of epidemiology in sub-Saharan Africa. Child Nerv Syst 30:137–146

Stefan DC, Rodriguez-Galindo C (2014) Pediatric hematology-oncology in countries with limited resources. A practical manual. Springer, New York

Wanyoike PK (2004) Posterior cranial fossa tumors in children at Kenyatta National Hospital, Nairobi. East Afr Med J 81(5):258–260

Chapter 19
Rare Childhood Cancers

This is a heterogeneous group of childhood cancers which can include low incidence tumors in human or adult tumors occurring in children. These tumors are mostly non-embryonic. Their incidence is higher among adolescents. The experience of a pediatrician may be limited and contribution of adult oncologist could prove beneficial.

In order to improve the knowledge about some of these tumors, data are collected in national or international registries.

Head and Neck Tumors

Nasopharyngeal Carcinoma

Carcinoma or nasopharyngeal lymphoepithelioma is a tumor that develops from the epithelium of the nasopharynx. These tumors have a high incidence in China, Southeast Asia, Alaska, and North Africa. They are extremely rare in the Southern part of the continent. This geographical distribution has led to incrimination to lifestyle-related risk factors including consumption of salted fish and meat. Predisposition is also reported in subjects with a HLA2 haplotype and HLA-B sin2 and AW19, BWA6, and B17. Furthermore the role of the Epstein Barr virus (EBV) is strongly suspected in the pathogenesis of this tumor. Patients with this type of cancer have high IgG and IgA directed against early EBV Ag or viral capsid. The viral genome is found at the level of malignant epithelial cells but not at the level of the infiltrating lymphocytes. Tumor cells express different genes of the EBV including EBNA1, LMP1, and EBER1.

D.C. Stefan, M. Harif, *Pediatric Cancer in Africa*,
DOI 10.1007/978-3-319-17936-0_19

Clinically, the tumor occurs usually in adolescence as a non-painful high cervical mass associated with cervical lymph nodes. The tumor may induce hearing difficulties, otitis, nasal obstruction, and epistaxis. The locoregional extension can infiltrate XIIth cranial nerve giving inducing dysphonia, or of VIth cranial nerve giving rise to diplopia. Unusually these tumors can be accompanied by a paraneoplastic syndrome (hypertrophic ostearthropathy, dematomyositis).

Pediatric forms are often extensive. Metastases may occur at the level of the lungs, bones, and bone marrow. The complete assessment includes an MRI. In absence of an MRI CT-scan contributes to the diagnosis. Distance metastases are ruled out by Chest radiography, abdominal ultrasound, CT-Scan, and bone scan. In case of skull base tumor infiltration, a cerebrospinal fluid analysis is indicated. Histopathology of nasopharyngeal carcinoma distinguishes type-I features or keratinizing squamocellular carcinoma often associated with alcohol and tobacco consumption but not the EBV type-II or squamous nonkeratinizing and type-III or lymphoepithelioma or undifferentiated carcinoma. Pediatric forms are almost exclusively of type-III.

Chemotherapy and radiotherapy are efficient in curing the disease.

Chemotherapy is recommended as the first-line treatment to reduce the size of the tumor and in this way also to reduce the dose and targeted volume of radiotherapy. The most used protocols combine cis-platinum, methotrexate, 5-fluorouracil paclitaxel and the carboplatin.

Esthesioneuroblastoma

This tumor originates from the olfactory nerve and has usually an intracranial extension. Clinical expression is usually anosmia, epistaxis, nasal obstruction, and cervical lymphadenopathies. The bone involvement with ethmoid and maxillary sinuses infiltration is commonly seen on CT-scan and/or MR.

The treatment combines surgery and irradiation. In extended forms, prolonged chemotherapy has shown a good and sometimes a complete response. It is however a rare tumor and not commonly known.

Juvenile Nasopharyngeal Angiofibroma

This is a malignant vascular tumor of the lateral wall of the nasopharynx with an extension to the adjacent structures including the sphenoid, orbital, maxillary, and the infratemporal fossa. It is found more frequently in patients suffering from a familial adenomatous polyposis. Clinical manifestations are characterized by epistaxis, cheek swelling, orbital tumor, and sometimes paralysis of cranial pairs.

Surgical resection is recommended in localized forms. Irradiation with or without surgery may be necessary.

Carcinoid Tumors

These tumors of epithelial origin can be benign or malignant and are mainly at the appendix. They are more frequent in girls and sometimes are found incidentally in the pathology of appendectomy for acute appendicitis. They derive from chromaffin cells and are capable of producing vasoactive peptides (5-hydroxytryptamine).

Clinical expression may be vasomotor disorders, diarrhea, and bronchoconstriction. Surgical resection is the treatment of choice for these patients.

Colorectal Carcinoma

It is one of the most common cancers in adults. Less than 1% of these cancers occur in the population of less than 20 years of age. In children the tumor is most of the time undifferentiated. Family polyposis, Gardner syndrome, Turcot, and other polyposis syndromes increase the risk of colorectal carcinoma.

Clinical expression is variable according to the tumor site and is associated frequently with abdominal pain, anorexia, anemia, constipation or diarrhea with hemorrhage or melena. It can also present with gastrointestinal perforation or intestinal obstruction. The diagnosis is facilitated by exploration which includes barium enema, CT-scan or colonoscopy to characterize the tumor and search for possible metastases. A High level of carcinoembryonic antigen is associated with a poor prognosis.

Surgery is the main treatment of colorectal carcinoma. In the rectosigmoidal locations treatment combining 5 Fluorouracil-based chemotherapy and irradiation can be used to make the tumor operable.

Gastrointestinal Stromal Tumors (GIST)

These tumors occur also mainly in adults. They derive from primitive mesenchymal cells having developed a proto-oncogene c-kit mutation. They are located in more than half of the cases at the level of the stomach but can also interest other digestive segments or be multifocal. Abdominal pain, bleeding, perforation or a palpable mass are the main presenting features. Surgical removal of the tumor when possible is the treatment of choice. Tyrosine kinase inhibitors have also proved their efficiency in this type of cancer.

Thoracic Tumors

Pneumoblastoma

This is an embryonic tumor of the lungs usually occurring in infants. The patient presents with respiratory signs of variable severity, sometimes with pneumothorax, fever, chest or abdominal pain. Histopathology features distinguish the cystic forms from solid and mixed types. Pleural or mediastinal infiltrations are associated with a poor prognosis. Purely cystic forms are of better prognosis and may progress to multilocular cyst. These forms occur at an earlier age.

Complete resection (lobectomy or pneumonectomy) is the main therapeutic option. It needs to be in conjunction with chemotherapy due to the risk of recurrence especially in mixed and solid forms. The recommended drugs are vincristine, actinomycin D, doxorubicin, cyclophosphamide, ifosfamide, and cis-platinum. Preoperative chemotherapy is also strongly indicated. The place of radiation therapy is debatable since the age of the patients is very young.

Askin Tumor

This malignant tumor of the chest wall belongs to the group of peripheral neuroectodermal tumors (PNET). It occurs with particular frequency in adolescents often in the paravertebral region with infiltration of mediastinal ganglia and the pericardium. The clinical presentation begins usually with chest pain, dyspnea, and a chest wall mass. Pathology examination shows round cell proliferation with expression of NSE in immunohistochemistry. As in Ewing sarcoma there is MIC2 expression. The prognosis of these tumors is pejorative with frequent recurrences after resection surgery and relative resistance to chemotherapy.

Thymoma

These are rare tumors of slow growth of the anterior mediastinum. They are more common in adults and can be associated with various autoimmune diseases including myasthenia, erhythroblasopenia, agammaglobulinemia, nephrotic syndrome, scleroderma, and dermatomyositis. These diseases can be initial mode of suspicion of the thymoma or occurring subsequently during the follow-up. Symptoms related to the thymoma are related to mediastinal compression.

Treatment is adapted to the tumor extension and histological aggressiveness. In localized forms, a surgical excision by median sternotomy may be sufficient.

Additional irradiation is recommended in histologically aggressive forms. Chemotherapy is indicated in steroid-resistant or metastatic cases. The usual drugs used include doxorubicin and the cis-platinum and more recently associations combining the carboplatin and taxol.

Bone Tumors

Chondrosarcoma

These tumors again occur mainly in adults. The pathologist should rule out chondroblastic osteosarcoma. They can develop in patients presenting with chondroma, exostosis, or chondroblastoma or could occur on a previously irradiated bone. The most common locations are the hipbone or the femur. Radiologic appearance is of lytic cortical breaking allure and infiltration of the soft parts. Histologically there are three grades of malignancy. The treatment is based on the surgical resection. Radiation therapy is proposed in inoperable forms. The prognosis is related to the quality of resection and histological grade.

Ameloblastoma

Ameloblastoma is a dysembryoplastic maxillary originating from odontogenic epithelium. It is a benign but potentially a locally aggressive. Liver and lung metastases are reported. This tumor seems more common in Africa and Asia. Surgical excision is the treatment recommended in the majority of cases.

Chordoma

Around 5% of chordomas are encountered in children. They originate from the remnants of the notochord. They essentially sit at the level of the base of the skull or coccyx and the sacrum. At the level of the base of the skull they give rise to cranial nerve paralysis and intracranial hypertension. In sacrococcygeal area they give rise to pain, constipation, and neurological disorders of the lower extremities. These tumors are not sensitive to chemotherapy. Surgical resection associated with postoperative radiotherapy remains the recommended treatment. Efficacy of Imatinib therapy has been recently reported.

Skin Cancers

Melanoma

It is a tumor of the second decade of life and occurs with more frequency in Caucasian patients. Its incidence seems to increase with more exposure to sun and the use of sunbeds. Congenital or infantile melanoma occurs at birth or during the first year. Risk factors are Xeroderma pigmentosum, Werner's syndrome, and immune deficiencies. There are the same recomandations for the diagnosis and treatment as in the case of melanoma in adults. The prognosis is associated with early dagnosis and complete removal of the tumor.In disseminated forms chemotherapy combining vincristine, actinomycin D, and cyclophosphamide have shown some degree of efficacity.

Gorlin Syndrome or Basal Cell Nevus Syndrome

This syndrome is caused by mutations in the PTCH1 gene at the chromosome 9q22. It is transmitted on the autosomal dominant mode and is characterized by the occurrence of carcinomas, odontogenic keratocysts of the jaw, palmoplantar hyperkeratosis, skeletal abnormalities, intracranial ectopic calcifications, and facial dysmorphia (macrocephaly, palatal cleft, and severe eye anomalies). Medulloblastoma occurs in 5% of patients with Gorlin syndrome. It is rather difficult to diagnose the syndrome in Africa.

Endocrine Tumors

These tumors are mostly benign and occur mostly sporadically but can be part of a syndrome of multiple endocrine tumors family.

Malignant Tumors of the Thyroid Gland

It is the most common malignant tumor of the endocrine glands. It is more common in adolescents and more common in girls.

Differentiated thyroid carcinoma is the most common histological type. Exposure to ionizing radiation and in particular at an early age is the main risk factor for occurrence of this tumor. Thyroid cancer has had a high incidence in regions exposed to radiation during the Chernobyl nuclear accident.

Asymptomatic anterior cervical mass is one of the first clinical manifestations. Satellite lymph nodes or lung metastases are sometimes present at diagnosis. These tumors are evaluated by ultrasound and CT-scan or MRI. Complete surgery is the main therapeutic option. Total thyroidectomy with lymph node resection gives the best chance of survival. In localized forms, a lobectomy or an isthmectomy may be sufficient. A complementary treatment with radioactive iodine could be considered in the event of residual tumor.

Medullary thyroid carcinoma is related to a mutation affecting the RET gene and is a part the multiendocrine neoplasms (MEN) syndrome type 2a or 2b. Early detection is possible when the anomaly of the RET gene is found in a context of familial predisposition. In other situations, the diagnosis is often made at the stage of lymph node, lung, liver, bone, or spinal cord metastasis. Surgery is the main therapeutic option. Therapies targeting tyrosine kinase also appear to bring benefit to these patients.

Pheochromocytoma

Pheochromocytomas and paragangliomas derive from neural crests. The pheochromocytomas are characterized by a secretion of catecholamines (epinephrine, dopamine, and norepinephrine) and their urinary metabolites (homovanillic acid, normetanephrin, and epinephrine). It sometimes occurs in a context of genetic predisposing syndrome in particular Von Hippel-Lindau syndrome, multiendocrine neoplasms syndrome type 2A or 2B and neurofibromatosis. High blood pressure is the main clinical expression related to catecholamine hypersecretion. Sometimes it is complicated by neurological or cardiac disorders, headache, palpitation, and drenching sweats. Other less specific symptoms may occur including orthostatic hypotension, syncope, visual disturbances, abdominal pain, or polyuria-polydipsia. Less often, the tumor is expressed as an abdominal mass. The tumor may be discovered during the monitoring of a patient with known cancer risk factor. The determination of plasma or urinary metanephrines is very sensitive to the diagnosis. The MiBG scintigraphy also has a diagnostic and extension evaluation. Surgery is the main therapeutic option. Radiotherapy and chemotherapy do not appear to improve survival.

Metastases Without Primary Tumor

This group corresponds to clinical situations where the tumor is revealed through metastases without clinical, radiological, or biological evidence of the primary tumor. Characterization of the malignant process can be difficult and requires immunohistochemistry and molecular biology. In most of the cases, these metastases are related to neuroblastoma, rhabdomyosarcoma, Ewing sarcoma, or malignant melanoma.

Key Features of Rare Tumors

- Rare tumors are usually of non-embryonic type and occur mostly in adolescents.
- Most of them are resistant to chemotherapy.
- According to the localization, these tumors can be found:
  - At the level of the head and the neck: carcinoma of the nasopharynx, olfactory esthesioneuroblastoma, and juvenile angiofibroma of the nasopharynx.
  - At the level of the abdomen: hepatoblastoma, carcinoides tumors, GIST or colorectal carcinoma.
  - At the level of the thorax: pulmonary blastoma, Askin tumors, and thymoma.
  - In the bones: chondrosarcoma, ameloblastoma, and chordoma.
  - Affecting the skin: melanoma or basal cell nevus syndrome.
  - Endocrine tumors involving different glands.
- Metastases without identified primary tumor can also be found and pose a problem of histopathological characterization.
- The diagnosis of rare tumors is sometimes diffcult as it requires a number of special investigations.

Suggested Reading

Daoud J, Ghorbal L, Siala W, Elloumi F, Ghorbel A, Frikha M (2013) Résultats thérapeutiques du cancer du cavum : y a-t-il une différence entre enfants et adultes? Cancer Radiothérapie 17:763–767

Ferrari A, Bisogno G, De Salvo GL, Indolfi P, Perilongo G, Cecchetto G (2007) The challenge of very rare tumours in childhood: the Italian TREP project. Eur J Cancer 43(4):654–659

Hadzic N, Finegold MJ (2011) Liver neoplasia in children. Clin Liver Dis 15:443–462

Janeway KA, Weldon CB (2012) Pediatric gastrointestinal stromal tumor. Semin Pediatr Surg 21:31–43

Ow TJ, Bell D, Kupferman ME, DeMonte F, Hanna EY (2013) Esthesioneuroblastoma. Neurosurg Clin N Am 24:51–65

The international pleuro-pulmonary blastoma registry. www.ppbregistry.org

Chapter 20
HIV-Related Malignancies

Case Presentation

A 6-year-old boy presents with a history of coughing for 4 months, as well as abdominal swelling for the last 3 weeks. His face and feet have also been slightly puffy. There is a history of episodes of diarrhea. He also complains of skin lesions on the abdomen that look like bruises. He has no history of night sweats, but has intermittent fever. There is no other relevant history. There is no known tuberculosis (TB) contact, but his mother is HIV-positive and on treatment. He has never had an HIV test though.

Findings on Examination

The patient is acutely ill and looks distressed. He has a respiratory rate of 44/min and a pulse rate of 120/min. His oxygen saturation in room air, as well as his blood pressure is normal.

Weight: 17.5 kg; Height: 108 cm.

Urine dipstick test: 2+ protein.

Pallor is present and he is clubbed. Facial and peripheral edema is noted. He has marked cervical, axillary, and inguinal lymphadenopathy. Nodular skin lesions (2×2 cm) with blue discoloration are found on the abdomen and left postauricular area. Several purple lesions are found on the hard palate.

Furthermore, he is tachypnoeic, dyspnoeic, and has intercostal recession. Stony dullness and decreased air entry are found at both posterior lung bases. The signs are much more pronounced on the right side.

D.C. Stefan, M. Harif, *Pediatric Cancer in Africa*,
DOI 10.1007/978-3-319-17936-0_20

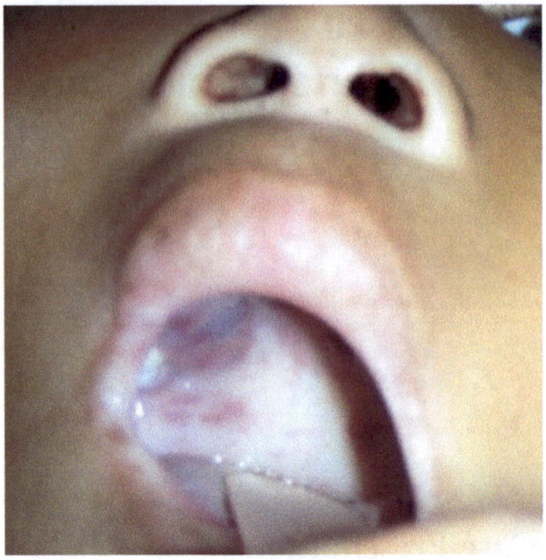

Fig. 20.1 Lesions on the palate

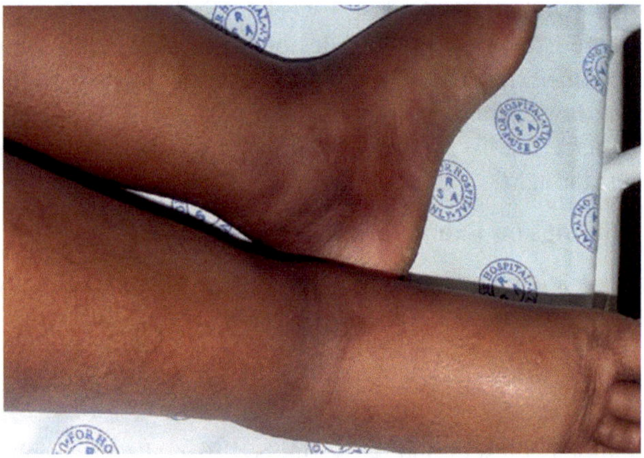

Fig. 20.2 Peripheral edema

On cardiovascular examination, a tachycardia is present, the peripheral pulse volumes are decreased and his apex is located in the 6th intercostal space, just lateral to the midclavicular line. The first and second heart sounds are normal; gallop rhythm is present, and an ejection systolic murmur is heard at the left sternal border.

Abdominal examination reveals marked distension of the abdomen. A fluid thrill and shifting dullness are noted. His liver is palpated 4.5 cm below the right costal margin, but there is no splenomegaly (Figs. 20.1, 20.2, and 20.3).

What Is Differential Diagnosis?

1. Infections, e.g., advanced HIV disease, cytomegalovirus (CMV), CMV, disseminated tuberculosis

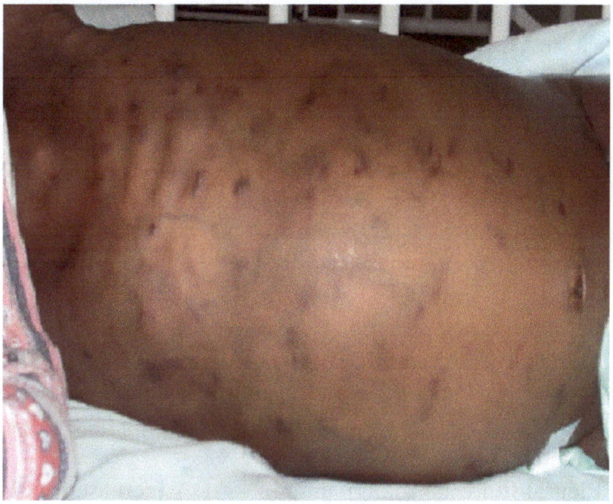

Fig. 20.3 Nodular, bluish discolored skin lesions, and abdominal distension

2. Neoplastic disease, e.g., Kaposi sarcoma, acute myeloid leukemia, neuroblastoma
3. Renal disorder, e.g., HIV nephropathy, nephrotic syndrome
4. Malnutrition
5. Vasculitic disorder

Most likely this child has advanced HIV disease (WHO stage III) with an opportunistic malignancy, i.e., Kaposi sarcoma (advanced stage) with skin and mucosal involvement as well as pulmonary and abdominal involvement. Malnutrition and anemia, most likely attributable to chronic disease and/or bone marrow infiltration, are also present. Tuberculosis will need to be excluded.

What Investigations Would You Like to Request?

1. Full blood and differential count, reticulocyte count and peripheral blood smear
2. Biochemistry: U&E, calcium, magnesium, and phosphate, total protein, albumin, bilirubin, AST, ALT, GGT, and LDH
3. HIV Elisa, CD4/CD8 subsets, HIV viral load
4. Blood culture, CRP, stool MCS
5. Urine protein/creatinine ratio
6. TB work-up: tuberculin skin test, chest X-ray, sputum or gastric washings for ZN and GeneXpert
7. Abdominal ultrasound
8. Skin biopsy (easiest access and least invasive)
9. Diagnostic pleural fluid/ascites analysis
10. Echocardiogram
11. Can consider an FNA of a lymph node
12. If Kaposi sarcoma is confirmed: bone marrow aspirate and biopsy, CT scan or MRI abdomen if available, CT chest if available

Herein listed are available results for your case scenario:

Wcc	Hb	MCV	Plt	N	L	Na	K	Ur	Cr	Ca	Mg	PO_4
11.5	7.4	97	86	2.5	7.9	131	4.0	2.9	27	2.2	0.8	1.2

CRP 85
Total protein 50 g/L, albumin 15 g/L
Bilirubin, liver enzymes normal
HIV Elisa positive
CD4 count of 17×10^6/L
Urine protein/creatinine ratio 0.13 g/mmol (normal <0.02 g/mmol)
FNA (lymph node): No malignant cells, inflammatory cells only, nonspecific findings
GeneXpert negative for *M. tuberculosis*
Blood and stool cultures negative
Pleural fluid: no malignant cells, ADA increased with a normal protein but raised LDH (exudate)
Bone marrow aspirate and biopsy: Depleted iron stores: erythroid hyperplasia
Echocardiogram: normal

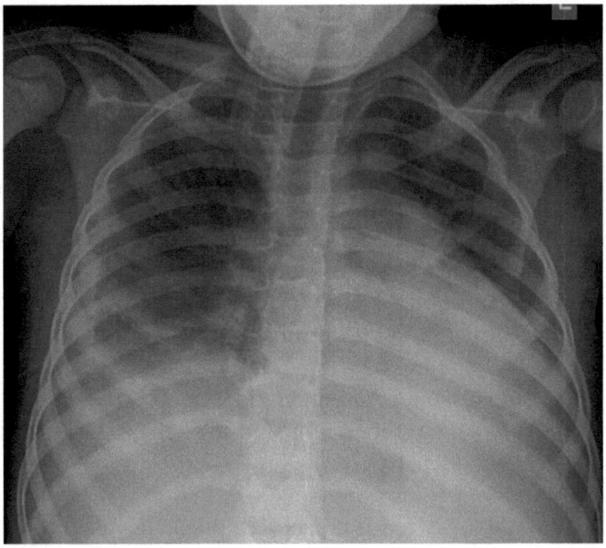

Fig. 20.4 Chest X-ray AP (erect)

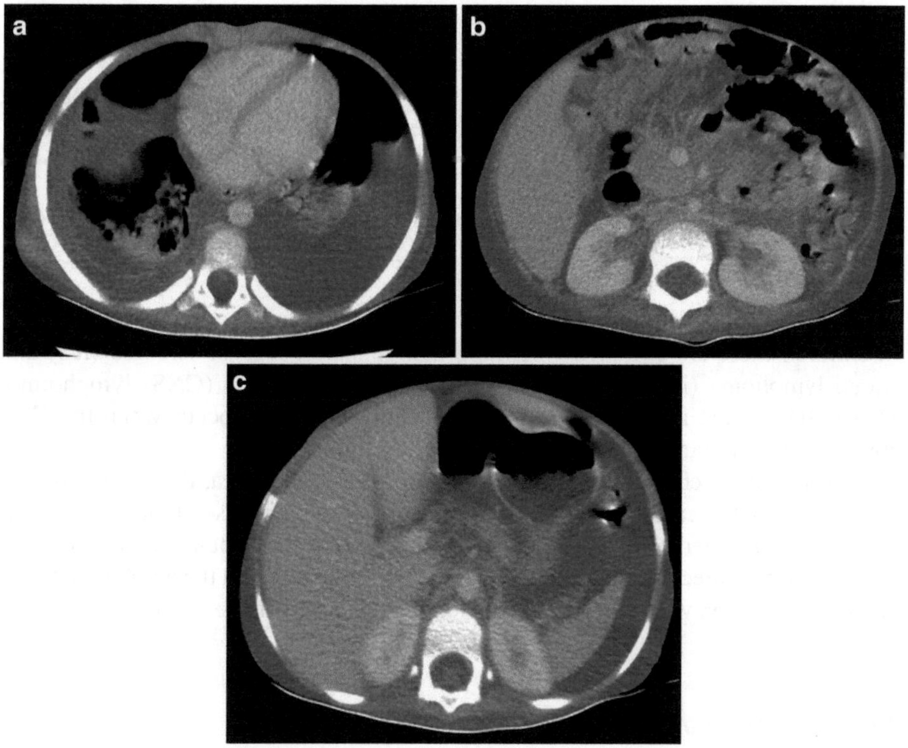

Fig. 20.5 (a–c) CT chest and abdomen. (a) CT chest shows bilateral effusions as well as underlying consolidation in the right lung. (b) CT abdomen shows para-aortic lymphadenopathy. (c) CT abdomen also shows ascites

Ultrasound Abdomen

A small amount of ascitic fluid is present. The liver appears normal in size and is homogeneous, while the kidneys are enlarged for age; other organs appear normal. No significant lymphadenopathy seen (Fig. 20.4).

Bilateral opacification, costophrenic angles obliterated, fluid meniscus seen on right, opacification/consolidation right middle and lower lobe. Cardiac thoracic ratio cannot be determined on this X-ray (Fig. 20.5a–c).

Other Findings of the Abdominal and Chest CT:

Loculated right-sided pleural effusion; possible empyema with collapse of the right lung

Left-sided pleural effusion with patchy consolidation suggestive of bronchopneumonia

Extensive thoracic and intra-abdominal lymphadenopathy

Skin Biopsy

Spindle-shaped cells arranged in fascicles are seen. Occasional mitoses are present. The morphological appearance is compatible with Kaposi sarcoma. Human herpes virus 8 (HHV8) positive.

Epidemiology of Kaposi Sarcoma

In children there are two AIDS-defining malignancies: Kaposi sarcoma (KS) and B-cell lymphoma (including primary central nervous system (CNS) lymphoma). These HIV-related malignancies (HIVRM) most frequently occur when the CD4 count is low, and far less frequent in children than in adults.

Globally, most children with HIV live in sub-Saharan Africa, thus it is expected that most pediatric cases of HIVRM will occur in Africa. Because of the introduction of antiretroviral therapy (ART), increased education of the population, and reduced transmission of infection from mother to child, it is expected that the number of newly diagnosed children with HIVRM will reduce considerably in the coming years.

Kaposi Sarcoma

Kaposi sarcoma is a mesenchymal tumor of multifactorial origin, which involves blood and lymphatic vessels. There are four recognized forms:

- The classical form: indolent, cutaneous involvement of the extremities (seen in elderly men from eastern Europe, the Mediterranean and the Middle East).
- The endemic African variant (mostly in men in the pre-HIV era), which may be indolent or aggressive.
- Iatrogenic (patients on immunosuppressive therapy); may regress if medication is stopped.
- The epidemic AIDS-related form (most common in sub-Saharan Africa); associated with HHV8 infection; aggressive behavior.

The development of the epidemic form of KS is attributable to the presence of HHV8, also known as the Kaposi sarcoma-associated virus as well as cytokine-induced growth in a child with immunosuppression. Although necessary, the mere presence of HHV8 is not sufficient for the development of KS. The seroprevalence of HHV8 among the general population varies geographically. The route of transmission is thought to include vertical and horizontal transmission, blood transfusion, and intravenous drug use as well as organ- or bone marrow transplantation. In endemic areas, the infection is probably acquired in childhood from seropositive family members; the seroprevalence rates increase with age, reaching as high as 80 %.

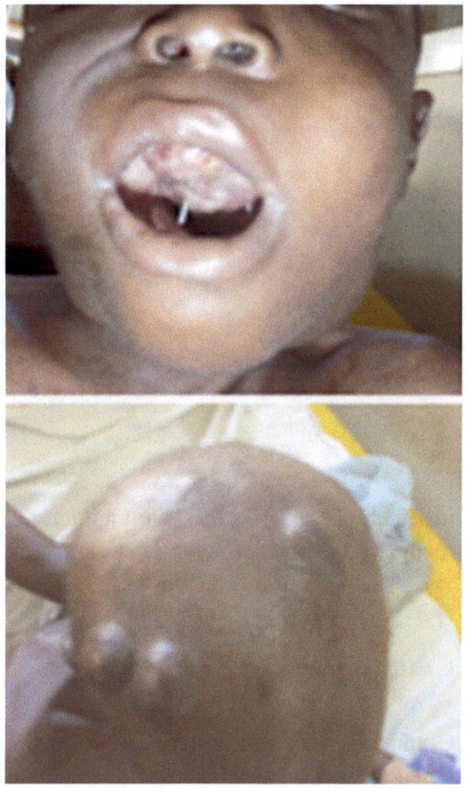

Fig. 20.6 Mucosal and skin involvement of KS

Clinical Characteristics

In immunocompetent children, HHV8 may be associated with a febrile, maculopapular skin rash, while in HIV-infected children a transient angiolymphoid hyperplasia occurs as part of the HHV8 seroconversion syndrome. The belief is that KS in young children is a manifestation of primary infection, whereas in older children KS occurs after primary infection (Fig. 20.6).

The presentation of epidemic KS has a wide spectrum, ranging from minimal disease that is discovered incidentally to aggressive disease with significant morbidity and mortality. The clinical presentation may be classified into lymphadenopathy, cutaneous, mucosal, visceral, and others.

Lymphadenopathic KS

This is the most common presentation of disease in children, which tends to occur in younger children with relatively higher CD4 counts. This is likely because of a recent HHV8 infection with rapid progression to malignancy. Lymph node

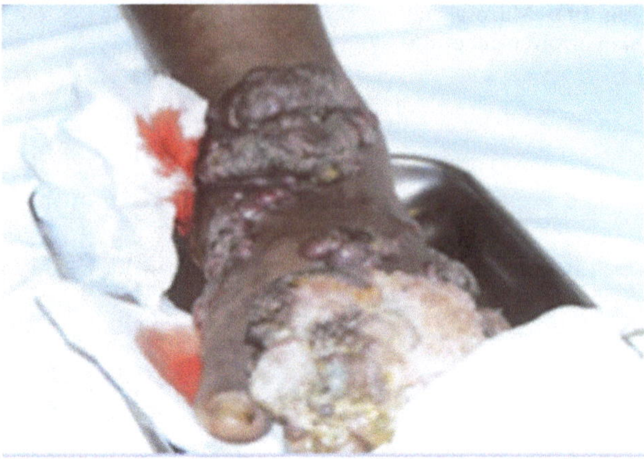

Fig. 20.7 Exophytic and fungating KS lesion

involvement may be the sole characteristic present. Massive lymph node enlargement and lymphedema may develop.

Cutaneous KS

Cutaneous lesions vary in size, characteristics, and number, ranging from a few isolated lesions to widespread cutaneous involvement. The lesions may be small (<1 cm) macular/papular lesions or large confluent nodules (≥10 cm). They appear to be dark, and almost black in dark-skin patients, and may also appear violaceous and hairy. This may occur linearly and symmetrically along skin tension lines, or may be randomly distributed. Although usually painless and non-pruritic, they may become painful. There may be associated edema. Plaque-like lesions also occur, often as a coalescence of multiple nodules. These lesions occur on the thighs, calves or feet soles and may be exophytic and fungating with breakdown of the overlying skin. These may ulcerate, bleed, or develop secondary bacterial infection, and lymphedema is often present (Fig. 20.7).

Mucosal Disease

Disease involving the oral cavity may be the initial presentation of KS. Oral lesions range from flat, red to violet papules to exophytic, ulcerative nodules. Lesions most commonly occur on the palate, oropharynx, and gingivae, but may involve any mucosal surface, i.e., the tongue, tonsillar pillars, mouth floor, pharynx, or trachea.

This may also become painful, bleed, or ulcerate if traumatized during normal chewing, and may become secondarily infected. If large, they may interfere with nutrition, speech, and breathing.

Laryngeal involvement may occur; the most common site being the epiglottis. Presenting symptoms of laryngeal KS may include pain, bleeding, dysphagia, speech abnormalities, and airway compromise.

KS involving the sclera is commonly missed. In the early stages of disease, it may appear as painless conjunctival injection, particularly at the canthi of the eyes, and is commonly treated as conjunctivitis. Red or purplish nodular lesions may also be seen involving the tarsal conjunctiva.

Visceral presentation includes pulmonary or gastrointestinal involvement and rarely other organs.

Pulmonary KS must be excluded in HIV-infected patients with respiratory symptoms or abnormal CXR findings, especially in the presence of cutaneous KS. Any intrathoracic structure may be involved, including lymph nodes, tracheobronchial tree, pulmonary parenchyma, and pleura. Common presenting symptoms include coughing, hemoptysis, shortness of breath, pleuritic chest pain, and fever. Physical examination may be normal or nonspecific.

Gastrointestinal involvement may occur in the absence of cutaneous disease and may in itself be asymptomatic. Symptoms include nausea, vomiting, abdominal pain, weight loss, upper and lower gastrointestinal bleeding or that of intestinal obstruction.

Less frequently, the heart, pericardium, kidneys, urogenital tract, and bone marrow may be involved. Involvement of the brain and intra-orbital structures is rare, likely owing to their lack of lymphatic structures.

Diagnostic Work-Up

A complete physical examination has to be performed, which also includes inspection of the skin, oral cavity and sclera to determine the extent of mucocutaneous involvement.

Laboratory Tests

Hematologic studies: Complete blood count (CBC) and reticulocyte count.

Biochemical studies: Renal function studies (blood urea nitrogen, creatinine, serum electrolytes, urinalysis), liver function tests, pleural fluid (often bloody) shows features of an exudate.

Virological: HIV Elisa and HIV viral load if possible, EBV, CMV, VZV, hepatitis A, B, C.

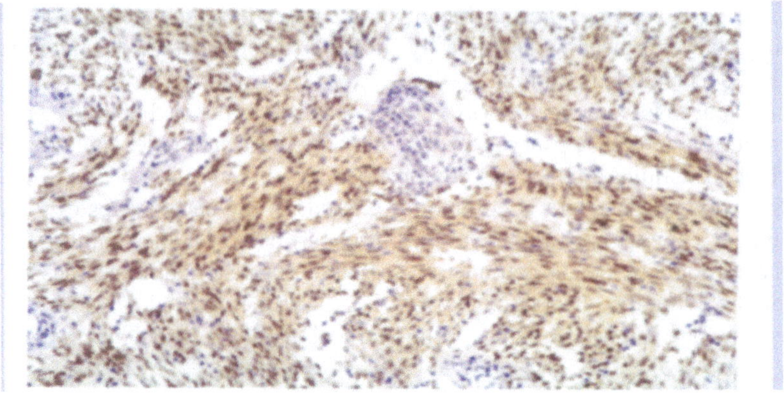

Fig. 20.8 Nuclear positivity for HHV in a lymph node

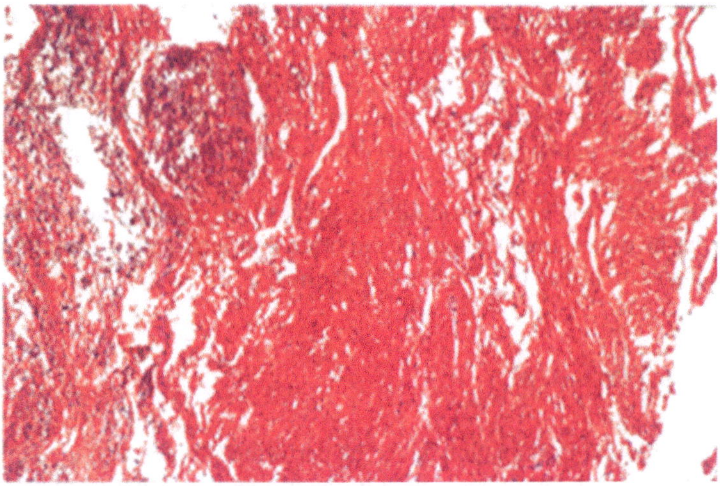

Fig. 20.9 Marked spindle cell and vascular proliferation with extravasation of erythrocytes

Immunological: CD4/CD8 subsets HIV viral load if possible.

Radiologic studies: An abdominal ultrasound and a chest radiograph are essential in a child with possible KS.

Histological: A biopsy of a lesion which is easily accessible should be performed, e.g., a skin or mucosal biopsy or a lymph node biopsy. Cytology of pleural fluid does not contribute to a diagnosis of KS. Microscopic characteristics of KS include an abundance of proliferating mononuclear inflammatory and spindle cells (Fig. 20.8), ill-defined vascular channels, hemorrhage, and edema (Fig. 20.9).

Table 20.1 AIDS Clinical Trial Group staging system for Kaposi sarcoma

Parameter	Good risk (all of the following symptoms)	Poor risk (any of the following symptoms)
Tumor bulk	Confined to the skin and/or lymph nodes and/or minimal oral disease (non-nodular KS confined to the palate)	Tumor-associated edema or ulceration, extensive oral KS, gastrointestinal KS, KS in other non-nodal viscera
Immune status	CD4 count >200	CD4 count <200
	CD4 percentage >15 %	CD4 percentage <15 %
Severity of illness	No history of opportunistic infection or thrush	History of opportunistic infection and/or thrush
	No B symptoms[a]	B symptoms[a] present
	Karnofsky Performance Status >70[b]	Karnofsky Performance Status <70
		Other HIV-related illness (e.g., neurologic disease, lymphoma)

[a]Unexplained fever, night sweats, involuntary weight loss (>10 %) or diarrhea for >2 weeks
[b]Patient is up and about most of the time and able to care for himself

Staging and Prognosis of Epidemic KS

The outcome for ART-naïve patients with epidemic KS is influenced, at least as much by the presence of other AIDS-related problems, as it is by the extent of KS. Thus, staging of epidemic KS also takes into account immune status and the presence of AIDS-related infections.

The AIDS Clinical Trial Group (ACTG) of the National Cancer Institute of Health developed a system that divides patients into good and poor risk groups based on three parameters:

- The extent of the tumor (T)
- The status of the immune system (I), as measured by the CD4 count or, in the case of children younger than 5 years, the CD4 percentage
- The extent of systemic involvement of KS (S)

Under each of these major headings, there are two sub groups identified by either a zero (good risk) or a 1 (poor risk) (Table 20.1).

Patients with a combination of advanced disease and constitutional symptoms (T_1S_1) have the worst prognosis, while those with minimal disease (T_0S_0) have the best prognosis. Important to note is that the advent of ART has affected the prognostic significance of the ACTG-staging system. Nasti et al. noted that patients on ART who develop KS, have less severe forms of disease compared to ART-naïve patients at the time of diagnosis. Thus, severity of immunosuppression, as reflected by the CD4 count is not an independent prognostic factor in the staging of epidemic KS.

The recommended management of HIV-positive children with KS, based on the above staging system, is presented in Table 20.2.

Table 20.2 Recommended management for HIV-positive children with KS

Severity of AIDS-KS	Management approach
T_0S_0 (focal disease in the absence of systemic illness)	Watchful waiting, consideration of CD4 count, viral load, and active opportunistic infections prior to ART initiation
T_0S_1 (early but mildly symptomatic KS, e.g., minimal cutaneous disease)	ART ± local therapy
T_1S_0 (early progressive AIDS KS)	ART
T_1S_1 disease	ART + chemotherapy
Extensive disfiguring skin lesions	
Widespread symptomatic cutaneous disease + edema	
Rapidly progressive disease	
Symptomatic visceral involvement	
Obstructive or painful oropharyngeal disease	
Inadequate response to HAART alone	
IRIS-associated KS	

Table 20.3 Chemotherapy drugs used in the treatment of Kaposi sarcoma

Chemotherapy agent	Dose
Vincristine	1,5 mg/m^2 intravenous bolus (max 2 mg)
Adriamycin/doxorubicin	20 mg/m^2 intravenous infusion over 1 h
Bleomycin	15 IU/m^2 intravenous bolus
Paclitaxel (for relapse disease)	100 mg/m^2 over 3 h with prednisone 1 mg/kg given just prior to the infusion

Approach to Therapy

Management of epidemic KS is not aimed at cure, rather it aims at palliation and control of KS progression. ART is the mainstay of treatment because the resultant immune restoration may be sufficient to induce remission. ART should be initiated promptly prior to referral to a pediatric oncology unit for staging and definitive management.

Chemotherapy

Several chemotherapy treatment regimens are used, which can include a single agent, double or triple chemotherapy depending on the availability of the drugs. The recommended regimen consists of Adriamycin, Bleomycin, and Vincristine (ABV). If ABV is used, it should be given 3–4 weekly; if BV is given it should be given 2-weekly for a total of 6–8 courses.

For limited disease and countries with limited resources, vincristine monotherapy is used. In more advanced disease, or if bleomycin is also available, a combination of vincristine and bleomycin is given (Table 20.3).

Relapsed Disease

Paclitaxel is reserved for patients who do not respond to ABV and for relapsed cases. This can be given as 100 mg/m^2 over 3 h every 2 weeks for 6 courses.

Antiretroviral Therapy

ART may be non-nucleoside reverse-transcriptase- or protease-inhibitor-based. Although protease inhibitors are thought to have specific antiangiogenic effects, the choice of ART regimen does not appear to influence KS outcome.

Local Therapy

Local therapy is not routinely recommended for children with KS. Though it is safe and can be used for selected asymptomatic patients if ART is not available, or as a palliative measure in patients with rapidly progressive mucocutaneous lesions.

Treatment modalities include cryotherapy with liquid nitrogen for focal skin lesions, surgical excision for focal, superficial mucocutaneous lesions, sclerotherapy, and intralesional therapy with vincristine or vinblastine. Radiotherapy is also not routinely recommended and is not widely available in developing countries.

Follow-Up During Treatment

During the chemotherapy phase, only a CBC and renal function are required before the start of each course. An echocardiogram is performed prior to the beginning of treatment with an anthracycline (adriamycin/doxorubicin), as a routine safety investigation. A maximum cumulative anthracycline dose of 250 mg/m^2 should not be exceeded.

Special attention must be paid to supportive care measures, especially in severely malnourished children, since they are more prone to develop treatment toxicity.

Follow-Up After Treatment

The follow-up after treatment includes intermittent clinical examinations (initially 6-weekly, then 3-monthly, etc.) as well as assessment of immune suppression, viral suppression, and comorbid conditions. Adherence to ART is important and patients and their caregivers should receive counseling. Imaging should be repeated at the end of treatment, if possible. With pulmonary involvement, chest X-ray or CT scan is indicated; for abdominal involvement, ultrasound, or CT scan. Other restaging investigations should be decided on based on the KS involvement at diagnosis.

Complications Related to Therapy

Complications related to the treatment are usually the side effects of the chemotherapy drugs (described in another chapter).

Kaposi Sarcoma IRIS

In some HIV-infected children, KS develops within a few weeks of commencing ART. This paradoxical exacerbation of opportunistic infections/conditions such as KS, despite immunologic recovery and favorable virological response to ART, is known as the immune reconstitution inflammatory syndrome (IRIS). In the management of IRIS-associated KS, ART should be continued and additional treatment modalities may be required.

HIV-Associated B-Cell Non-Hodgkin Lymphoma

Case Presentation

A 12-year-old boy presents with abdominal pain and distension for 3 weeks and a 2-day history of ptosis of his left eye. He also has a painful, swollen left mandible and is struggling to open his mouth. He is known with HIV infection, but is not on ART.

Weight: 27 kg; Height: 88 cm.

Findings on Examination

On examination he appears chronically ill and wasted. There is pallor, generalized lymphadenopathy and oral thrush as well as dermatitis of the left ear lobe. The left-sided mandible appears swollen. Dental caries are present, but no tooth abscess. The abdomen is distended with several palpable masses as well as hepatosplenomegaly. He is awake and alert and has no signs of raised intracranial pressure. Ptosis of his left eye is noted as well as cranial nerve VI palsy on the left. There are no other focal signs. On respiratory examination, he does not have signs of distress, but the air entry on the right is decreased, with stony dullness present. No abnormal findings were found on cardiovascular examination.

What Is Differential Diagnosis?

Neoplasm: B-cell lymphoma (Burkitt, diffuse large B-cell), Hodgkin lymphoma, large cell anaplastic lymphoma, lymphoblastic lymphoma, leukemia.
Infections: HIV, disseminated tuberculosis.

Which Investigations Would You Request?

CBC, reticulocyte count, and peripheral blood smear.
Biochemistry: U&E, calcium, magnesium, phosphate, uric acid, total protein, albumin, bilirubin, AST, ALT, LDH, GGT.
Virological: HIV viral load, hepatitis A, B, and C, VZV, CMV, EBV.
Immunological: CD4/8 subsets.
Chest X-ray.
Abdominal ultrasound (and CT or MRI abdomen if available).
CT brain.
FNA of abdominal mass or may consider cytology and flow cytometry of pleural fluid.
Bone marrow biopsy.
CSF cytospin (after the CT brain).
Bone scan.

Herein listed are available results for your case scenario:

Wcc	Hb	MCV	Plt	N	L	Na	K	Ur	Cr	Ca	Mg	PO_4	Uric acid
3.8	9	81.7	678	2.86	0.38	135	5.5	12	88	2.0	0.9	2.8	0.65

HIV viral load: 667,535 copies/ml (log 5.8).
CD4 count: 107×10^9/L.

Abdominal Ultrasound

Multiple well-defined hypoechoic lesions of various sizes in left and right lobes of the liver (40–80 mm). Multiple hypoechoic lesions in the porta hepatis as well as between the spleen and left kidney (3–5 cm) are demonstrated. Kidneys are normal (Figs. 20.10 and 20.11).

Enhancing lesion seen in midbrain.

Fig. 20.10 Chest X-ray

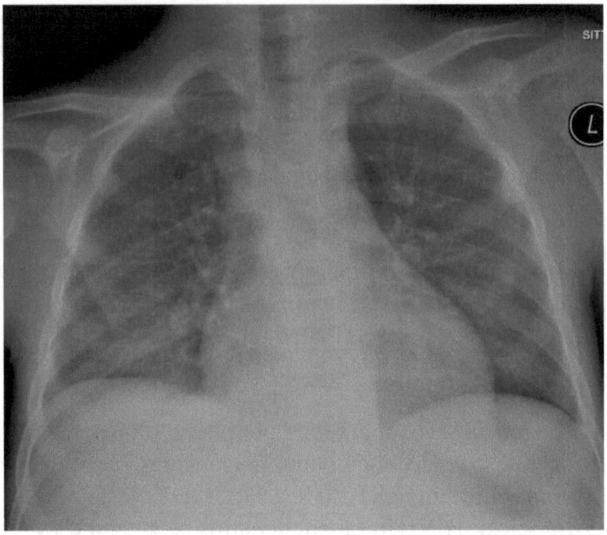

Fig. 20.11 CT brain

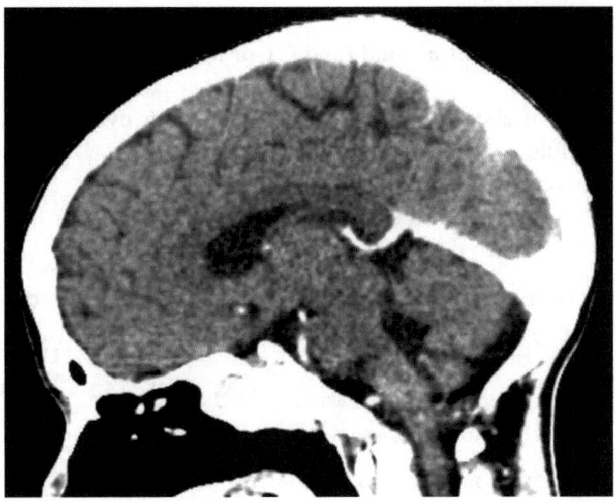

Multiple large round hypodense lesions in liver and spleen. Lymphadenopathy present throughout the abdomen; the largest inferior to the pancreas. Several hypodense regions in the liver (Fig. 20.12a–c).

Thickened dilated central abdominal bowel loop. Large soft tissue mass lateral to the sigmoid colon, as well as a lytic lesion in the left (not visible on this image).

FNA of abdominal mass: consistent with Burkitt lymphoma.

Bone marrow biopsy: no evidence of infiltration.

Pleural fluid: compatible with Burkitt lymphoma.

CSF cytospin: no infiltration.

Bone scan: lytic lesion in left ischium.

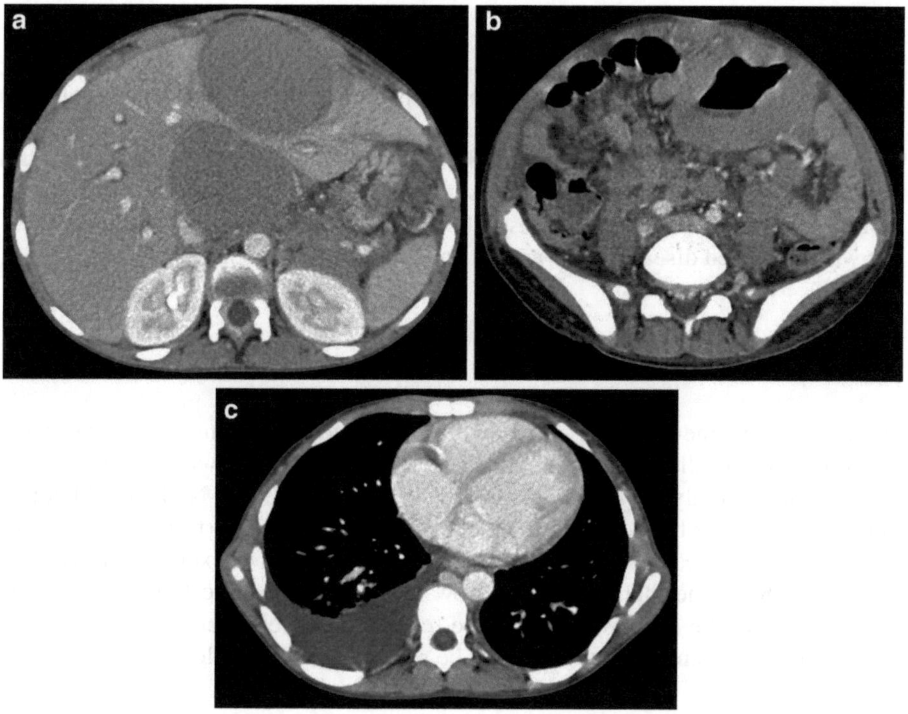

Fig. 20.12 (**a**) CT abdomen. (**b**) Ischium. (**c**) Large right-sided pleural effusion is seen

B-Cell NHL

There is a 1200-fold higher relative risk for high-grade B-cell NHL among HIV-infected children, compared to HIV-negative children. In infected children, this malignancy arises because of failure of the immune system to eradicate lymphocytes, which are latently infected with EBV.

Burkitt lymphoma (BL) is a highly proliferative B-cell tumor that includes three variants: endemic (affecting children in equatorial Africa and New Guinea), sporadic (children and young adults throughout the world), and immunodeficiency-related (primarily in association with HIV infection). Constitutive activation of the c-myc oncogene on chromosome 14 through its translocation from this locus onto chromosome 8, 2 or 22, is the key factor in the oncogenesis of Burkitt lymphoma.

Diffuse large B-cell lymphoma (DLBCL) is the most common B-cell NHL among HIV-infected children, in whom it tends to be more indolent. Other histological forms of B-NHL include immunoblastic lymphoma and primary CNS lymphoma (PCNSL).

Clinical Presentation

Abdominal lymphadenopathy/mass remains the most common presentation of HIV-related B-NHLs. Extranodal disease occurs relatively more frequently in this population compared to HIV-negative children and involves sites such as the central nervous system (CNS), bone marrow, sinuses, adrenal gland, kidney, heart, lungs, and mediastinum. The disease tends to be aggressive and children commonly present with advanced disease (CNS and/or bone marrow involvement).

Diagnosis

While awaiting the diagnosis, preventative measures for tumor lysis syndrome (hyperhydration, allopurinol) should be started for patients with bulky disease. Because of its highly aggressive nature, the diagnosis of B-cell NHL should not be delayed. An urgent biopsy of the suspicious mass should be performed in the most appropriate, most feasible, and least invasive way (lymph node excision, ultrasound-guided biopsy, bone marrow biopsy, flow cytometry of ascitic fluid, etc.). Local sedation should be used where possible, especially in children with mediastinal involvement. The child should urgently be referred to the oncology unit for appropriate management.

Investigations

Hematological: CBC and reticulocyte count (may be abnormal with one or more cell lines depressed suggestive of bone marrow involvement).

Biochemistry: renal function, calcium, magnesium, phosphate, total protein, albumin, bilirubin, liver enzymes including LDH, uric acid.

Because of the significant risk of tumor lysis syndrome, biochemistry should be monitored frequently, at least 12 hourly if possible in the setting of bulky disease.

Immunological and virological investigations: as described above.

Radiological investigations:

Chest X-ray
Abdominal ultrasound (Table 20.4)

Differential Diagnosis

1. Infections: viral (Parvo, EBV, CMV), tuberculosis, malaria
2. Other neoplasms: leukemia (ALL or AML), Hodgkin lymphoma, other NHLs (Anaplastic large cell lymphoma, lymphoblastic lymphoma), rhabdomyosarcoma, neuroblastoma, leiomyosarcoma

Table 20.4 Initial assessment of HIVRM and minimal investigations required for the diagnosis

History	Weight loss, fatigue, edema, lymphadenopathy, weight loss, pallor, abdominal distension or other visible mass, vomiting, pain, skin and mucosal lesions, petechiae/ecchymoses, respiratory symptoms (cough, dyspnea, hemoptysis, etc.), change in level of consciousness, focal neurological signs, raised intracranial pressure
Clinical examination	Malnutrition, lymphadenopathy, pallor, edema, abdominal distension, blue/purple skin and oral lesions, hepatosplenomegaly, palpable mass, respiratory distress (tachypnea, dyspnea, consolidation, pleural effusion, airway obstruction, etc.), altered level of consciousness, focal neurological signs, raised intracranial pressure
Hematology and biochemistry	Anemia, thrombocytopenia, leukopenia or leukocytosis, high LDH, renal dysfunction, liver dysfunction, features of tumor lysis syndrome (hyperkalemia, hyperphosphatemia, hypocalcemia, renal dysfunction, uricemia)
TB work-up	Tuberculin skin test, gastric washings, sputum
Viral studies	HIV viral load, CD4 count/percentage
	EBV, CMV, VZV, hepatitis (non-contributory)
Radiological investigations	Abdominal ultrasound, chest X-ray
Pay attention to possible tumor lysis syndrome in a HIV-positive child with BL	

Table 20.5 St Jude (Murphy) staging system for non-Hodgkin lymphoma

Stage	Description
I	One tumor or involved lymph node (excluding abdomen and mediastinum)
II	Disease limited to one tumor with regional lymph node involvement or ≥2 tumor/nodal areas on one side of the diaphragm or completely resected gastrointestinal tumor ± regional lymph node involvement
III	Tumor/lymph node involvement on both sides of the diaphragm; also any intrathoracic disease, extensive abdominal disease or paraspinal/epidural mass
IV	Bone marrow and/or CNS involvement

Staging and Prognostic Factors

Age, site of disease, chromosomal abnormalities, tumor burden, and response to therapy are the most important prognostic factors. The St Jude (Murphy) staging system is most commonly used (Table 20.5).

Approach to Therapy

There are several regimens available for the treatment of B-NHL, but the LMB regimen, developed by the French group, is the most widely used. In this regimen, patients are stratified as group A (resected stage I or abdominal stage II disease), group B (unresected stage I/II disease), and group C (with CNS or bone marrow involvement). Another commonly used regimen was developed by the BFM

(Berlin-Frankfurt-Munster) group. Both regimens yield very good outcomes for early stage disease and moderate outcomes for advanced disease. Supportive care during the regimen is very important, since significant treatment-related toxicity may occur. Dose reductions should not be routinely employed.

In some developing countries, it is not feasible to use an intensive chemotherapy regimen like LMB because of a lack of supportive care. Thus, modified protocols for Burkitt lymphoma have been developed for use in Africa. In Malawi, the 28-day regimen for Burkitt lymphoma only contains intravenous and oral cyclophosphamide as well as intrathecal methotrexate and the outcome after four cycles is about 50 %. The French-African Pediatric Oncology group (GFAOP) designed two less intensive treatment plans based on the LMB 89 protocol. The 3-year overall survival for the patient cohort was 61 %.

Primary CNS Lymphomas

PCNSL occur almost exclusively in HIV-infected children and have been reported to make up to 20 % of AIDS-related lymphomas in some studies. The African studies report a much lower incidence, most probably because of the challenges of diagnosis.

PCNSL tend to be cerebral and present with symptoms of raised intracranial pressure, such as headaches and vomiting. Affected children may present with convulsions, ataxia, gait disturbances, and neuropsychiatric symptoms. The main stay of treatment is steroids, high dose methotrexate, and radiotherapy in children.

Leiomyosarcoma

Leiomyosarcoma (LMS), a smooth muscle tumor, is the second most common malignancy seen in HIV-infected children in the developed world, but is often not reported as frequently in African children. The relative risk for the development of LMS in an HIV-infected child compared with a non-infected child is 10,000. In the case of HIV infection, this tumor appears to be associated with EBV infection. In these children, lesions occur in various anatomical locations, including the gastrointestinal tract (GIT), liver spleen, lung, and CNS.

The pulmonary lesions are often visible as nodules on chest CT, whereas the GIT tumors present with evidence of obstruction, abdominal pain, and bloody diarrhea.

The course of this disease is highly variable with indolent tumors (more likely leiomyomas) that probably do not necessitate intervention in some children and are very aggressive, disseminated tumors in others.

Incidental Malignancies

The spectrum of incidental malignancies is similar to those in HIV-negative children.

The Importance of HIV Status in Children with Cancer

The need to establish the HIV status of children with a malignancy cannot be overemphasized, as immunosuppression may complicate treatment resulting in increased toxicity and treatment interruptions, which could compromise the outcome. However, chemotherapy doses should not be modified purely because a child is HIV-positive. Furthermore, many children with cancer will be exposed to blood products and thus the small risk of HIV transmission mandates documentation of HIV status at the time of diagnosis. All HIV-positive children diagnosed with a malignancy, should receive ART. The regimen instituted should not contain zidovudine, as this is known to cause marrow suppression and would thus exacerbate chemotherapy-induced cytopenias, especially anemia. Tuberculosis, frequently associated with HIV infection, should be excluded and treated appropriately if present.

Outcomes of Treatment of HIV-Infected Children with Cancer

The outcomes of cancer treatment in this population are much improved for children who have access to ART, with an estimated 5-year overall survival for a South African cohort of 45.2 % for Burkitt lymphoma, 67.4 % for Kaposi sarcoma, and 69.6 % for incidental malignancies.

In Africa

HIV-related malignancies remain common childhood cancers in sub-Saharan Africa and they are relatively easy to diagnose. Most children present with advanced disease, huge tumors, severe malnutrition, and associated comorbidities. A thorough nutritional evaluation is required as well as exclusion of other associated infections. Patient outcomes are still inferior to those of patients without HIV disease. The lack of availability of chemotherapeutic agents in some African countries contributes to poorer outcomes. Good supportive care is required during the treatment phase since treatment-related toxicity is likely to occur.

Suggested Reading

Biggar RJ, Frisch M, Goedert JJ (2000) Risk of cancer in children with AIDS. AIDS—Cancer Match Registry Study Group. JAMA 284(2):205–209

Caselli D, Klersy C, de Martino M et al (2000) Human immunodeficiency virus-related cancer in children: incidence and treatment outcome—report of the Italian Register. J Clin Oncol 18(22):3854–3861

Fatahzadeh M (2012) Kaposi sarcoma: review and medical management update. Oral Surg Oral Med Oral Pathol Oral Radiol 113(1):2–16

Ganem D (2010) KSHV and the pathogenesis of Kaposi sarcoma: listening to human biology and medicine. J Clin Invest 120(4):939–949

Harif M, Barsaoui S, Benchekroun S, Bouhas R, Doumbé P, Khattab M, Ladjaj Y, Moreira C, Msefer-Alaoui F, Patte C, Rakotonirina G, Raphael M, Raquin M, Lemerle J (2008) Treatment of B-cell lymphoma with LMB modified protocols in Africa—report of the French-African Pediatric Oncology Group (GFAOP). Pediatr Blood Cancer 50:1138–1142

Hengge UR, Ruzicka T, Tyring SK et al (2002) Update on Kaposi's sarcoma and other HHV8 associated diseases. Part 1: epidemiology, environmental predispositions, clinical manifestations, and therapy. Lancet Infect Dis 2(5):281–292

Jacobson CA, Abramson JS (2012) HIV-associated Hodgkin's lymphoma: prognosis and therapy in the era of cART. Adv Hematol 2012. doi:10.1155/2012/507257

Molyneux EM, Rochford R, Griffin B, Newton R, Jackson G, Menon G, Harrison CJ, Israels T, Bailey S (2012) Burkitt's lymphoma. Lancet 379:1234–1244

Mueller BU (1999) Cancers in children infected with the human immunodeficiency virus. Oncologist 4(4):309–317

Orem J, Otieno MW, Remick SC (2004) AIDS-associated cancer in developing nations. Curr Opin Oncol 16(5):468–476

Spina M, Carbone A, Gloghini A, Serraino D, Berretta M, Tirelli U (2011) Hodgkin's disease in patients with HIV infection. Adv Hematol 2011:7p

Chapter 21
Characteristics of Cancers in the Neonatal Period

Case Presentation

Youssef is 15-days-old neonate boy. He is brought by his mother because of abdominal distension. No past medical history was reported during the pregnancy. Examination shows a huge abdominal mass.

Abdominal ultrasound (Fig. 21.1) found heterogeneous hepatomegaly and suspected right suprarenal mass. Abdominal CT (Fig. 21.2) confirmed the diagnosis.

- What is the most likely diagnosis?
- What are the investigations required to confirm the diagnosis?
- What is the treatment and prognosis in this case?

Cancer is rare in the neonatal period and has special epidemiology features and unique presentations. The care of neonates requires taking into account organic immaturity and sensitivity to chemotherapy. In Africa, there are sparse reports on cancer in neonates.

Epidemiological Profile

The most common cancers in the newborn are neuroblastoma representing almost 50 % of cases, leukemia, renal tumors, and sarcomas. These cancers might be related to predisposing genetic factors or conditions acquired during pregnancy.

D.C. Stefan, M. Harif, *Pediatric Cancer in Africa*,
DOI 10.1007/978-3-319-17936-0_21

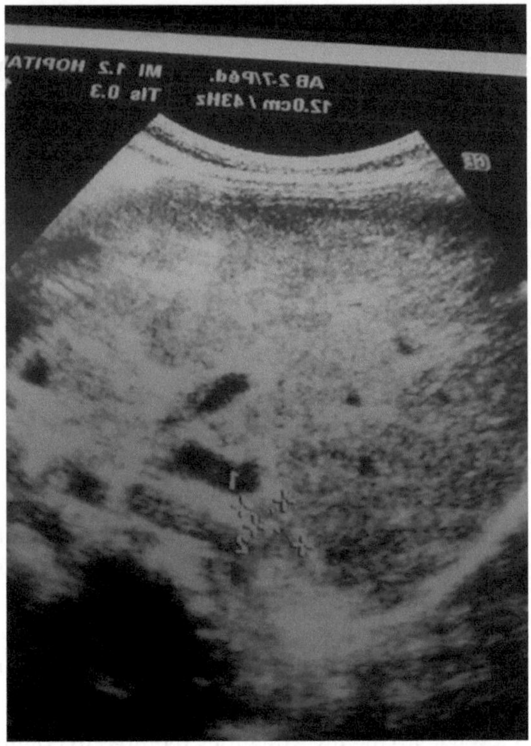

Fig. 21.1 Abdominal ultrasound

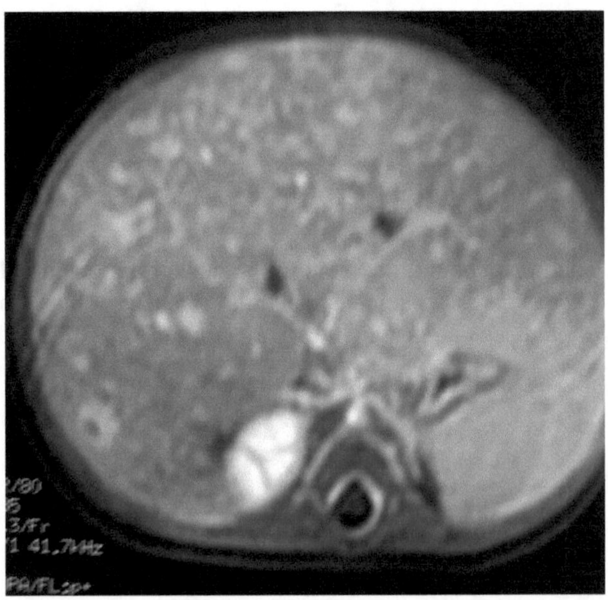

Fig. 21.2 Abdominal CT-Scan

Some molecular abnormalities associated with cancer are found with a high frequency at this age. These are the MLL gene abnormalities in acute lymphoblastic leukemia, abnormalities of the WT1 in Wilms tumor, and abnormalities of the RB1 in retinoblastoma. In neuroblastoma, amplification the n-Myc gene might be present.

Adaptation of Chemotherapy Treatement for use in Neonates

Diagnostic and therapeutic approach must take into account the physiological peculiarities of this neonatal period and, in particular, hepatic and renal immaturity that contribute significantly to pharmacokinetic changes of drugs. These patients should be treated in a neonatology unit or pediatric oncology where different expertise, supportive care, and adequate monitoring are available.

Chemotherapy is highly toxic during the first 30 days of life. Vincristine is neurotoxic, toxicity which can manifest as convulsions, hypotonia, feeding difficulties, or a flaccid paralysis. Nephrotoxicity and myelotoxicity are also often more prominent at this age. In most protocols, dose reductions are recommended to prevent or reduce these toxicities.

Peculiarities of Some Neonatal Cancers

Neuroblastoma represents almost half of the cases of cancer in this age. Its incidence is however underestimated because spontaneous regression is common. Thus, tests of systematic screening by searching for urinary catecholamins are no longer required.

Neuroblastoma during the first 30 days (actually the first 6 weeks) is often localized or stage IVs and rarely amplifies the N-Myc gene. The prognosis is usually favorable as the tumor regresses spontaneously. Clinical manifestations are associated with a huge hepatomegaly, skin lesions, and sometimes bone marrow infiltration. Biopsy and/or high urinary catecholamine level confirm the diagnosis. Close observation without treatment intervention may be recommended if the patient is stable and disease localized.

Chemotherapy is used in disseminated disease or in case of life-threatening respiratory or abdominal compression. Seldom low doses of irradiation (450 cG) can be added. Surgical removal of adrenal tumor is an option to be considered but usually done 6–12 months later.

Lymphoblastic leukemia at this age has a poor prognosis being often associated with the MLL gene rearrangements. The patients present with high leukocyte count, infiltration of the central nervous system, and lack of expression of CD10. They respond poorly to initial treatment.

Acute myeloblastic leukemia in neonates is associated with a greater frequency of M4 and M5 types, with significant leukocytosis, skin, and the central nervous system involvement.

Most of the renal tumors are due to mesoblastic nephroma or Bollande tumor. Only surgical treatment is recommended for these tumors. Few recurrences are reported. The rare cases of Wilms tumors have a similar prognosis similar to those of the older child.

Key Points

- Cancer is rare in the neonatal period and most likely associated with predisposing genetic factors.
- Neuroblastoma is the most common neonatal cancer and has good prognosis.
- Transient leukemia is associated with Down syndrome.
- Chemotherapy has high toxicity at this age and dose reduction should apply.

Suggested Reading

Moore SW, Satge D, Sasco AJ et al (2003) The epidemiology of neonatal tumours. Report of an international working group. Pediatr Surg Int 19:509–519

Orbach D, Sarnacki S, Brisse HJ et al (2013) Neonatal cancer. Lancet Oncol 14:e609–e620

Reaman GH (2003) Biology and treatment of acute leukemia in infants in treatment of acute leukemias. In: Pui CH (ed) New directions of clinical research. Humana, Totowa, pp 73–83

Chapter 22
Cancers in Adolescence

Cancer in adolescent is not common. The probability of developing cancer prior to age 20 varies slightly by sex. A newborn male has 0.32 % probability of developing cancer by age 20, (i.e., a 1 in 300 chance). Similarly a newborn female has a 0.30 % probability of developing cancer by age 20, (i.e., a 1 in 333 chance).

The age-specific incidence rates of cancer showed the most common cancer below the age of 15 years to be represented by leukemia and above 15 years by lymphoma. The second most common cancer in young children is represented by brain tumors and leukemia in adolescents.

This information is specific for developed countries and does not correspond with the African reality which in most cases is not known.

Cancer in Adolescence in Africa

Most pediatric units in Africa treat children with cancer below the age of 13 years or in some cases below 15 years. Most African hospitals do not have dedicated units for the treatment of cancer in adolescence.

The profiles of cancers include different forms of leukemia (including chronic leukemia), lymphomas, bone tumors, and sarcomas.

Some of the required investigations are not always available (scintigraphy, MRI, etc.) or are expensive and unaffordable. The basic radiography compliments the blood tests and is in most cases sufficient for an accurate diagnosis.

The treatment of the adolescents with cancer is complicated by the psychological mental and physical transformations associated with age and is associated with a late diagnosis and poor outcome.

D.C. Stefan, M. Harif, *Pediatric Cancer in Africa*,
DOI 10.1007/978-3-319-17936-0_22

A special attention must be given to sharing news and information related to the disease and also to ensure a correct and sustained pain relief and palliation program.

Cancer in adolescents is characterized by an epidemiological profile approaching that of the adult. Its occurrence during psychological and physical transformation poses specific problems. According to the organization of care, these patients can be treated in pediatric oncology or adult's oncology unit. Patients may then have for the same disease, but different therapeutic approach and different outcome. In some countries, dedicated units to this age group are created to adapt care and environment to this population.

Epidemiological Data

The incidence of cancer in adolescents is higher than in children. Some cancers secondary to environmental factors similar to those of the adult are observed with a high incidence. The most frequent cancers are lymphomas, sarcomas, leukemias, germ cell tumors, and tumors of the central nervous system. The distribution of these cancers is also different from that observed in the youngest child. Non lymphoblastic leukemias and chronic myeloid leukemia are significantly more common at this age. The rhabdomyosarcomas represent only a quarter of the tumors of soft tissue. Synovial sarcoma, liposarcoma, and other soft tissue tumors are more common. Large cell lymphomas are also more frequent than lymphoblastic or Burkitt's lymphomas observed in the younger child. Embryonic tumors are exceptional. In Africa, non-Hodgkin lymphoma seems significantly less frequent than in the younger children.

Clinical Expression

A significant delay diagnostic is common at this age. This is due to the desire for independence of the teenagers, taking away their parents and especially mothers from their health problems. Other factors related to the psychological changes in adolescents contribute to the delay in consultation including shyness or a sense of invincibility. The disease also makes them vulnerable and pushes them to return to their dependence on their parents.

Special Needs

Adolescence is a critical period in life with specific challenges. Care of adolescents requires taking into account increased needs for information on the disease and its treatment. Side effects and in particular the alopecia may be poorly tolerated by girls. At this age, the description of the symptoms and signs is often accurate. Usually, there is less use of sedation for diagnostic investigations or for the treatment given the increased compliance.

Various studies have shown that treatment outcomes are significantly better when teenagers and young adults are treated with pediatric protocols. However, there is less success compared to younger children with a reduced survival rate in a number of tumors in adolescents.

Key Points

Cancer is more common in adolescents and its features are close to young adult cancer.

Delayed diagnosis is frequent because of psychological disruptions at this age amongst other many causes.

Treating adolescents with cancer following pediatric protocols give better results than those of the adults in many cases.

Requirements in providing comprehensive information regarding the disease, treatment, complications, side effects, survival and psychological support are particularly pronounced at this age.

Suggested Reading

Magrath I, Epelman S (2013) Cancer in adolescents and young adults in countries with limited resources. Curr Oncol Rep 15(4):332–346

Mbika Cardorelle A, Okoko A, Nika E, Nsondé Malanda J, Ngolet L (2011) Cancers du grand enfant à Brazzaville. Arch Pediatr 18(11):1227–1232

Penson RT, Rauch PK, McAfee SL et al (2002) Between parent and child: negotiating cancer treatment in adolescents. Oncologist 7(2):154–162

Pollock BH, Krischer JP, Vietti TJ (1991) Interval between symptom onset and diagnosis of pediatric solid tumors. J Pediatr 119(5):725–732

Chapter 23
General Principles of Cancer Chemotherapy

Chemotherapy is an extremely important component of childhood cancer treatment. It has dramatically transformed the prognosis of most malignant childhood tumors, which are usually chemotherapy-sensitive. The relative tolerance of children to chemotherapy compared with adults also contributes to good patient outcomes. In addition, modern chemotherapy includes new agents which selectively target tumor cells, thus limiting toxicity.

Prior to initiating a chemotherapy protocol, a definitive diagnosis should be established and a printed pathology/hematology report should preferably be available. Adequate information must be provided to the patient and/or the parents about the disease, its treatment and treatment-related complications. Chemotherapy should then be initiated by a specialized medical team according to a specific treatment protocol. While receiving chemotherapy, the patient should be seen regularly to assess treatment response, as well as to monitor for immediate and late treatment-related toxicity after completion of treatment.

Tumor Growth and Sensitivity to Chemotherapy

Chemotherapy drugs have an anti-mitotic action which is more pronounced in cells that have a high rate of cell division. The rate of tumor growth varies from one tumor to another, but also in different parts of the same tumor. This is mainly due to genetic, but also external and internal variables in the particular microenvironment.

Various models explaining tumor growth have been proposed. According to the Gompertzien model, growth takes place through an initial slow phase, followed by exponential proliferation and then a significant decrease in proliferation once the tumor mass reaches a critical volume. Growth is thus based on a sigmoid curve. The slowdown is explained by the mismatch between availability of metabolic building blocks and the metabolic needs of tumor cells, leading to anoxia and tumor necrosis.

D.C. Stefan, M. Harif, *Pediatric Cancer in Africa*,
DOI 10.1007/978-3-319-17936-0_23

A significant fraction of tumor cells will then enter the quiescent cell phase (G0) and become insensitive to chemotherapy. This type of resistance is termed the kinetic type.

The proliferation of tumor cells may also be affected by genetic mutations, which lead to cellular resistance (the genetic type of resistance) with selection of a cell clone with a proliferative advantage. Metastatic lesions, which occur after multiple cell divisions, as well as large tumors are also more likely to be more resistant to chemotherapy. According to the mathematical model of Goldie and Coldman, when a tumor is detected, it already contains resistant clones, of which the magnitude depends on the frequency of genetic mutations and of the tumor mass.

Other mechanisms of tumor resistance to chemotherapy include modification of the chemotherapy receptor and metabolic inactivation or excretion of the active molecule of the drug. The tumor cell may also be able to repair chemotherapy-induced damage.

Chemotherapy resistance may occur to several different agents simultaneously. The acquisition of this multi-drug resistance (MDR) is due to the expression of p-glycoprotein and/or multi-drug resistance-associated protein on the tumor cell membrane. The presence of these two proteins is associated with a poor treatment response and prognosis.

Chemotherapy Mechanisms of Action

The induction of apoptosis is one of the predominant mechanisms of action. Apoptosis is a physiological cell death in which the cell condenses and fragments without altering surrounding tissues and without causing an inflammatory reaction. The cell cycle is divided into four phases (Fig. 23.1). The critical check points at which the cell has to either undergo DNA repair and continue the process of division or activate apoptosis, lie between phases G1 and S and phases G2 and M. At these critical points, the cell requires the interaction of cyclins and enzymes called cyclin-dependent kinases to regulate these processes.

Anti-mitotic drugs may be phase independent or have an effect only in certain phases of the cell cycle. For example, cytarabine is phase S-dependent, while

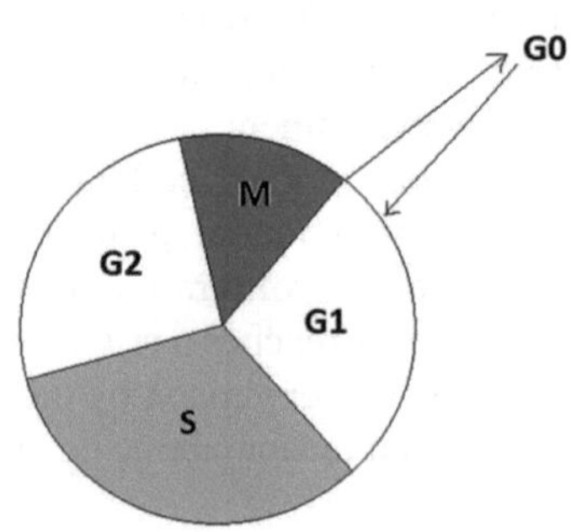

Fig. 23.1 Cell cycle. Phase S (DNA synthesis), phase M (mitosis), and phases G1 and G2 (Gap). Cells that are not in this mitotic cycle are in phase G0 (rest phase)

Table 23.1 Classification of the major chemotherapy agents used for childhood cancer

Alkylating agents	*Chemotherapy agents*
Nitrogen mustards	Chlorambucil, chlormethine, cyclophosphamide, ifosfamide, melphalan
Hydrazines and triazines	Procarbazine, dacarbazine, temozolomide
Nitrosureas	Carmustine, lomustine
Metal salts	Carboplatin, cisplatin
Alkylsulfonates	Busulfan
Antimetabolites	
Folate antagonists	Methotrexate
Purine antagonists	Fludarabine, 6-mercaptopurine, 6-thioguanine
Pyrimidine antagonists	5-Fluorouracil, cytarabine, gemcitabine
Topoisomerase inhibitors	
Camptothecin derivatives	Topotecan, irinotecan
Epipodophyllotoxins	Etoposide, teniposide
Other	Bleomycin
Anthracyclines	Daunorubicin, doxorubicin (synonym adriamycin), epirubicin, idarubicin.
Spindle poisons	
Vinca-alkaloids	Vincristine, vinblastine, vindesine, vinorelbine
Other	Paclitaxel
Other	
Asparaginase, Tretinoin (ATRA)	

vincristine only affects cells in phase M. Depending on their mechanism of action, the chemotherapy drugs are classified into four major groups: the alkylating agents, topoisomerase inhibitors, the antimetabolites, and the plant alkaloids (Table 23.1).

Alkylating agents are drugs that have the property to transfer an alkyl group to proteins that bind together to form the double helix DNA structure. DNA synthesis is impaired due to this alkylation process, but the alkylating agents are active in all phases of the cell cycle. They are important in the treatment of slow-growing cancers, but are also used widely in the treatment of leukemia, lymphoma, sarcoma, neuroblastoma, nephroblastoma, retinoblastoma, osteosarcoma, Ewing sarcoma, germ cell tumors, and brain tumors.

Antimetabolites also interfere with DNA synthesis and are S phase-dependent. Their activity is dependent on rapid cell proliferation. Some have a structural analogy with physiological molecules (folic acid, purine or pyrimidine antagonists), while others have an inhibitory effect on enzymes necessary for DNA synthesis.

Inhibitors of topoisomerases play a major role in the restructuring (coiling and uncoiling) of DNA for transcription, replication, and mitosis. Depending on their mechanism of action, these drugs are grouped into camptothecin derivatives inhibiting topoisomerase I (topotecan and irinotecan) and the epipodophyllotoxins (etoposide and teniposide) inhibiting topoisomerase II.

Anthracyclines are also known as antitumor antibiotics and were derived from the Streptomyces species. The mechanism of action occurs via multiple pathways,

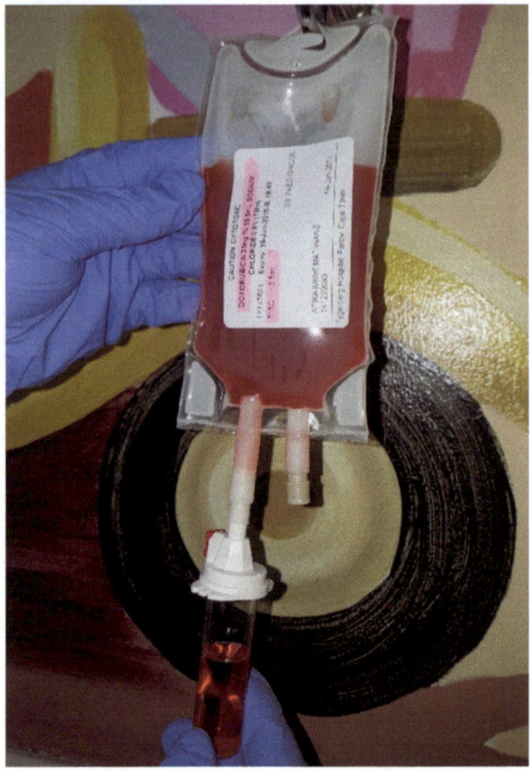

Fig. 23.2 Anthracyclines most often have a characteristic *red/orange* color. Mitoxantrone has a blue color

such as impaired DNA synthesis, DNA intercalation, inhibition of topoisomerase I, induction of apoptosis, the generation of free radicals and an anti-angionetic action. These drugs are usually red or orange in color (Fig. 23.2). It is important to limit the cumulative dose of anthracyclines in order to reduce the risk of cardiotoxicity.

Spindle poisons bind to microtubules, which interfere with the formation of the tubules. They are phase M-dependent.

Recent developments: Research in the field of cancer drugs have different focus areas, e.g. reduction in toxicity, improving efficacy, and the development of novel agents. Liposomal anthracyclines have been developed in order to reduce the cardiotoxicity of this class of drugs. Asparaginase conjugated to polyethylene glycol (PEG-asparaginase) reduces immunogenicity and has a longer half-life. New classes of drugs specifically targeting tumor cells have emerged, e.g. rituximab, targeting tumor cells expressing CD20 on their surface, and many other monoclonal antibodies.

Most cancer drugs are metabolized by the liver and eliminated via urinary excretion. For this reason, it is essential to determine renal and hepatic function prior to starting treatment, as well as intermittently during treatment. In the case of renal or hepatic insufficiency, dosages should be adjusted. Drug interactions must also be taken into account. For example, the use of anti-convulsants increases the catabolism of some chemotherapeutic agents.

First-line treatment protocols typically involve combination therapy, while monotherapy is sometimes used in metronomic or palliative therapy. The goal of combination therapy is to overcome drug resistance by targeting tumor cells in various ways.

Pharmacological Data

To understand and adapt chemotherapy treatment, it is important to know the behavior of each drug once it has been administered, e.g. bioavailability, distribution, biotransformation, and excretion. The bioavailability of drugs given by mouth may vary from one individual to another, as well as in the same individual at different points in time. Hepatic metabolism can significantly reduce the bioavailability of some drugs (e.g. 6-mercaptopurine). Several drugs are transported bound by albumin. A decrease in albumin will thus result in a high concentration of free drug and consequently more toxicity. Furthermore, third space dissemination (ascites, pleural effusion) is responsible for a decrease in drug clearance and greater toxicity. This is noted in particular when high-dose methotrexate is administered to patients with non-Hodgkin lymphoma. Drug clearance may also be reduced in the case of renal or hepatic failure (Table 23.2) and doses of certain drugs should be adjusted as indicated in Table 23.2.

Inherited or acquired impaired hepatic metabolism may cause major toxicity. In patients with a deficiency of thiopurine methyl transferase, an enzyme that degrades azathioprine and 6-mercaptopurine, these drugs are the cause of excessive toxicity at normal doses. Drugs metabolized by microsomal P450 in the liver have a reduced clearance when ketoconazole or anti-retroviral drugs are administered concomitantly and increased clearance in case of simultaneous treatment with anti-convulsants. Examples of such drugs include cyclophosphamide, the vinca-alkaloids, and the epipodophyllotoxins.

Table 23.2 Chemotherapy drugs that require dose adjustment in renal or hepatic failure

Renal failure	Liver disease
Bleomycin	Daunorubicin
Carboplatin	Doxorubicin
Cisplatin	Epirubicin
Cyclophosphamide	Idarubicin
Etoposide	Vincristine
Hydroxyurea	Vinblastine
Ifosfamide	Vinorelbine
Methotrexate	
Nitrosoureas	
Topotecan	

Administration of Chemotherapy

Chemotherapy is usually administered in timed cycles in order to allow normal tissues to regenerate in between cycles. Usually the more intensive the chemotherapy, the longer the time interval between treatment cycles. In more recent years, dose-dense chemotherapy protocols have been studied to determine whether outcome would be improved, for example giving chemotherapy cycles 2 weekly instead of every 3 weeks with supportive granulocyte colony stimulating factor. Several cycles are needed to eliminate the disease. The disappearance of clinical and radiological signs that signifies remission, does not equate to cure since continued chemotherapy is required in order to eradicate all undetectable tumor cells.

When protocols are designed, the method of administration and dose of a drug are also important factors to take into account. For example, methotrexate is given intravenously at high doses in order to achieve better central nervous system (CNS) penetration in the treatment of acute leukemia and is also given intrathecally to eradicate leukemic blasts in the cerebrospinal fluid and prevent CNS relapse.

The method of administration of chemotherapy drugs is varied according to what preparation of the drug is available. Chemotherapy regimens for leukemias and non-Hodgkin lymphomas include oral, intravenous, intramuscular, and intrathecal drugs. Hodgkin lymphoma and solid tumors are usually treated only with intravenous chemotherapy. Asparaginase may be given intravenously or intramuscularly, but the incidence of anaphylaxis is significantly reduced when given intramuscularly, thus most pediatric oncology units use the intramuscular route. Whenever asparaginase is being administered, a trolley should be prepared with the necessary drugs and equipment to treat anaphylaxis, if it should occur. The patient should also be observed for at least 1 hour. Glucocorticosteroids are equally effective whether it is given orally or intravenously. In some countries it may be difficult to obtain oral dexamethasone, thus the intravenous form may be used.

Chemotherapy should preferably only be administered in a pediatric oncology unit where staff have been trained to handle these drugs. After the required chemotherapy drugs have been prepared in a sterile manner in a laminar flow box by a trained pharmacist or other experienced healthcare worker, the drug name, dose, volume, method of administration, patient details, date prepared, and expiration time should be checked by two persons. The administration should take place as soon as possible, since some agents such as cyclophosphamide and dacarbazine expire rapidly. Most other agents are stable for 8 hours after preparation. Protection against light may be necessary for some agents, such as dacarbazine. The period of administration is very important, since toxicity may be increased by a longer infusion time (e.g. doxorubicin). Therefore, the treatment protocol should be followed meticulously regarding prescription and administration instructions. The information on the drug pamphlet should also be studied carefully.

It is extremely important to remember that only three drugs may ever be administered via the intrathecal route: methotrexate, cytarabine, and hydrocortisone (given to prevent chemical arachnoiditis). In some treatment protocols, vincristine

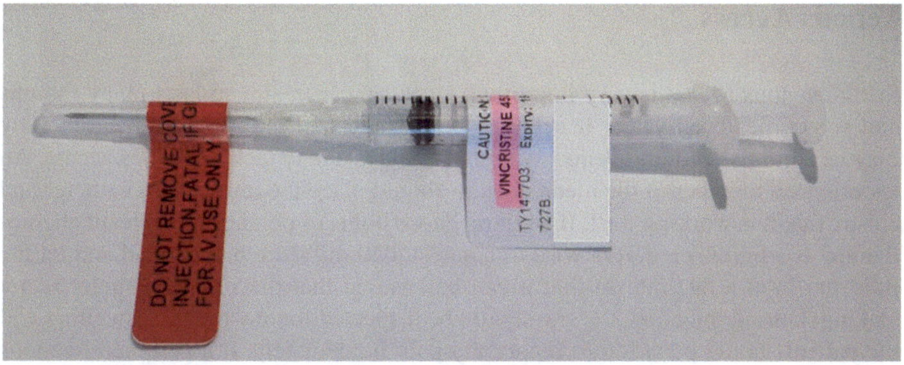

Fig. 23.3 Syringes with vincristine should be clearly marked with a bright colored sticker to prevent inadvertent intrathecal administration

and methotrexate are administered on the same day. The utmost care should be taken not to administer vincristine intrathecally, since that is invariably fatal. The vincristine should be kept separate in a different plastic bag or container and should be marked clearly with a bright colored sticker (Fig. 23.3).

Staff handling chemotherapy should be adequately trained in the correct handling of these drugs. Gloves not penetrable by chemotherapy should be worn. If chemotherapy-impenetrable gloves are not available, double latex gloves may be used. Tablets should not be crushed or manipulated in open areas. If a chemotherapy drug is spilled, it should be cleaned immediately. If it should come into contact with the skin or eyes, the affected area should be washed or rinsed immediately. Bodily secretions should be handled correctly and disposed of in the chemotherapy waste bin. Parents should also be taught how to handle oral chemotherapy and bodily secretions appropriately at home.

Some drugs require concomitant intravenous fluids (hyperhydration), such as cyclophosphamide, ifosfamide, intravenous methotrexate, high-dose cytarabine (≥ 1 g/m^2) and cisplatinum. Mesna is usually given together with ifosfamide (and sometimes cyclophosphamide) in order to prevent hemorrhagic cystitis. Leukovorin is given after a methotrexate infusion to supply substrate for folate production in order to rescue normal cells. Urine alkylinization when methotrexate is administered, is used to limit renal failure induced by methotrexate. Lubricating eye drops and piridoxine are given together with high-dose cytarabine to prevent toxicity.

A patient receiving an infusion of a chemotherapeutic drug, or who has received a drug intrathecally or intramuscularly, should be observed very carefully for signs of anaphylaxis, hypotension, fever, fluid overload, hematuria, nausea, and vomiting or any other side-effect. Most units provide conscious sedation for the administration of intrathecal chemotherapy, since children need to have this painful procedure multiple times. Each unit should thus have a protocol for the care of patients who receive sedation.

Venous Access

Secure venous access is very important, since cancer treatment lasts many months and sometimes even years. It needs to be ensured that intravenous chemotherapy may be administered intravenously without delays due to lack of venous access. An experienced member of the medical team should place the intravenous catheter and ensure that it is working well. If an intravenous bolus of potentially vesicant chemotherapy is administered, it is wise to connect a 50 millilitre bag of fluid and let the fluid run in at a fast rate so that it can be ensured that the venous catheter is not leaking. During injection, the site should be inspected for any redness, swelling and the patient should be asked to report any pain immediately. If a peripheral venous catheter is in situ for several days, it should be inspected often for any signs of thrombophlebitis or leaking.

For patients with poor venous access, it may be advisable to insert a central venous catheter (CVC). A jugular, subclavian or femoral central venous pressure (CVP) line may be inserted if short periods of venous access are needed or while the placement of a CVC is being awaited. Another short-stay option is a peripherally inserted central catheter (PICC) line. The most commonly used CVCs however, are Broviac lines and portocaths or ports. Broviac lines exit the chest wall anteriorly and thus breach the skin barrier. A port is completely submerged under the skin. For this reason, the risk of infection is lower with a port. Port needles are very expensive though and this may limit the use of ports in developing countries. All central catheters must be handled in a sterile manner.

Chemotherapy Toxicity

The medical team must know the side-effect profile of each chemotherapy agent very well in order to prevent, monitor, and recognize adverse events.

Bone marrow suppression is the main and most important side-effect; also the most common cause for delays in chemotherapy administration. The drugs most frequently causing myelosuppression in Pediatric oncology is shown in Table 23.3. The severity of myelosuppression is influenced by the dose of the chemotherapy agent, bone marrow reserve, intensity of the treatment protocol, and individual pharmacokinetics. The lowest peripheral blood counts are usually seen 7–10 days after administration of chemotherapy. Leukopenia, specifically neutropenia, predisposes the patient to infection with the highest risk for neutropenia below 0.5×10^9/L and extended periods of neutropenia. Granulocyte colony stimulating factor (GCSF) may be used in selected cases of febrile neutropenia or as part of some treatment protocols to prevent neutropenia and treatment delays. Anemia and thrombocytopenia may require supportive blood- and blood-product transfusions.

Nausea and vomiting are common if no preventative anti-emetic therapy is given. The mechanism of nausea and vomiting is stimulation of the serotonin (5-hydroxy-

Table 23.3 Chemotherapy drugs with a high potential of hematopoietic toxicity

Actinomycin D	Idarubicin
Cytarabine	Ifosfamide
Busulfan	Mercaptopurine
Carboplatin	Mitoxantrone
Cisplatin	Nitrosureas
Cyclophosphamide	Teniposide
Daunorubicin	Thioguanine
Doxorubicin	
Dacarbazine	
Etoposide	
Hydroxyurea	

Table 23.4 Emetogenic potential of chemotherapy agents used in treating childhood cancers (HD=high dose)

Level of emetogenic risk	Percentage of patients who experience nausea and vomiting (%)	Drugs
Level 4 (high)	>90	Cisplatin, HD cyclophosphamide, Dacarbazine, Dactinomycin
Level 3 (moderate)	30–90	Carboplatin, Cyclophosphamide, Daunorubicin, Doxorubicin, Idarubicin, Ifosfamide, HD Cytarabine (Ara C), Epirubicin, Irinotecan
Level 2 (Low)	10–30	Cytarabine, Etoposide, Gemcitabine, Methotrexate, Mitoxantrone, Paclitaxel, Topotecan
Level 1 (Minimal)	<10	Vinblastine, Vincristine, Vinorelbine, Fludarabine, Bleomycin, 2-Chlorodeoxyadenosine, Rituximab

tryptamine) receptors at the level of the vagal and splanchnic nerves. Inhibitors of these receptors, such as ondansetron and granisetron, are very effective anti-emetic agents. Table 23.4 lists chemotherapy drugs with varying emetogenicity.

Other common side-effects include temporary hair loss, mucositis (Table 23.5), diarrhea, constipation, and abdominal and bone pain. Other toxicities include renal, neurological (Table 23.6), hepatic, pulmonary (Table 23.7) and cardiac side-effects, as well as skin manifestations. The routes of elimination, some drug interactions, precautions and side-effects are summarized in Table 23.8.

Gonadal toxicity that may lead to infertility is observed especially with alkylating agents. It is dose-dependent and is more readily seen in boys.

Table 23.5 Chemotherapy drugs causing mucositis

Actinomycin D	Fluorouracil
Cytarabine	Idarubicin
Busulfan	Ifosfamide
Bleomycin	Methotrexate
Cyclophosphamide	Mercaptopurine
Daunorubicin	
Doxorubicin	Mitoxantrone
Epirubicin	Nitrosureas
Etoposide	Procarbazine
Etoposide	Thioguanine
Hydroxyurea	

Table 23.6 Chemotherapy drugs with a potential for neurological toxicity

Cytarabine	Nitrosureas
Asparaginase	Pentostatine
Carboplatin	Procarbazine
Cisplatin	Tretinoin
Fluorouracil	Vinblastine
Ifosfamide	Vincristine
Interferon	Vinorelbine
Methotrexate	

Table 23.7 Chemotherapy drugs with a potential for pulmonary toxicity

ATRA	Ifosfamide
Cytarabine	Mercaptopurine
Azathioprine	Methotrexate
Bleomycin	Melphalan
Busulfan	Nitrosureas
Cyclophosphamide	Procarbazine
Etoposide	Vincristine
	Vinblastine

Secondary cancers may occur following treatment with alkylating agents, epipodophyllotoxins and anthracyclines. The risk is higher in association with radiotherapy. Secondary cancers usually occur 5 years after treatment.

Summary

- Chemotherapy should be given according to a standard treatment protocol after a definitive diagnosis has been made.
- It must preferably be administered in a pediatric oncology unit by trained healthcare workers.
- The main mechanisms of action are interference in cell division and DNA synthesis, as well as induction of cell apoptosis.

Table 23.8 Main chemotherapy agents (drug pamphlets should still be consulted for complete information)

Drug	Mechanism of action/metabolism	Major side-effects	Precautions/Drug Interactions
Alkylating agents			
Cyclophosphamide	Activation in the liver by oxidative microsomal P450; metabolites include acrolein which causes bladder toxicity. Urinary excretion	Myelosuppression Hemorrhagic cystitis Headache Nausea/vomiting Alopecia Stomatitis Sterility More rarely: Inappropriate ADH (SIADH) Secondary cancer	Prevention of cystitis by good diuresis. At high doses: preventative administration of Mesna Phenobarbital, phenytoin, and other drugs that stimulate hepatic P450 may increase toxicity. Digoxin levels are reduced by cyclophosphamide
Dacarbazine (DTIC)	Activation in the liver by oxidative microsomal P450. Especially urinary elimination Action not phase-dependent	Myelosuppression, Nausea/vomiting Pain at injection site Alopecia, photosensitivity Rarely: Diarrhea, stomatitis, thrombosis, anaphylaxis	Phenobarbital, phenytoin, and other drugs that stimulate hepatic P450 reduces the effectiveness of dacarbazine
Ifosfamide	Activation in the liver by oxidative microsomal P450; metabolites include acrolein (bladder toxicity) and chloroacetaldehyde (neurological toxicity). Urinary excretion	Myelosuppression, hemorrhagic cystitis Neurotoxicity: dizziness, confusion, ataxia, lethargy and rarely coma nausea/vomiting, alopecia Stomatitis Urticaria, Hyperpigmentation, Renal tubular acidosis, SIADH	Cystitis: Prevent by hyperhydration and Mesna Phenobarbital and phenytoin increase toxic metabolites. Cimetidine and allopurinol increases the toxicity of ifosfamide
Nitrosureas	Effect is cycle-independent Fat-soluble molecules with good brain penetration	Myelosuppression, Nausea/vomiting Stomatitis, esophagitis, alopecia, interstitial lung disease Dizziness, ataxia	Cimetidine reduces the degradation of the nitrosureas
Procarbazine	Activation in the liver by oxidative microsomal P450. Hepatic degradation and urinary elimination	Myelosuppression, nausea/vomiting, flu-like symptoms, Hypersensitivity, hyperpigmentation Rarely neuropsychiatric disorders, photophobia, papilledema	Hypertension, Fever, convulsion if association with tricyclic antidepressants

(continued)

Table 23.8 (continued)

Drug	Mechanism of action/metabolism	Major side-effects	Precautions/Drug Interactions
Cisplatinum	Long plasma half-life (close to 3 days) and remain several months in tissues. Mainly urinary excretion	Renal toxicity Peripheral neuropathy Ototoxicity Nausea/vomiting Hypokalemia, hypomagnesemia	Hyperhydration Monitoring of creatinine, electrolytes (magnesium, calcium) Inhibits the elimination of bleomycin, etoposide, methotrexate, and ifosfamide Other nephrotoxic agents (e.g., amikacin) increase the risk of nephrotoxicity
Carboplatin	Half-life 2–3 hours Urinary excretion	Myelosuppression Nausea/vomiting Peripheral neuropathy, Ototoxicity Hypersensitivity reaction	Adjust dose according to creatinine clearance: Creat clearance ≥60 mL/min: dose = 360 mg/m^2 Creat Clearance 41–59 mL/min: Dose = 250 mg/m^2 Creat clearance ≥16–40 mL/min: dose = 200 mg/m^2
Antimetabolites			
Cytosine arabinoside (Ara C)	Urinary excretion	Myelosuppression Nausea/vomiting Mucositis, diarrhea, Arachnoiditis (intrathecal injection) Neurotoxicity (lethargy, confusion, ataxia) Conjunctivitis AraC syndrome: fever, myalgia, flu-like symptoms, bone pain, and maculopapular rash	Prevention of conjunctivitis by eye drops (for high-dose AraC) Hyperhydration for high dose AraC Higher risk of pancreatitis in association with L-asparaginase Toxicity increases if association with cisplatinum, hydroxyurea, and methotrexate Causes reduced effectiveness of gentamycin and digoxin

(continued)

Table 23.8 (continued)

Drug	Mechanism of action/metabolism	Major side-effects	Precautions/Drug Interactions
5-Fluorouracil	Half-life 10–20 min, mainly hepatic degradation	Myelosuppression, mucositis, diarrhea. Conjunctival irritation, photosensitivity, pigmentation of the infusion site veins, neurological disorders	Toxicity is increased if given together with leucovorin, methotrexate, trimetrexate Allopurinol inhibits the activation of the fluorouracyl and reduces its effectiveness
Hydroxyurea	Crosses the blood–brain barrier Short half-life Urinary elimination	Myelosuppression, Sometimes nausea and vomiting, mucositis, diarrhea Skin rash, erythema, Hyperpigmentation Alopecia	
6-Mercaptopurine (6MP)	6 MP is slowly degraded in the liver, mainly by xanthine oxidase	Myelosuppression Anorexia, nausea, vomiting, reversible cholestasis, photosensitivity	Allopurinol (xanthine oxidase inhibitor) may cause increased toxicity
Methotrexate (MTX)	Elimination is mainly urinary The half-life is 8–10 hours Significantly slower elimination in the case of effusion, leading to greater toxicity	Myelosuppression, stomatitis, renal failure At high dose: nausea, vomiting, renal tubular necrosis Acute encephalopathy, chronic leucoencephalopathy Intrathecal: aseptic meningitis, myelopathy, and encephalopathy	Folinic acid is an inhibitor of MTX. It is routinely given together with alkaline hyperhydration to reduce the toxicity of high-dose MTX Drugs carried by albumin (sulfonamides, aspirin, etc.) increase the free form of MTX and its toxicity L-Asparaginase and thymidine inhibit the activity of MTX Nonsteroidal anti-inflammatory drugs, penicillin, cephalosporins, phenytoin, and probenecid decreased renal excretion of MTX and increase the toxicity Trimethoprim is also an inhibitor of dihydrofolate reductase and may also increase the risk of toxicity. Should thus be avoided in the week of MTX administration

(continued)

Table 23.8 (continued)

Drug	Mechanism of action/metabolism	Major side-effects	Precautions/Drug Interactions
6-Thioguanine (6TG)	6-TG is degraded in the liver regardless of xanthine oxidase	Myelosuppression Stomatitis, diarrhea Nausea/vomiting Sinusoidal obstruction syndrome	
Anti-mitotic antibiotic			
Actinomycin D	Relative long half-life Biliary and urinary excretion	Myelosuppression Nausea/vomiting Alopecia Acne Hyperpigmentation Mucositis Rarely: hepatitis, anaphylaxis	
Bleomycin	Urinary excretion	Lung disease that can lead to fibrosis, especially in association with radiotherapy Hypersensitivity: fever, chills, pruritus, urticaria Hyperpigmentation and skin lesions Anorexia, mucositis	Phenothiazines increase the toxicity of bleomycin by competition at the level of the microsomal P450 Radiation therapy and oxygen increase pulmonary toxicity
Anthracyclines (Daunorubicin, doxorubicin, Idarubicin, Epirubicin, Mitoxantrone)	Quickly metabolized by the liver Also biliary excretion Some chromogenic derivatives are eliminated by the kidney sometimes giving a reddish color to the urine	Myelosuppression Congestive cardiomyopathy related to the formation of free radicals Cardiotoxicity is cumulative dose-dependent Mitoxantrone is less cardiotoxic Alopecia Nausea/vomiting	Cardioprotection by dexrazoxan may be considered when higher cumulative doses are used. Monitor left ventricular ejection fraction 6-MP increases the risk of hepatotoxicity

(continued)

Table 23.8 (continued)

Drug	Mechanism of action/metabolism	Major side-effects	Precautions/Drug Interactions
Spindle poisons			
Vinblastine, Vincristine, Vindesine, Vinorelbine	Vinorelbine is a semisynthetic derivative of vinblastine Activation in the liver by oxidative microsomal P450 Hepatic degradation and essentially biliary excretion	More frequent and more severe neurological toxicity with vincristine: Hypoesthesia, paresthesia, areflexia, mandibular pain, constipation that can evolve into paralytic ileus, optic atrophy, convulsion Moderate leukopenia especially with vinorelbine Rarely: nausea, vomiting, SIADH	Phenobarbital, calcium channel blockers, cimetidine, metoclopramide and drugs inhibiting P450 liver increase the production of metabolites. Vincristine reduces the level of phenytoin and digoxin. Filgastrim, administered concomitantly increase the risk of neuropathy L-asparaginase reduces the clearance of vincristine and must be administered 12–24 hours after vincristine
Inhibitors of topoisomerases			
Etoposide (VP16) Teniposide (VM26)	It is carried by albumin and may have greater toxicity in the case of hypoalbuminemia Hepatic metabolism and urinary excretion	Myelosuppression Nausea/vomiting Alopecia	Intravenous infusion must be given over an hour to avoid hypotension Concomitant administration of calcium channel blockers or methotrexate increases the toxicity of VP16
Topotecan	Topotecan undergoes activation in the plasma Urinary elimination	Myelosuppression Nausea/vomiting Alopecia Arthralgia Abdominal pain, microscopic hematuria	

(continued)

Table 23.8 (continued)

Drug	Mechanism of action/metabolism	Major side-effects	Precautions/Drug Interactions
Other agents			
L-asparaginase	Enzyme extracted from Escherichia coli or Erwinia chrysanthemi Short half-life No liver metabolism or renal elimination	Allergic reactions (chills, skin rash, urticaria, fever, laryngeal spasm, anaphylactic shock) usually occurring within 1 hour following administration More common in the case of intravenous injection Neurological disorder (cerebral thrombosis) Disorders of hemostasis (Deficiency of antithrombin, protein C and S) Nausea/vomiting Pancreatitis Hepatitis	In case of allergy it is recommended to use Asparaginase extracted from Erwinia chrysanthemi L ' Asparaginase blocks the action of methotrexate L-asparaginase reduces the clearance of vincristine and must be administered 12–24 hours after
All-trans retinoic acid (ATRA)	Indicated in acute promyelocytic leukemia Induces differentiation of promyelocytes into normal myelocytes Metabolism at the level of the hepatic P450 system Urinary and digestive elimination	ATRA syndrome: Leukocytosis, dyspnea, fever, pulmonary infiltrates, weight gain, pleurisy, pericarditis Toxicity of vitamin A: fever, headache, dryness mucocutaneous, cutaneous rash, conjunctivitis. Hypercholesterolemia	In case of ATRA syndrome: corticosteroids Drug interactions with drugs inhibiting or stimulating the hepatic cytochrome P450 system
Imatinib Dasatinib	Hepatic metabolism and eliminated primarily in the stool	Myelosuppression Nausea/vomiting Water retention: peri-orbital edema, pleurisy	Plasma levels changed by drugs affecting hepatic CYP3A4 (cyclosporine, ketoconazole, itraconazole)

- Depending on their mechanism of action, the main classes of agents are the alkylating agents, antimetabolites, topoisomerase inhibitors, anthracyclines, spindle poisons, and other.
- Chemotherapy agents are highly toxic and should be handled with care by medical staff who has taken the necessary precautions when handling these drugs.
- Measures to prevent or limit toxicity include hyperhydration, urine alkalinization, and the administration of leukovorin, mesna, lubricating eye drops and pyridoxine.
- Patients should be monitored carefully for acute and long-term side-effects.
- The main acute side-effects are myelosuppression, nausea and vomiting, mucositis, diarrhea, constipation, abdominal and bone pain and temporary hair loss.
- Long-term toxicity is to be taken into consideration and include infertility and the risk of a second cancer.
- Newer chemotherapy drugs have less toxicity, since they specifically target tumor cells.

Suggested Reading

Adamson PC, Bagatelli R, Balis FM, Blaney SM (2014) General principles of chemotherapy. In: Pizzo PA, Poplack GD (eds) Principles and practices of paediatric oncology, 6th edn. Lippincott Williams & Wilkins, Philadelphia, pp 279–355

http://chemoth.com/types

Neuss MN, Polovich M, McNiff K, Gilmore TR, LeFebvre KB, Schulmeister L, Jacobson JO (2013) Updated American Society of Clinical Oncology/Oncology Nursing Society Chemotherapy Administration Safety Standards Including Standards for the Safe Administration and Management of Oral Chemotherapy. Oncol Nurs Forum 40(3):225–233

Safe handling of hazardous chemotherapy drugs in limited-resource settings (2013). A WHO and PAHO publication. www.paho.org

Taşkin-Tok T, Gowder S Anticancer drug—friend or foe. Chapter 9. http://www.intechopen.com/books/pharmacology-and-therapeutics

Chapter 24
Febrile Neutropenia

Case Presentation

A 2-year-old boy known with acute lymphoblastic leukemia (ALL), presented with a 1-day history of fever, 7 days after completing the induction phase of chemotherapy. His mother also reported lesions in his mouth and refusal to eat.

Findings on Examination

The patient appeared irritable and acutely ill.

Weight: 14 kg; Height: 85 cm.

Observations: temperature 38.7 °C, pulse rate 125/min, respiratory rate 33/min, oxygen saturation 98 % in room air.

Pallor was present and ulcers were seen on his tongue and buccal mucosa.

There was no lymphadenopathy, but petechiae were noted on his trunk and limbs; no active bleeding was present. He was mildly dehydrated.

Respiratory examination: except for mild tachypnea, no other abnormalities were noted.

Abdominal and neurological examinations were normal, except for the irritability.

What Is Your Initial Diagnosis Based on the Available Information?

A 2-year-old boy, post-ALL induction (expected to be neutropenic at this stage), with fever, mucositis, anemia, and most likely thrombocytopenia.

D.C. Stefan, M. Harif, *Pediatric Cancer in Africa*,
DOI 10.1007/978-3-319-17936-0_24

What Other Information (History, Clinical, or Other) Is Important to Obtain to Make a Complete Assessment?

Does this patient have a central venous catheter (CVC) in situ?
Has he had exposure to someone with an infection and if so, which type of infection?
Any recent infection and antibiotic use, while receiving induction chemotherapy?
When was he discharged from hospital, i.e. could this be a hospital-acquired infection?
What medication is he currently taking?
What is his cardiovascular status: blood pressure, adequate peripheral circulation (capillary refill time, warm peripheries, pulse volume, etc.)?
Ask his mother for a recall of oral intake and urine output over the last 24 h.
Is he indeed neutropenic or not?

His full blood count showed the following:

WCC	Neutro	Lymph	Hb	Plt	Na	K	Urea	Creat	CRP
1.9	0.43	1.0	7	19	138	3.8	9	55	255

What Is the Most Likely Diagnosis Now?

ALL post-induction phase
Febrile neutropenia
Pancytopenia
Mucositis
Mild dehydration with pre-renal failure picture on biochemistry

Which Special Investigations Should Be Performed in Cases of Febrile Neutropenia?

Full blood and differential count
Infective markers—C-reactive protein (CRP) or procalcitonin (PCT)
Blood cultures—peripheral and from central venous catheter
Urine dipstix—urine culture if clinically indicated or if dipstix abnormal
Urea, creatinine, and electrolytes
Blood cross-match (patient is pale, has a tachycardia and fever; so a transfusion may be indicated)

The following should be performed only if indicated by history or clinical examination:

Stool culture (MCS, viruses, and parasites)—if diarrhea or dysentery present
Chest X-ray—if signs of a lower respiratory tract infection

Table 24.1 Classification of neutropenia

Mild	$1–1.49 \times 10^9$/L
Moderate	$0.5–0.99 \times 10^9$/L
Severe	$<0.5 \times 10^9$/L

Lumbar puncture—if signs and/or symptoms of meningitis/encephalitis
Echocardiogram—if signs of infective endocarditis

How Is Neutropenia Classified and What Is the Definition of Febrile Neutropenia in Children?

For the diagnosis of febrile neutropenia, severe neutropenia needs to be present (Table 24.1).

Fever:

There are several definitions of fever. The most common definitions used in febrile neutropenia are:

1. A sustained temperature of ≥38 °C for at least 1 h duration more than once in 24 h, or a single oral temperature of >38.3 °C
2. Two consecutive temperatures of ≥38 °C for 2 h or an oral temperature of ≥38.5 °C

What are the risk factors and pathophysiology of febrile neutropenia in children?

A functional immune system is made up of the innate and the humoral (or adaptive) immune systems. The innate system includes physical barriers (skin and mucosa), phagocytic cells, and cytokine responses, while the humoral (adaptive) component refers to the T-lymphocyte-mediated immune system, where specific pathogens are targeted. Both these systems are affected by the malignancy itself and/or the treatment.

Humoral (Adaptive) System

Besides causing reduced erythropoiesis and megakaryopoiesis, hematological malignancies and bone marrow infiltration caused by solid tumors, also result in reduced production of functional white blood cells (phagocytic cells and lymphocytes). Chemotherapeutic agents and radiotherapy cause further bone marrow suppression of all cell lines, aggravating the immune deficiency.

The resultant neutropenia leads to abnormal (inadequate) phagocytosis and the lymphopenia causes an abnormal pathogen-specific response (generated by T-lymphocytes) with an increased risk for viral and bacterial infections.

Innate System

Because chemotherapeutic agents act on all rapidly dividing cells, it results in impaired mucosal function and mucosal lesions, therefore, causing a breach in the mucosal barrier and increasing the risk of bacterial invasion. Overgrowth of intestinal flora further increases the risk of acquiring an infection.

The use of indwelling central venous catheters disrupts the skin and is a foreign body, therefore increasing the susceptibility to bacterial infections in particular.

Most children with cancer in developing countries are malnourished, which further reduces the immune function (both innate and humoral (adaptive) systems). Children with HIV infection are of course, also immune suppressed because of the presence of the virus.

The patient's cardiovascular examination reveals good peripheral circulation with warm peripheries, a good capillary refill time of 2 s and a blood pressure of 110/65 mmHg.

Should he be admitted to hospital? (Motivate your answer).

Yes, all children with febrile neutropenia in developing countries should be admitted to hospital. Febrile neutropenia is a medical emergency with a high mortality rate if not managed appropriately.

This patient most likely has severe neutropenia after the ALL induction; he also has mucositis, thus the risk for infection is very high and empiric intravenous antibiotics should be initiated for febrile neutropenia. Since he has mild dehydration and his oral intake is reduced, he will also require intravenous fluids and/or nasogastric feeding.

In developed countries, some low-risk cases of febrile neutropenia are treated on an outpatient basis. This can only be done if appropriate monitoring can take place at home, if appropriate oral antibiotics are available, and the caregivers have transport to return to hospital should the child worsen.

Which Other Systemic Areas/Sites Should Specifically Be Examined and Why?

Skin: cellulitis, rash (maculopapular, petechial,or vesicular), wound infection, thrombophlebitis

Nails: fungal or other infection

Perineum and perianal area: anal fissure, cellulitis, or abscess

Central venous catheter site: signs of tunnel/exit site infection

Ear, nose, and throat: signs of an upper respiratory tract infection (otitis media and sinusitis) should be sought, the oropharynx should be examined for the presence of a dental abscess, as well as mucositis (erythema, ulcers)

Respiratory: signs of a lower respiratory tract infection (tachypnea, respiratory distress, cyanosis). Be aware of Pneumocystis jerovecii pneumonia, especially if the patient was not on trimethoprim/sulphamethoxazole (Bactrim) prophylaxis

Cardiovascular: signs of infective endocarditis, especially if a central line is present
Gastrointestinal: signs of *Clostridium difficile* colitis or typhlitis
Urogenital: pyelonephritis or perirenal abscess
Neurological: signs of a meningitis or shunt infection, if shunt is present

What will your initial management be?

The patient should be nursed in strict isolation, as far as possible, to prevent spread of the existing infection and to prevent a hospital-acquired infection. He should have at least 4-hourly observations taken, with clear instructions to the nurse when the doctor should be called for abnormalities, e.g., hypotension, tachypnea, etc. The patient should ideally also be regularly assessed by a doctor, since septicemia may progress rapidly.

Intake and output, as well as hydration and circulatory status should be assessed often. A soft, bland diet should be offered (including cold foods such as ice cream and yoghurt) as well as oral nutritional supplements. If the patient continues to refuse oral intake, nasogastric feeding should be commenced. Intravenous fluid may be necessary in case the dehydration worsens or the oral or nasogastric fluids are not tolerated.

Adequate analgesia should be provided: the WHO pain ladder should be followed by giving paracetamol first, followed by weak opioids (tilidine, codeine) and stronger opioids (morphine) if paracetamol alone is ineffective. Other alternatives include clonidine and ketamine. Tilidine is given sublingually and is highly effective, but may cause a burning sensation in the mouth because of the mucosal lesions. Unfortunately the availability of tilidine is currently limited in some countries. Nonsteroidal anti-inflammatory agents should preferably be avoided, because of a risk of potential platelet dysfunction.

A mouth wash should be used regularly: normal saline or a chlorhexidine mouthwash (e.g., Andolex). Strongly consider adding aciclovir, since herpes simplex virus is often found in patients with mucositis.

Broad spectrum intravenous antibiotics should be started as soon as possible; the choice will depend on the individual unit's microbiological audit results. Initially, gram-positive and gram-negative organisms should be covered by the antibiotic regimen. An example of an empiric regimen would be a beta-lactam antibiotic with *Pseudomonas* cover (such as piperacillin/tazobactam) and an aminoglycoside (e.g., amikacin). Monotherapy with ceftazidine or cefepime may also be chosen.

The patient has a Broviac line in situ. *Would this change your choice of antibiotic therapy?*

If there are signs of a tunnel infection (erythema, induration, and tenderness of the skin overlying the tunnel), vancomycin should be added to treat a possible methicillin-resistant Staphylococcus aureus infection. Infection of the exit site should also be treated as such. The vancomycin could be downscaled to a more appropriate antibiotic once the antibiotic sensitivity profile is known.

If a tunnel infection is present, the line should be removed as soon as possible. In the case of a superficial exit site infection, the line may be kept in situ, provided that the patient is improving.

After 48 h the patient still has an oral temperature of 38 °C. The oral lesions have improved and he has a good oral intake.

What would your management be now?

Do a thorough clinical examination looking for a source of infection. This should be performed daily in any patient with febrile neutropenia. Bear in mind that an abscess may be difficult to identify, since patients with severe neutropenia are unable to form puss. The following blood tests should be repeated: full blood and differential counts, blood culture (both peripheral and central) and CRP and/or procalcitonin. Other cultures may be performed based on (new) clinical findings.

Because he shows clinical improvement, the results of the investigations can be awaited before making a change to the antibiotic regimen. However, if there is no improvement in the clinical condition and fever persists, vancomycin should be added after 48 h, or earlier, if the suspicion of a staphylococcal infection is raised. An antifungal agent should be empirically added after 72 h, or earlier, in the case where a fungal infection is suspected. The choice of an antifungal agent would depend on local sensitivities.

If the patient clinically deteriorates or develops signs of septicemia at any time, the antibiotics should immediately be changed to cover for resistant organisms and/or hospital-acquired organisms, e.g. meropenem or ciprofloxacin.

For an overview of the spectrum of organisms covered by commonly used antibiotics see Table 24.2, and for suggested antibiotic choices for specific clinical scenarios, see Table 24.3. Table 24.4 shows the organisms most commonly encountered in febrile neutropenia.

Table 24.2 Overview of spectrum of organisms covered by antibiotics commonly used in pediatric oncology (neg-negative; pos-positive)

Class	Agent	Spectrum	Doses
Antibiotics			
Cephalosporins	Ceftriaxone	Gram-neg bacilli (including *Pseudomonas aeruginosa*)	100 mg/kg/day once daily dose (Max 2 g)
	Ceftazidime	Gram-neg bacilli (including *Pseudomonas aeruginosa*) and Gram-pos	100 mg/kg/day IV in 3 divided doses (Max 6 g)
Carbapenem	Imipenem	Gram-neg bacilli	50 mg/kg/day IV in 4 divided doses (Max 4 g)
	Meropenem	Gram-neg and -pos bacilli Anaerobic organisms	20 mg/kg 8 hourly or 40 mg/kg 12 hourly for severe infection

(continued)

Table 24.2 (continued)

Class	Agent	Spectrum	Doses
Aminoglycosides	Amikacin	Gram-neg bacilli	1 wk–10 years: 25 mg/kg day 1, then 18 mg/kg/day. >10 years: 20 mg/kg day 1, then 15 mg/kg/day (Max 1 g)
Glycopeptides	Vancomycin	Gram-pos cocci	25 mg/kg stat, then 15–20 mg/kg 8 hourly (Max 3 g)
Extended spectrum penicillin	Piperacillin and Tazobactim	Gram-neg bacilli Anaerobic organisms	>9 months: 100 mg/kg 8 hourly (Max 3.375 g per dose)
Antifungals			
Amphotericin B	Amphotericin B	Extended spectrum	0.1 mg/kg IV test dose—then 0.6–1 mg/kg/day over 6–8 h
Triazoles	Fluconazole	*Candida*	10–12 mg/kg IV daily for systemic infection
Antiviral			
	Aciclovir	Herpes simplex	Immunodeficient patients: 4 wks–12 years: 500 mg/m^2 8 hourly; >12 years: 10 mg/kg 8 hourly Cutaneous herpes: 250 mg/m^2 (birth–12 years), 5 mg/kg 8 hourly IV
		Varicella zoster	400 mg (<2 years) or 800 mg (>2 years) 5× per day
	Ganciclovir	Cytomegalovirus, Herpes simplex, Varicella zoster, Human Herpes virus 6	5 mg/kg 12 hourly for 2–3 weeks, then 5 mg/kg daily
Anti-pneumocystis			
	Trimethoprim/sulphametoxazole	Pneumocystis jirovecii	20 mg/kg IV in 4 divided doses

Table 24.3 Suggested antibiotic choices for specific clinical problems

Scenario/problem	Choice of antibiotics
Always	ß-lactam active against *P. aeruginosa* ± aminoglycoside
Cellulitis around a catheter or other suspected staphylococcal infection	Add a glycopeptide
Perianal abscess, necrotic gingivitis or typhilitis	Add anaerobic cover (piperacillin, tazobactam, imipenem, third- or fourth-generation cephalosporin plus metronidazole)
Severe mucositis	Optimal coverage of streptococci + aciclovir
Cutaneous cellulitis	Optimal coverage of *S. aureus* and *P. aeruginosa*. If significant resistance rate to oxacillin in institution: add glycopeptide
Diarrhea	Toxin detection of *C. difficile* and add metronidazole

Table 24.4 Most common organisms associated with febrile neutropenia

Organism	Details	Common clinical spectrum
Gram-positive		
Staphylococci	Cocci in clusters	CVC infections, infective endocarditis
S. epidermidis	Catalase +, coagulase–, facultative anaerobe	Skin infections, septic arthritis, endocarditis, pneumonia
S. *aureus*	Cocci in clusters, catalase +, coagulase +	
α-hemolytic Strep (*S. pneumoniae*)	Gram-pos cocci in chains	Pneumonia, otitis media, sinusitis, meningitis
Enterococcus (*E. faecium*)	Cocci in pairs (diplococcic)/short chains Commensal organisms	Urinary tract infection, bacteremia, infective endocarditis, diverticulitis, meningitis
Bacillus (*B. cereus*)	Aerobic bacilli—spore-forming Heat-stable toxin	Food poisoning—vomiting 6 h after exposure
Clostridium (*C. difficile*)	Bacilli, obligate anaerobic, spore-forming Enterotoxin A & B	Pseudomembranous colitis, toxic megacolon, bowel perforation
Gram-negative		
Enterobacteriaceae		
E. coli	Rod, facultative anaerobe (gut flora) Some strains produce toxins	Urinary tract infection, gastroenteritis, septicemia
K. pneumoniae	Rod, facultative anaerobe, encapsulated (normal flora of skin, mouth, and intestine)	Hospital-acquired—ventilator-associated pneumonia, urinary tract infection, wound infection, and septicemia
Enterobacter	Rod, facultative anaerobe	Hospital-acquired pneumonia, wound sepsis, epticemia
Serratia	Rod, facultative anaerobe	Hospital-acquired pneumonia, wound sepsis, septicemia
P. aeruginosa	Bacillus, aerobic, environmental organism Human carriage increases with hospitalization	Septicemia, destructive skin complications (ecthyma gangrenosum) osteomyelitis, septic arthritis, meningitis
Stenotrophomonas maltophilia	Bacillus, normal environment soil and water colonize moist areas—ICU/immunocompromised	Septicemia, pneumonia
Anaerobes	Non-sporing anaerobes—endogenous (normal flora)	Generalized intra-abdominal sepsis after spontaneous perforation
Fungi		
Candida		Oral mucositis, pharyngitis, esophagitis, septicemia

(continued)

Table 24.4 (continued)

Organism	Details	Common clinical spectrum
Aspergillosis		Pneumonia—progressing to septicemia. Other sites—paranasal sinuses, skin, CNS and eye
Viruses		
Herpes simplex virus (HSV)		HSV-1 vesicular gingivostomatitis, pharyngitis, tonsillitis, keratoconjunctivitis, primary skin infection, encephalitis
Varicella		Chicken pox (varicella)—pneumonia, post-infectious encephalitis, shingles (recurrence)
Cytomegalovirus		Pneumonitis, retinitis, colitis
Epstein Barr virus (EBV)		Lymphadenopathy
Adeno		Pharyngitis, pharyngoconjunctival fever, pneumonia, pertussis-like syndrome, keratoconjunctivitis, hemorrhagic cystitis
Influenza		Flu, pneumonia
Parainfluenza		Flu, croup, bronchiolitis, bronchopneumonia, acute epiglottitis
Rotavirus		Diarrhea

Suggested Reading

Behrman RE, Kliegman RM, Jenson HB (2000) Nelson textbook of pediatrics. Part XVI. Infectious diseases, 16th edn. WB Saunders, Philadelphia, pp 793–986

Fever in children with chemotherapy-induced neutropenia. http://www.uptodate.com. Accessed 12 April 2015

Gea-Banacloche J (2013) Evidence-based approach to treatment of febrile neutropenia in hematologic malignancies. ASH Edu Book 2013(1):414–422

Hakim H, Flynn PM, Knapp KM, Srivastava DK, Gaur A (2009) Etiology and clinical course of febrile neutropenia in children with cancer. J Pediatr Hematol Oncol 31(9):623–629

Lehrnbecher T, Phillips R, Alexander S, Alvaro F, Carlkesse F, Fisher B et al (2012) Guideline for the management of fever and neutropenia in children with cancer and/or undergoing hematopoietic stem-cell transplantation. JCO 30(35):4427–4437

Chapter 25
Blood Transfusion in Pediatric Oncology

Case Presentation

Amina, a 5-year-old girl with a weight of 15 kg, was diagnosed with acute lymphoblastic leukemia. She presented with a fever of 40 °C, severe pallor, and petechiae on her lower limbs. On admission, her hemoglobin level was 5.5 g/dL, the platelet count was 12×10^9/L, and the white cell count 3×10^9/L.

Which blood products would you order and how much?
How should the transfusion be documented and monitored?

Cancer itself, and cancer treatment, are the main factors that lead to increased blood loss and impaired hematopoiesis. Very often, transfusion with blood products is lifesaving and an indispensable component of supportive care. Advances in supportive transfusion with blood products have significantly improved the management, outcome, and quality of life of children with cancer. However, transfusion is associated with an increased risk of morbidity and mortality when good practice rules regarding the choice of product, prescription, administration, and monitoring are not adhered to (Table 25.1). The decision regarding blood-product transfusion should always take into consideration the benefit/risk ratio for the patient.

From a pathophysiological perspective, anemia and thrombocytopenia may be caused by the following:

- Bone marrow infiltration by the tumor
- Antimitotic action of the chemotherapy and/or radiotherapy
- Blood loss from surgical procedures or tumor and non-tumor-related hemorrhage
- Or very occasionally an autoimmune phenomenon
- And focal or disseminated intravascular coagulation

D.C. Stefan, M. Harif, *Pediatric Cancer in Africa*,
DOI 10.1007/978-3-319-17936-0_25

Table 25.1 Important considerations and tasks before, during, and after transfusion

Stage of the transfusion procedure	Recommendations
Pretransfusion	*Consider*
	The primary diagnosis and any comorbid conditions
	The full blood count results
	The indication for the transfusion
	The urgency of the transfusion (life-threatening clinical situation, symptoms and signs of cardiac failure, ongoing blood loss, etc
	Tasks
	Obtain informed consent/assent
	Ensure compatibility testing is performed correctly (important that a specimen is obtained from the correct patient)
Order/prescription	*Tasks*
	Complete the blood order form meticulously
	Calculate the number of units required
	Prescription should include:
	Patient name, folder number, date of birth
	Time, date, and ward name
	Type of product and the number of units
	Duration and rate of transfusion
	Name and signature of the prescribing physician
Transportation	Blood products should be transported without delay in an insulated box containing ice packs for packed red blood cells, and without ice packs for platelets and fresh frozen plasma
Reception of product at the bedside	*Check*
	Transport conditions (temperature, duration, etc.)
	Type of product and expiration date
	Integrity of the product and appearance (e.g. color)
	Compatibility with the blood group of the recipient
Final pretransfusion control at the bedside	*Important checks for each product and unit*
	Patient name, date of birth, folder number (patient should state their own details if possible)
	Type of product
	Identification number on the product and the request form
	Patient blood group and Rh status
	Time and date of expiry
	The control card with the above information should be kept in the medical/nursing file of the patient (medicolegal implication)
During transfusion	Before starting the transfusion, the vital signs should be documented. After starting the transfusion, the patient should initially be monitored every 15 min; then every 30 min thereafter. All vital signs, as well as urine output must be recorded. Critically ill patients should be monitored every 15 min

(continued)

Table 25.1 (continued)

Stage of the transfusion procedure	Recommendations
After transfusion	*Documentation*
	Repeat all vital signs and document urinary output
	Complete the transfusion information sheets and record all incidents or reactions
	Report transfusion incidents or reactions immediately when it occurs
	Efficacy
	Assess the clinical effect of the transfusion
	Consider performing a ward Hb or full blood count/clotting profile if needed
In case of a transfusion reaction	Stop the transfusion immediately
	Change the drip set and infuse normal saline
	Notify a doctor immediately
	Record all vital signs and urinary output
	Repeat all identification and compatibility checks
	Provide supportive or definitive care depending on the severity of the reaction
	Notify the blood bank and return all blood products
	Complete the necessary notification forms and obtain the required blood samples from the patient

General Principles of Transfusion

Once a decision has been made that a transfusion is required, the doctor has the responsibility of explaining to the child (if he/she is old enough and able to understand) and/or to his parents the indication for, as well as the benefits and potential risks of the transfusion, and to obtain their consent and assent. The doctor should be able to justify the decision and be able to answer any questions about possible alternatives. This process should be documented in the patient file.

The entire healthcare team has the medicolegal responsibility of ensuring that compatibility testing was performed, and that the correct product was ordered and issued for the correct patient. Two appropriately qualified team members (a doctor and registered nurse or two registered nurses) should check the details on the blood product against the patient details at the bedside in order to ensure that the product is administered to the patient it was intended for. Information should be read aloud by one person and checked by the other. The expiry date of the product should also be checked prior to administration, as well as the quality of the product, e.g. temperature, color, etc. All these processes should also be documented on a pretransfusion chart. If any inconsistencies are noted, the blood bank should be informed and the product should be returned.

The transfusion should be initiated in an aseptic manner and should be infused via a blood recipient set (containing a filter) at the correct rate. The patient should then be monitored carefully and frequently (initially every 15 min; then every 30 min). Any reaction should be reported immediately and the transfusion should be stopped, after which supportive care or other treatment should be provided immediately. Furthermore, it is recommended that parallel administration of medications or fluids other than normal saline, calcium-free balanced salt solutions (Plasmalyte, Balsol, modified Ringer's lactate), 4 % albumin, plasma protein fractions and ABO-compatible plasma should be avoided if possible, otherwise a second intravenous line should be started.

Blood should be warmed when a massive transfusion is being administered (>50 mL/kg), when infants receive >15 mL/kg of a blood product, an exchange transfusion is performed, for patients with high-titre cold hemagglutinins and when transfusion occurs via a central line. A specific blood warming apparatus should be used; microwave oven heating may cause extensive hemolysis and can result in a disastrous and potentially fatal transfusion reaction.

In addition to the usual procedures for ordering, checking, and monitoring blood products, the presence of significant immunosuppression in the recipient calls for additional measures, including leukodepletion and irradiation of blood products.

Leukodepletion reduces the incidence of viral infection transmission (in particular cytomegalovirus (CMV)), platelet allo-immunisation, sensitization to transplant antigens in a pretransplant setting and febrile non-hemolytic transfusion reactions. Leukoreduction is recommended in all patients with cancer. Leukodepletion is performed routinely in developed countries, but is only available on request in most countries in Africa due to a significant additional cost. Patients on chronic transfusion programs, those at risk for CMV infection, infants, as well as critically ill, cardiac surgery or severe trauma patients should receive leukodepleted products.

Irradiation of blood products is recommended for patients with severe T-lymphocyte immunodeficiency syndromes, patients receiving a stem cell transplant (from the time of conditioning), before and after stem cell harvest for future autologous transplant, patients receiving HLA-selected platelets or donations from family members, patients with Hodgkin lymphoma, patients receiving fludarabine or cladribine and patients with aplastic anemia receiving anti-thymocyte globulin. This is done in order to prevent graft versus host reactions which may occur in patients with immunosuppression and where the donor and patient share an HLA haplotype. This reaction is mediated by the donor T lymphocytes that proliferate in the recipient and cause cellular damage. It may occur after the transfusion of packed cells, whole blood, granulocytes and platelets. In developing countries where access to radiotherapy is limited, irradiation of blood products is very challenging and sometimes impossible.

Transfusion of Specific Blood Products

Transfusion of Packed Cells

Anemia occurs very frequently in children with cancer and significantly contributes to a deterioration in their quality of life. The decision retransfusion should take into consideration the clinical tolerance of the anemia, existing comorbidities (in particular cardiac and respiratory disease), as well as the presence of risk factors such as hemorrhage and infection. Most guidelines advise to transfuse packed cells when the hemoglobin level is below 6–7 g/dL. If the hemoglobin is 6–8 g/dL and the patient appears to be symptomatic of the anemia (symptoms of anemia or signs of cardiac failure) or has risk factors as mentioned, a transfusion is also advised. If acute blood loss is estimated to be more than 30 % of the blood volume, packed cells should be ordered.

The quantity of blood to be transfused is a function of the actual hemoglobin level of the patient and the desired hemoglobin level. The amount of blood to be transfused is often estimated using the following formula: (desired hemoglobin—patient's hemoglobin) × weight (kg) × 3. The required volume of packed cells can also be calculated as 15–20 mL/kg and should then be rounded off to the unit of blood product closest in volume.

From another perspective, considering the hematocrit of the unit of packed cells to be transfused is usually around 55 %, 10 mL/kg of packed cells are expected to increase the patient's hemoglobin level by 2–2.5 g/dL in the absence of concomitant bleeding.

Transfusion with packed cells should be administered over 4–6 h, considering the amount of blood to be transfused, the mechanism of the anemia, as well as signs and symptoms of anemia. In anemia of slow onset, there is a risk of cardiocirculatory decompensation due to volume overload. Packed cells can usually be administered over 4 h, but in cases of potential volume overload, e.g. patients with symptoms and signs of cardiac failure, it should be administered over 6 h and care should be taken to monitor the fluid balance of the patient.

When *hyperleukocytosis* (a white cell count of 100×10^9/L and higher) is present, the increased blood viscosity may lead to leukostasis, which may impair the function of vital organs such as the lungs and brain. A transfusion with packed cells could aggravate this phenomenon by rapidly increasing the hematocrit and therefore the viscosity. Thus, in the case of hyperleukocytosis, transfusion with packed cells should only be considered when absolutely necessary, and should as far as possible be postponed until the white cell count is reduced through hyperhydration and definitive treatment of the cancer.

Washed red cells are used for patients who have developed severe allergic transfusion reactions which are not prevented by the administration of antihistamines prior to transfusion, patients with an IgA deficiency with anti-IgA antibodies present and neonates with necrotizing enterocolitis and exposed red cell T crypt antigen. Red cells which have been stored and irradiated should also be washed to avoid a high potassium concentration.

Whole Blood

Whole blood is rarely used and has to be fresh, otherwise the different components deteriorate rapidly and will result in an ineffective transfusion. The two indications are exchange transfusion in neonates and in cases of massive bleeding.

Platelet Transfusion

Thrombocytopenia also occurs commonly and imparts a risk of bleeding. The risk increases with the severity of thrombocytopenia, the presence of infection, clotting factor deficits due to liver involvement or disseminated intravascular coagulation, as well as factors related to the specific malignancy. Life-threatening hemorrhage is rarely observed when the platelet count is above $20 \times 10^9/L$.

The strategy of prophylactic platelet transfusion is still debatable. It is important to consider the benefits and risks, including the risk of infection and the risk of developing allo-immunization, which could lead to ineffective transfusions. Most authors recommend prophylactic transfusion when the platelet count is below $10 \times 10^9/L$. A higher transfusion threshold of $20 \times 10^9/L$ may be employed when infection, disseminated intravascular coagulation, or other risk factors are present.

The decision to transfuse platelets prior to invasive procedures is determined by the expected risk of bleeding. Platelet transfusion prior to a bone marrow aspiration and biopsy is not necessary, since compression is usually sufficient to obtain hemostasis.

There are different opinions regarding transfusion prior to a lumbar puncture. Most sources recommend a platelet count of at least $100 \times 10^9/L$ for a diagnostic lumbar puncture in acute lymphoblastic leukemia to avoid a traumatic tap and the risk of introducing blasts into the cerebrospinal fluid. Some institutions do not give platelet transfusions prior to a lumbar puncture, but most recommend a threshold of $20–30 \times 10^9/L$. For intramuscular injections, a platelet count of $20 \times 10^9/L$ is considered to be safe. The majority of invasive procedures can be performed safely with a platelet count of above $50 \times 10^9/L$. In the case of major surgery, neurosurgery or eye surgery however, it is recommended to transfuse platelets if the count is less than $100 \times 10^9/L$.

There are two types of platelet products available: a platelet concentrate derived from whole blood of five donors (pooled unit), which contains a minimum of 2.4×10^{11} platelets per unit and a platelet concentrate derived via apheresis from a single donor (apheresis or single donor unit), which contains $3–8 \times 10^{11}$ platelets per unit. An apheresis unit corresponds to 6–10 pooled units. Platelets can also be HLA-matched in cases of allo-immunization.

Platelet concentrates can be kept for 5 days at temperatures ranging from 20 to 24 °C, while being slowly agitated.

The usual recommended dose is 15–20 mL/kg, rounded off to the closest unit. Higher doses are justified in the case of severe bleeding. The efficacy of a platelet

Table 25.2 Measurement of the efficacy of platelet transfusion

Percent platelet recovery (PPR):
PPR = (PC postT−PC preT)($\times 10^9$/L) × blood volume (weight (kg) × blood volume (L)[a])/number of platelets transfused ($\times 10^9$/L) × 100
Corrected count increment (CCI):
CCI = (PC postT−PC preT) ($\times 10^9$/L) × BSA (m^2)/Number of platelets transfused ($\times 10^{11}$/L)

PC postT platelet count after transfusion (1–24 h), *PC preT* platelet count before transfusion, *BSA* body surface area in m^2

[a]Total blood volume = 0.08 L/kg for a child; 0.085 L/kg for a neonate. PPR: ineffective platelet transfusion if <30 %. CCI: ineffective platelet transfusion if <7500

transfusion depends on the initial platelet count and the presence or absence of concomitant platelet consumption and bleeding. The efficacy is assessed based on the clinical status of the patient and post-transfusion platelet count. If the latter is $<5 \times 10^9$/L or has not risen at all, the transfusion has been ineffective.

The efficacy of platelet transfusion can also be assessed by estimating the percent platelet recovery (PPR) or corrected count increment (CCI) which both takes into consideration the platelet count before and after the transfusion, as well as the count in the transfused unit (Table 25.2) and the posttransfusion platelet count. These formulas cannot be used if the platelet dose is unknown.

Ineffective transfusion can be due to excessive consumption during disseminated intravascular coagulation, severe bacterial or viral infection, splenomegaly or less often sinusoidal obstruction syndrome and graft versus host disease. Treatment with amphotericin B and other antibiotics such as vancomycin and sulphonamides can also lead to ineffective transfusion. Less commonly, it may be immune-modulated. ABO incompatibility can contribute to ineffectiveness, but more often this is due to antiplatelet or anti-HLA antibodies which are more likely to be present in patients who frequently receive platelet transfusions.

Platelets should be transfused rapidly, usually over 30 min, via a platelet administration set. Platelets should be group-specific as far as possible, but ABO nonidentical platelets may also be used if group-specific platelets are not available. Rh-D negative platelets should be administered to all girls; if not available, anti-D immunoglobulin should be given following platelet transfusion.

Fresh Frozen Plasma Transfusion

Fresh frozen plasma (FFP) contains all clotting factors and transfusion is thus indicated for certain isolated clotting factor deficiencies (factors VII, VIII, and IX deficiencies excluded). It is also used for warfarin reversal, disseminated intravascular coagulopathy, and vitamin K deficiency. The usual dose is 10–20 mL/kg. ABO compatibility is necessary to prevent reactions. Patients susceptible to fluid overload should be monitored carefully.

Cryoprecipitate

Cryoprecipitate is made by thawing FFP; it is the cold insoluble fraction of FFP. It contains factor VIII and von Willebrand factor, fibrinogen, fibronectin, and factor XIII. It only has a few indications: the treatment of hypofibrinogenemia (congenital or acquired) or dysfibrinogenemia, factor XIII deficiency and massive transfusion. The recommended dose is 5 mL/kg which should be rapidly infused.

Massive Blood Transfusion

The definition of massive blood loss is blood loss equal to one blood volume within 24 h, or 50 % blood volume loss over 3 h. If this is identified in a patient, the massive transfusion protocol of the local blood bank should be activated. This ensures rapid provision of different blood products. It usually includes group O emergency blood, FFP, and platelets. A hemoglobin level of 8–9 g/dL should be aimed for. If hypofibrinogenemia occurs (often due to dilution), cryoprecipitate should also be administered.

Complications of Blood Transfusion

Complications related to a blood product transfusion may be associated with short- or long-term mortality or morbidity. The term "transfusion reaction" refers to any potentially adverse sign or symptom that is noted after the start of a transfusion with any blood product. The mechanism of the adverse event may be immunologic or infectious in nature or related to volume overload. Strictly observing the rules of preparation, ordering, administration, and monitoring can prevent or facilitate early detection of these complications.

Hemolytic Accidents

Adverse events related to ABO incompatibility are severe and may result in significant mortality and morbidity. The recipient's immune system will react to ABO incompatible donor cells by producing IgG and IgM antibodies, as well as complement activation, which leads to rapid hemolysis. Clinically symptoms and signs may occur within 10–15 min of starting the transfusion. Severe pallor, anxiety, dyspnoea, fever, rigors, nausea, and vomiting, lower back or chest or flank pain occur, followed by oliguria, shock (hypotension), hemoglobinuria with renal failure and disseminated intravascular coagulation, depending on the amount of incompatible blood that was transfused, is usually noted.

Extravascular hemolytic reactions also occur after transfusion of incompatible blood when an atypical IgG antibody is present (e.g. anti-Kell and anti-Duffy). This reaction may be mild (only mild anemia and jaundice noted 2–10 days after transfusion) or severe (acute onset of anemia and jaundice).

If a hemolytic transfusion reaction is suspected, the transfusion should be stopped immediately, the infusion set changed and normal saline should be infused while a doctor is notified urgently. The patient details, known blood group and the blood group of the transfused product should be checked. The required blood specimens should be sent to the blood bank and the report form completed. A positive direct Coobs test confirms the immunologic nature of the accident. Other laboratory investigations will confirm hemolysis. If severe hemolysis is present, disseminated intravascular coagulation with or without renal failure may also develop. Supportive care should be provided and hemodialysis may be required in severe cases.

The outcome of acute hemolytic events depends on early diagnosis, which helps to limit the amount of incompatible blood transfused.

Transfusion-Related Respiratory Distress Syndrome

This syndrome, which is also known as TRALI (Transfusion-Related Acute Lung Injury), is a major cause of mortality and morbidity and is caused by leucoagglutinins in the donor plasma. This reaction is often not recognized and correctly diagnosed. It occurs a few hours after transfusion and is characterized by difficulty in breathing which can lead to respiratory distress and hypoxia requiring mechanical ventilation. Hypotension and fever may also be noted. The chest X-ray shows signs of pulmonary infiltration without vascular congestion. Corticosteroid therapy has no proven benefit; supportive care and ventilation, if needed, are advised. This complication fortunately seems to be rare in children.

Febrile Non-hemolytic Transfusion Reactions

This reaction is fairly commonly seen (especially in patients who have had multiple transfusions) and should be a diagnosis of exclusion. It develops due to pyrogenic cytokines released by recipient white cells. Leukodepletion has significantly reduced the incidence of this complication. Fever can occur during or within 1–2 h following the start of the transfusion. Headache, muscle aches, malaise, rigors, tachycardia, and hypertension may also be noted. The fever usually subsides after termination of the transfusion. Subsequent transfusions should be leukodepleted.

Allergic Reactions

Allergic reactions are due to the presence of allergens to plasma proteins in the donor's plasma. Histamine release takes place and variable clinical expression may occur, ranging from itching or urticaria to angioedema or cardiorespiratory involvement. It is most commonly seen with plasma transfusion and less often during platelets transfusion. The transfusion should be stopped immediately, infusion set changed and normal saline administered. The usual reaction protocol should be followed. Antihistamines may be administered.

Anaphylactic reactions are more severe and may be related to IgA deficiency. Supportive therapy includes intravenous fluid, adrenaline, steroids, and oxygen. Following stabilization, patients need to be tested for IgA deficiency.

Transfusion-Associated Circulatory Overload

Transfusion-associated circulatory overload (TACO) usually occurs as a result of rapid and massive transfusion in a patient with underlying heart disease or chronic anemia. Clinical expression is similar to that of TRALI, but signs of cardiac failure are also noted. Supportive care, as well as treatment for cardiac failure is indicated. This is a preventable reaction, since the fluid balance status of patients at risk should be monitored during transfusion and rapid and massive transfusions avoided as far as possible.

Transfusion-Associated Graft Versus Host Disease (TA-GvHD)

This very rare complication is usually observed in immune-compromised children transfused with non-irradiated blood. It may also occur when a recipient receives a blood product from someone with an identical HLA haplotype. Leukodepletion does not prevent TA-GvHD. It occurs 10–14 days following transfusion and fever, nausea/vomiting, marked jaundice, diarrhoea, and a maculopapular skin rash are present. Pancytopenia may complicate the picture. Unfortunately this type of reaction has a very high mortality rate. Diagnosis may be dependent on a skin or liver biopsy. The treatment includes chemotherapy.

Post-transfusion Purpura

Post-transfusion purpura is rare and is a result of antibodies (HPA1a or HPA5a) against donor platelets. It usually occurs in females. Significant thrombocytopenia is seen 9–10 days following transfusion. Patients usually present with mucocutaneous bleeding. It is treated with intravenous immunoglobulin and high-dose platelets, if necessary. Plasma exchange may also be considered.

Infectious Complications

Careful selection of donors and systematic screening for infectious markers has significantly reduced the risk of transfusion-related infectious complications. There is however a small residual risk due to blood products collected from donors during the silent phase of infectious diseases, but also to a very small possibility of false negative results.

The main microorganisms involved in post-transfusion hepatitis are hepatitis B and C viruses. Cytomegalovirus (CMV) and Epstein Barr virus (EBV)-related hepatitis are usually mild. Post-transfusion hepatitis may be acute, clinically silent, or symptomatic; but can also progress to chronic hepatitis, cirrhosis, and hepatocellular carcinoma.

Transmission of CMV can lead to various clinical diseases, including retinitis, nephritis, interstitial pneumonia, neurological involvement or cytopenia. It can either be a primary infection or reactivation of an existing infection. Leukodepletion of transfused products significantly reduces the risk of CMV transmission. It is good practice to select seronegative derivatives when transfusing a patient due to hematopoietic stem cell transplant.

Transmission of HIV infection has dramatically reduced with the introduction of systematic screening for anti-HIV1 and -2 antibodies. Screening for the viral genome further reduces the risk by allowing the detection of HIV-infected donors in the seronegative window period.

Bacterial infections remain a cause of significant morbidity and mortality. Microbial contamination by skin microflora can occur during blood collection, or during processing at the blood bank. Preservation of blood products and platelets in particular, since platelets are stored at ambient temperature, contribute to microbial proliferation. Microorganisms often identified include *Yersinia enterocolitica* and *Staphylococcus epidermidis*. The clinical severity is determined by the bacterial load of the inoculum and the clinical state of the patient. Any suspicion should trigger immediate termination of the transfusion, microbiological investigation via cultures of the transfused blood and the patient's blood and treatment with broad spectrum antibiotic should be started.

Very occasionally, other infectious agents are reported. These include human herpes virus 8 (HHV8) infection, parvovirus B19 infection, West Nile virus, as well as infection with a spongiform encephalopathy agent (a variant of Jacob Creutzfeldt disease).

Iron Overload

This complication is seen in patients who have had multiple transfusions. It is however very rare in the field of pediatric oncology. Iron accumulation may involve the liver, heart, and pancreas. A ferritin level is a good surrogate marker of iron overload, but other diagnostic means include hepatic or cardiac MRI or liver biopsy. Treatment of iron overload involves chelation with desferrioxamine or oral chelating agents (e.g. desferasirox), if available.

Alternatives to Blood Transfusion

Designated donations are not encouraged any more in countries where blood products from the general population are considered to be very safe, since the risk for infection is similar due to meticulous testing. It should also be avoided in cases where a bone marrow transplant may be a future treatment option. Acute normovolemic hemodilution, as well as intra- and postoperative blood recovery are options for patients undergoing surgery. Several pharmacological agents are available for use to limit blood loss and increase hemoglobin levels in certain cases: local hemostatic products (e.g. thrombin sprays and fibrin glue), desmopressin, tranexamic acid, and erythropoietin. The safety of bovine hemoglobin in children has not been established, it is not widely available and has significant side-effects.

Key Points

- Transfusion is a major therapeutic and supportive intervention in pediatric oncology, but it is important to assess the benefit/risk ratio on a case-by-case basis.
- The choice of blood product should take into consideration the clinical context, etiology of the anemia and/or thrombocytopenia, as well as concurrent conditions and risk factors.
- Informed consent and assent should be obtained prior to a transfusion.
- It is important in all cases to strictly observe the rules of compatibility testing, ordering, prescription, transport, quality control of the product, and patient identification.
- Careful monitoring during a blood product transfusion is required.
- In case of a transfusion-related reaction, the transfusion should be stopped immediately and the responsible doctor and the blood bank should be notified.
- Reactions due to ABO incompatibility are the most severe and result in significant mortality and morbidity.
- Other reactions include transfusion-related acute lung injury (TRALI), febrile non-hemolytic transfusion reaction, allergic reaction, bacterial contamination, transfusion-associated circulatory overload, extravascular hemolytic reaction, graft versus host disease, and post-transfusion purpura.
- There is a risk of infectious complications (HIV 1 and 2, hepatitis B and C, syphilis).
- Patients on a chronic transfusion program should be monitored for secondary iron overload.

Suggested Reading

British Committee for Standards in Haematology, Blood Transfusion Task Force (2003) Guidelines for the use of platelet transfusions. Br J Haematol 122:10–23

Gibson BE, Todd A, Roberts I, Pamphilon D, Rodeck C, Bolton-Maggs P, Burbin G, Duguid J, Boulton F, Cohen H, Smith N, McClelland DB, Rowley M, Turner G (2004) Transfusion guidelines for neonates and older children. Br J Haematol 124:433–453

Harrison E, Bolton P (2011) Serious hazards of transfusion in children (SHOT). Paediatr Anaesth 21(1):10–13

Kneyber MC (2011) Red blood cell transfusion in paediatric critical care. Clin Lab 57(3–4):263–266

Murray NA, Roberts IA (2004) Neonatal transfusion practice. Arch Dis Child Fetal Neonatal Ed 89(2):F101–F107

Paananen P, Arola MO, Pelliniemi TT, Salmi TT, Lähteenmäki PM (2009) Evaluation of the effects of different transfusion trigger levels during the treatment of childhood acute lymphoblastic leukemia. J Pediatr Hematol Oncol 31(10):745–749

Sharma S, Sharma P, Tyler LN (2011) Transfusion of blood and blood products: indications and complications. Am Fam Physician 83(6):719–724

WP Blood Transfusion Service and the South African National Blood Service (2014) Clinical guidelines for the use of blood products in South Africa, 5th edn. South African National Blood Service, Cape Town

Chapter 26
Nutrition for Children with Cancer in Africa

Case Scenario

A 2-year 4-month-old girl diagnosed with AML on admission presented with a weight-for-height ratio that appears clinically normal and on par with the age-appropriate stages of development. See measurements below. Further investigation of her Road to Health booklet (RTHB) or individual growth chart shows her birth weight was 3 kg and she since followed her own expected normal growth curve. The RTHB shows she started to present with failure to thrive (FTT) 2 months ago and according to the mother this is caused by an unexplained loss in appetite.

Measurements	Interpretation
Birth weight: 3 kg	On 0 *z*-score
Birth Length: 47 cm	Just above the-2 *z*-score
Weight-for-height at birth	On the 0 *z*-score
Head circumference at birth: 35 cm	Just above the 0 *z*-score
Admission weight: 13.0 kg	Above 0 *z*-score
Admission length: 87 cm	Just below 0 *z*-score
Weight-for-height at admission	On the +1 *z*-score
What other information would you like to have?	
Description of growth trends wrt weight and length/height	Following normal growth curve since birth with slight plato/FTT in the last 2 months of life
MUAC on admission: 14.4 cm	Normal

D.C. Stefan, M. Harif, *Pediatric Cancer in Africa*,
DOI 10.1007/978-3-319-17936-0_26

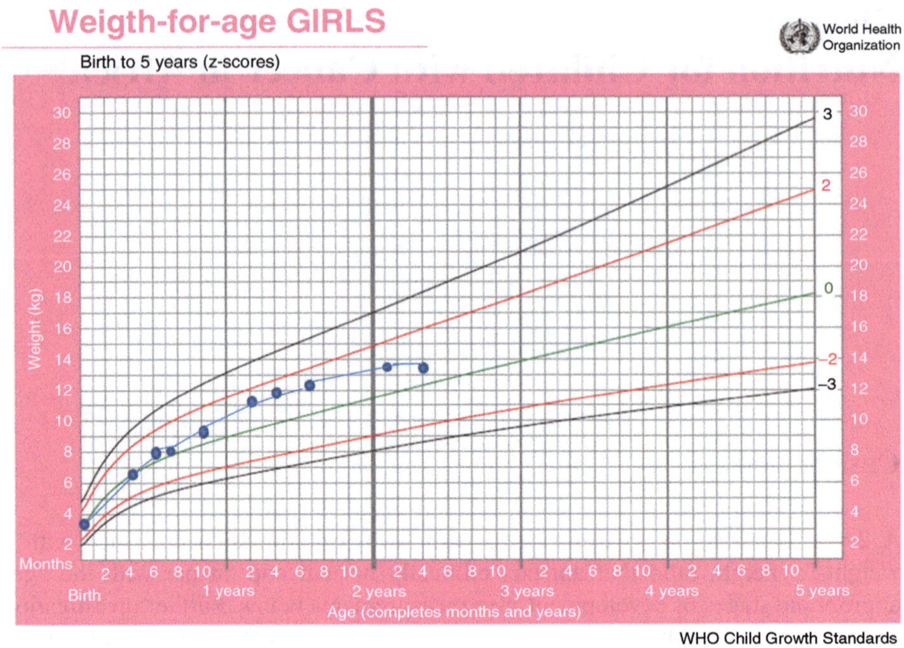

Introduction: The Role of Nutrition

Children with cancer are especially at risk for developing malnutrition because they require elevated substrate needs as a result of the disease and its treatment [1, 2]. At the same time, they need to grow and develop optimally, and therefore, have even higher nutritional needs to facilitate the process [2, 3]. An optimal nutritional status in children has also been described to help them better recover from illness and trauma [1].

Malnutrition can affect tolerance of cancer therapy (disturbed drug metabolism), increase the risk of comorbidities (decreased immune function and delayed wound healing) and ultimately, adversely influence overall survival and prognosis [1, 2, 4]. The younger the child, the more severe the effects of malnutrition can be [5].

Therefore, nutrition plays a very important role in the management of the child with cancer!

What Is Malnutrition?

The term malnutrition is a very unspecific description of an impaired nutritional state, and is characterized by either a deficiency or excess intake of energy that has a negative impact on a person's clinical outcome [2]. Malnutrition, that encompasses

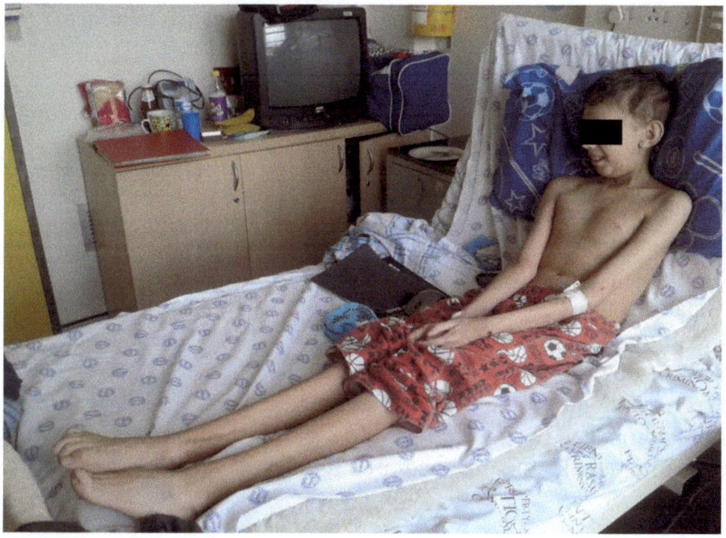

Fig. 26.1 Prevention of malnutrition is important to facilitate growth in young children and adolescents

both extremes of the weight spectrum, if not present at diagnosis, may develop throughout the course of treatment [3, 4].

The occurrence of malnutrition in children with childhood tumors is multifactorial, and the prevalence will vary according to its vague definition and different diagnostic techniques used to assess nutritional status [2, 4] (Fig. 26.1).

Factors that Influence Nutritional Status [4]

(a) Cancers associated with high risk of developing malnutrition

- Advanced disease during initial intense treatment
- Wilms tumor (metastatic) and Neuroblastoma
- Soft tissue sarcomas (Ewing or Rhabdomyosarcoma)
- Some non-Hodgkin lymphoma and advanced Hodgkin disease
- Relapsed Leukemia
- Acute Myeloid Leukemia
- Poor prognosis ALL (infants diagnosed <12 months, certain chromosomal abnormalities)
- Brain tumors, especially those with decreased level of consciousness

(b) Low-risk nutrition based on less intensive chemotherapy protocols

- Good prognosis ALL
- Non-metastatic solid tumors

- Advanced diseases in remission during maintenance treatment

(c) Factors that can further deplete nutritional stores

- Anorexia—either related to treatment-induced nausea and vomiting or to presence of psychological factors
- Infection
- Stomatitis/Mucositis
- Diarrhea
- Nausea and vomiting
- Malabsorption
- Blood loss and iron deficiency
- Renal damage and nutrient loss
- Mechanical gut problems
- Xerostomia and dysgeusia
- Psychological factors like acquired food aversion, depression

Mechanisms of Weight Loss

Anorexia is defined as the loss of a desire to eat. Cachexia is a syndrome of progressive and profound wasting of equal amounts of lean body mass and body fat in relation to total body weight [2] and associated with both anorexia and metabolic alterations [3]. The metabolic and body composition changes in cancer cachexia are similar to those in people with polytrauma, acute sepsis, burns, and AIDS [2]. In contrast to simple starvation, wasting induced by cancer cachexia cannot be prevented or reversed by increasing nutrient ingestion alone [2].

The pathogenesis of malnutrition during chronic diseases, such as cancer, is the direct result of diminished intake, enhanced losses (like malabsorption) and increased needs [1]. Changes in metabolism of macronutrients take place, which results in a net energy loss clinically that presents as weight loss, particularly lean body mass [1, 2]:

- Increased lipid breakdown via lipolysis that result in depletion of fat stores
- Altered (energy consumptive) carbohydrate metabolism
  - The body uses glucose from dietary sources as well as glucose gained from the liver converting muscle-derived proteins via gluconeogenesis, which results in increased energy expenditure
  - Increased Cori cycle—glucose is transformed into lactate by the tumor and recycled by the liver at a high energy cost
- Insulin resistance and elevated secretion of growth hormone occur
- Increased total body protein turnover (likely mediated by cytokines), reduced muscle protein synthesis, and increased hepatic protein synthesis that result in loss of lean body mass.

Nutrient deficiencies tend to develop over a period of time, and the extent will depend on the patient's substrate reserves [1]. Metabolic changes are not necessarily uniformly altered in all patients with cancer [2]. A review by Bauer et al. investigated studies that suggested the changes in macronutrient metabolism can be attributed to a cancer-host rivalry. They discovered that recent trials do not support this theory indicating no positive correlation between tumor size or extension and the severity of host depletion [2].

Which aspects would one consider when assessing the nutritional status of a newly diagnosed child with childhood cancer, such as this 28-month-old patient?

Assessment of Nutritional Status

Children living with childhood cancer are at higher risk of developing malnutrition during cancer treatment than adults, because they have higher nutritional requirements to facilitate optimal growth and development [3]. Some children may already present with malnutrition at diagnosis, but others may develop this during the course of their treatment. Determining a patient's nutritional status at diagnosis is important as it has prognostic implications [5]. Therefore, nutritional assessment is an important part of caring for this patient population, and imperative to recognizing and preventing the development of malnutrition by implementing early nutritional interventions before cancer treatment starts and further depletes stores [2, 5]. Assessing a patient's nutritional status is tough because there is no gold standard and little information is still available on formal comparisons of different measures on how to best define nutritional status [1].

Anthropometry

Nutritional assessments previously relied heavily on height and weight measurements. However, these measurements may be misleading because of large masses of solid tumors masking a patient's real weight, influencing the weight-for-height ratio. Other factors influencing weight include edema, organ congestion, and amputations, as seen in osteosarcoma cases [1, 2, 4].

Measurement of body compartments provides useful information at diagnosis, and presents additional information from that obtained through anthropometry and subjective nutritional assessments. Changes in body composition can also occur as a direct result of chemotherapy treatment, resulting in a reduction in lean body mass and an increase in fat mass. Body composition can affect the distribution, absorption,

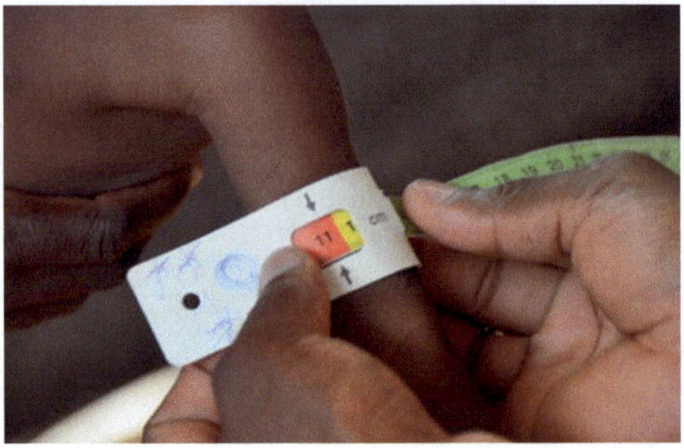

Fig. 26.2 Measuring the mid-upper arm circumference

metabolism, and elimination of cytostatic drugs. Steroids may also increase fat mass and cause insulin resistance [2] (Fig. 26.2).

The upper limbs are not usually directly affected by edema or tumor mass and arm anthropometry can be used as an additional method to provide an accurate evaluation of body composition [1, 4]. Biceps and triceps skinfold measurements provide an estimate of the body's fat reserves, whereas calculating the arm muscle area will help estimate muscle protein reserves. Measuring the mid-upper arm circumference (MUAC) is another cost-effective and reliable way to assess nutritional status and proven most practical as this can be performed anywhere [1, 4].

General consensus supports that one marker alone is not sufficient to fully evaluate nutritional status and diagnostic criteria should be used together [4, 5]. Recommendations are that arm anthropometry, together with weight or height indexes are completed in all patients with solid tumors and repeated weekly during the course of their treatment [1, 4]. The RTHB is a valuable tool to assess a patient's pre-tumor growth trends in children <5 years old [4]. In 2010, the World Health organization (WHO) released new standardized growth charts based on *z*-scores for interpreting growth and identifying malnutrition [6, 7].

Monitoring schedule for anthropometrical evaluations

Daily	Weight
Weekly	Height/length
	MUAC
	Triceps, biceps, and subscapular skinfolds. Indirect calorimetry
Monthly	Head circumference
	Trends in % EWA, % EWH, % EHA and *z*-scores

Classification of Nutritional Status Based on Anthropometrical Findings [6]

Tables 26.1 and 26.2.

Table 26.1 The new WHO classifications using *Z*-scores

Z-scores	Classification
Length/height for age:	
Above 3	Child very tall—rarely endocrine disorder
Below 2	Stunted
Weight for age:	
Below 2	Underweight
Below 3	Severely underweight
Weight for L/H:	
Above 3	Obese
Above 2	Overweight
Above 1	Possible risk of overweight
Below 2	"Wasted"
Below 3	"Severely wasted"

Table 26.2 The MUAC reference ranges for moderate-to-severe malnutrition, ages 6 months to 14 years [7]

Infants 12 months	MUAC < 110 mm	Severe malnutrition
	MUAC < 115 mm	Moderate malnutrition
Children 1–5 years	MUAC < 110 mm	Severe malnutrition
	MUAC < 135 mm	Moderate malnutrition
Children 6–9 years	MUAC < 135 mm	Severe malnutrition
	MUAC < 155 mm	Moderate malnutrition
Children 10–14 years	MUAC < 160 mm	Severe malnutrition
	MUAC < 185 mm	Moderate malnutrition

Overweight (Not Common in Africa) [5]

The detrimental effects of obesity in children are well described and may include the development of hyperlipidemia, hypertension, diabetes and insulin resistance, hepatic steatosis, cholelithiasis, sleep apnea, and orthopedic abnormalities. While having increased risk for developing chronic diseases of lifestyle later in life, they are also proposed to be more susceptible to certain cancers (esophagus, colon and rectum, and breast when postmenopausal). In obese children and adolescents with childhood cancer, there are also risks for over- or underdosing with treatment that could result in poorer treatment outcome and greater toxicities. In pediatric acute myeloblastic leukemia (AML), obese patients have a higher treatment-related mortality and inferior survival compared to those who are not obese.

Survivors of common childhood malignancies are at risk for adult-onset diseases such as obesity that is in turn associated with a high risk for cardiovascular and endocrine diseases [2] (Table 26.3).

Table 26.3 Criteria for overweight and obesity [6]

BMI-for-age	Classification
Above +2 SD	Obesity (at 19 years: >30 kg/m^2)
Above +1 SD	Overweight (at 19 years: >25 kg/m^2 for girls)
Below −2 SD	Thinness
Below −3 SD	Severe thinness

Screening Tools for Early Detection of Malnutrition [8]

Although many malnutrition screening tools exist there are no screening tools specifically designed for the assessment of oncology patients.

The Screening Tool for Assessment of Malnutrition in Pediatrics (STAMP) was developed in the UK and is quite useful for nutritional assessment of the general at-risk patient. This can be downloaded from the website www.stampscreeningtool.org.

A work group formed at the Royal College of Nursing (2010) compiled a supplementary diagnostic section to STAMP, specific to pediatric oncology and suggested this section replace section one of the original STAMP tool. To note: This supplementary section was not audited or evaluated by the time of publication. They recommend one should combine the score for this tool with the STAMP score for nutritional intake, weight, and height. A total score of >4 should be referred to the dietician for further nutritional management [3] (Table 26.4).

Biochemistry

Select biochemical markers commonly used to interpret a patient's nutritional status may be influenced by the disease state (including sepsis and infections) and chemotherapy treatments received, thus bearing restricted usefulness in reporting malnutrition [2, 4]. These markers include plasma protein, serum albumin, pre-albumin, retinol-binding protein, transthyretin, and transferrin [2]. Claims have been made that pre-albumin may have better validity than albumin for children presenting with ALL and solid tumors [1, 4]. Hemoglobin and hematocrit are also affected by the disease state, specifically leukemia, lymphomas, and Hodgkin's disease [4]. Some studies suggest that serum creatinine levels may be a good substitute for measuring lean body mass especially in the absence of DXA scans [1].

Common chemotherapy side-effects include diarrhea and vomiting, which could lead to severe micronutrient and electrolyte losses. These deficiencies should be monitored and corrected according to the progression of the side-effects [2].

Table 26.4 Supplementary tool for identifying malnutrition in pediatric oncology patients, for use with the STAMP document (step one) [3]

High nutritional risk (definite nutritional implications: score 3)	Low nutritional risk (possible nutritional implications: score 2)
• Advanced disease during initial intense treatment	• ALL—regimen A patients
• High-risk neuroblastoma	• Non-metastatic solid tumors
• Stage 3 and 4 Wilms tumor	• Retinoblastoma
• Rhabdomyosarcoma	• Hodgkin's disease
• Ewing sarcoma/primitive neuroectodermal tumor (PNET)	• Germ cell tumors
• Osteosarcoma	• Advance diseases in remission
• Medulloblastoma/CNS PNET	• During maintenance treatment
• Nasopharyngeal tumors	
• B-cell non-Hodgkin's lymphoma	
• Acute myeloid leukemia	
• Acute lymphoblastic leukemia (ALL)	
o Infant and toddlers	
o Regimen B and C patients	
o Relapsed ALL	
• Bone marrow transplant patients	
• High-dose therapy and PBSCT patients	

Biochemical measurements can be very useful to measure the risk for developing of, and severity of present refeeding syndrome. Patients identified with severe malnutrition should be monitored and appropriate feeding and electrolyte/trace element replacement protocols followed to prevent and manage the incidence of refeeding, especially in the use of parenteral nutrition (Fig. 26.3 and Table 26.5).

Clinical Examination

A detailed clinical assessment should include a medical history, specifically focusing on factors that could exacerbate risk for malnutrition like the stage and type of tumor, intensity of planned anti-cancer therapy and the presence or absence of remission [4].

Expected clinical signs, also based on anthropometrical and biochemical findings, may include depleted muscle mass, fat stores (over or underweight), micronutrient deficiencies, and changes in body composition including edema. The nutritional plan can be modified to treat nutrition-related clinical signs. A critical approach to the clinical assessment may divulge information not forthcoming in anthropometrical or biochemical data, for example trends in the extent of muscle wasting (Fig. 26.4).

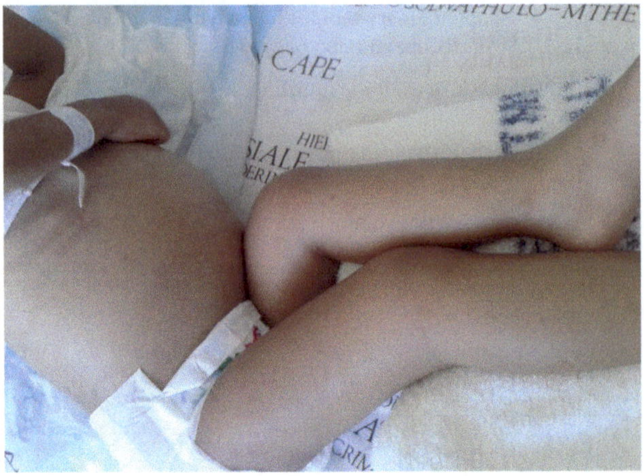

Fig. 26.3 Severe edema may influence biochemical markers

Table 26.5 Monitoring schedule for patients with cancer [3, 4]

Parameter	Hospitalized patients		Outpatients on oral or enteral
	Parenteral nutrition	Oral/enteral feeds	
Electrolytes, glucose	Daily	Weekly	Monthly
Urea, Creatinine	Weekly	Weekly	Monthly
Calcium, phosphorous, magnesium	Daily to weekly	Weekly	Monthly
Triglyceride	Weekly	Monthly	As indicated
LFTs	Weekly	Weekly	Monthly
Trace elements	Monthly	As indicated	As indicated
Carnitine	Monthly	As indicated	As indicated
Vitamin levels	Monthly	As indicated	As indicated

Diet History

Hospitals should essentially respond to the particular needs of this patient population, because of the severe negative impact poor nutritional intake will have on nutritional status, treatment tolerance, and ultimately prognosis [3]. Performing a detailed assessment of a patient's diet history will provide one with crucial information to help compose an individualized nutritional plan. The process will engage both parents/caregivers and child in the "treatment" process, cementing the importance of nutrition and promoting compliance when implementing different nutritional strategies throughout the course of treatment. Overreporting of food intake often occurs in families from low-income households who may be afraid to share the true extent of their circumstances. Critically assess information gleaned and compare to anthropometry, biochemical and clinical investigations to formulate your opinion.

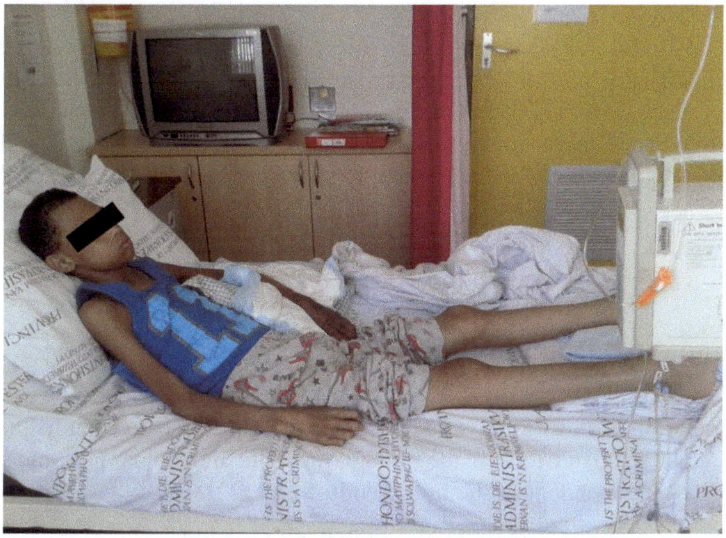

Fig. 26.4 An example of a patient who is severely wasted with pitting edema on lower limbs that may potentially mask the severity of the malnutrition

Caregivers are a great source of practical information that one can share in turn with newly diagnosed patients. Such information includes recipes for poor appetite and home diet food fortification, practical information to treat food aversions, low-cost options for meals high in protein and energy, etc.

Garofolo et al. suggests the following concepts as important information to include when performing a diet history [9]:

- Appetite or recall of actual intake at home.
- Presence of a limited or monotonous diet.
- Acquired food aversions and specific food intolerances.
- Use of nutritional supplements at home.
- Recent changes in weight and activity levels.
- Treatment-related complications.
- Treatment schedules and sleeping periods that interfere with mealtimes.
- Other medications that affect appetite or GIT function.
- Prolonged periods of neutropenia.
- Developmental status, feeding milestones, and swallowing function.
- Family history, parental and sibling growth patterns.
- Social history.

The patient's dietary preferences and taste fatigue may vary during the course of treatment and hospitalization and frequent follow-up is recommended to adjust the nutritional plan accordingly.

The nutritional assessment of this patient is complete and shows that even though she may have an optimal nutritional status at diagnosis she may be at high risk for developing malnutrition because of the type of cancer that has been diagnosed as recent reduction in appetite and FTT. What would your nutritional goals be for such a patient to prevent malnutrition?

Nutritional Goals and Objectives

The formulation of nutritional strategies begins at diagnosis to establish the essential role of adequate nutrition in the mind of the child and the parents, and should be implemented independent of the initial body weight [2].

- Maintenance of body stores as close to ideal as possible.
- Minimization of wasting and preservation of lean body mass.
- Promotion of appropriate growth and development.
- Providing good quality of life.
- Early detection of malnutrition and at-risk patients.
- Minimize treatment-related side-effects.
- Nutrition education.

The Role of the Dietician

A multidisciplinary approach, including the dietician, will ensure optimal care and patient outcomes by meeting nutritional goals. Nutrition education is an important part of the treatment process and forms the basis of nutritional support. The significance of adequate nutrition support (from diagnosis throughout treatment) should be explained to the patient and their families as early as possible to improve nutritional care and compliance. Nutrition information to be provided should include [3]:

- Importance of maintaining the child's nutritional status during the course of treatment.
- Potential side effects of treatments that may interfere with oral intake.
- Practical advice to deal with cancer treatment-related issues and when to refer to the dietician.
- Guidelines on high energy/high protein foods especially during periods of poor intake and weight loss.
- The variety of nutritional support options available and indications for implementation.
- General food safety guidelines.

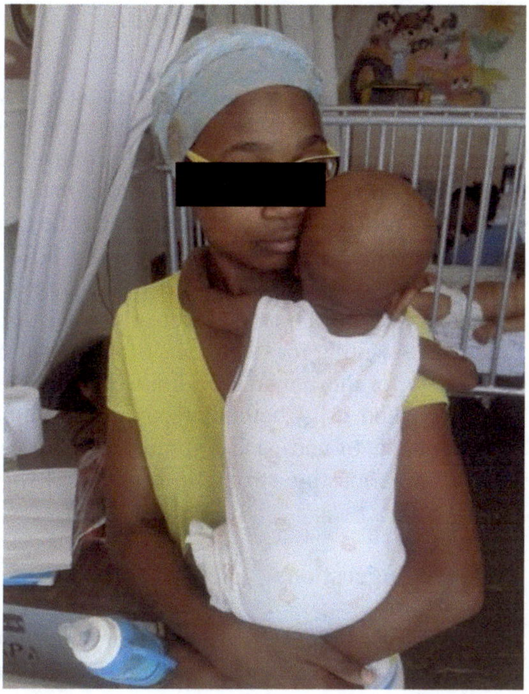

Fig. 26.5 A mother concerned with her child's waning appetite

Nutrition education should not only be restricted to the patients and their families/caregivers, but be extended to include all ward staff that come into close contact with your patient. Staff members, such as nurses, are often one's eyes and ears to spot problems and concerns when the dietician and doctors are not around, especially after hours. They provide invaluable information when interpreting patients' symptoms, i.e., reasons for refusal to eat meals or providing accurate information that the patient may have withheld previously. They also ensure continuation of care after hours, for example starting night feeds/encouraging eating bed-time supplements (Fig. 26.5).

One week since admission the mother expresses her concern to the doctor that her child is experiencing a further drop in appetite and refusing to eat solid foods provided by the hospital her diet mainly consists of fluids like juice and milk. Her weight drops with 500 g to 12.5 kg (3.8 % weight loss). Her MUAC is still 13 cm.

Dealing with Inadequate Intake

The pediatric oncology patient experiences a variety of dietary problems during hospitalization [3]. The diet is the center of their day and one of the few things in their environment they can potentially control. Caregivers often opt to spend a lot of money in a desperate attempt to improve their child's dietary intake, often focusing on favorite foods (like chips) that may not be considered a "healthy" food choice, as poor dietary habits are quick to form.

Food intake can be hampered by changes in mood/depression, unappetizing appearance of meals, smells from the food trolley that may put them off, limited time to eat, waiting for treatments of investigations, limited/repetitive menu options (especially for those who are admitted for long periods of time) and food that is not freshly cooked [3]. Chemotherapy can also hinder optimal oral intake by causing frequent bouts of nausea and vomiting. Some patients also report taste changes that leave them requesting strong flavored food [3].

Practical Suggestions

Equipping ward staff with the necessary nutrition background and ward-based tools will help them make nutrition-based decisions to improve a patient's intake when the dietician is not available:

- Provide a good knowledge base for the type of ward diets available to in-patients, including appropriate dietary changes that could be made to accommodate taste and consistent changes as the patient's condition either deteriorates or improves.
  - Staff should be made aware of all the different ward diets available from the main kitchen. They should ideally be able to order different types of meals anytime throughout the day at ward level when dietary changes are requested or deemed necessary. Thereby preventing patients from having to wait hours or sometimes a full day/weekend before the necessary change is made by the dietician, resulting in poor intake.
  - Examples of different types of ward diets include—normal ward diet, soft diet, semi (puree) diet, full fluid or clear fluid diets, high protein diets (also High Protein fluid available), diabetic diets, baby/toddler/peds diets.
  - Extra food items can be added to the standard meals available to promote exposure to a larger variety of foods to prevent taste fatigue and ultimately poor oral intake (especially for those frequently admitted and used to the basic hospital menu). Examples include serving dry cereals instead of cooked porridge, stocking items acceptable for a more traditional diet like amasi.
  - Check with your Food service unit and dietician which changes your institution is able to make.
- Provide a good knowledge base of all available enteral products used for both enteral feeds (NGT, pegs, jejunostomy feeds) and as oral supplements.

- There is a host of products on the market that can help improve a patient's nutritional intake. Government institutions are usually restricted to tender approved products but different flavors of supplements are available from most companies that should provide a variety of options for patients from which to choose. Ideally, patients with inadequate oral intake should be given the choice of which flavor product they would like to enjoy daily to help prevent taste fatigue. In my experience taste satiety can develop very quickly and early on in treatment.
- Certain characteristics of feeds are more acceptable to some individuals than others based on their usual intake and preferences at home. A patient's preference may also vary between chemotherapy sessions, as potential taste changes occur and even depends heavily on mood changes. Doing a taste test to compare product characteristics may be very helpful when prescribing supplements. Being familiar with the products could help you motivate a patient to take the supplements as prescribed. Patients are usually able to tell you whether they prefer certain aspects regarding meal options or supplements like sweet vs. bland tastes during the course of their hospitalization. Look for criteria such as products that are the sweetest vs. the blandest (taste changes/aversions), the smoothest vs. the thickest (swallowing problems), the most concentrated (high osmolarity), which products may be acceptable to patients who are used to a more traditional diet, i.e., denser supplements such as amazi.
- To note: Semi-elemental products are lightly flavored (usually vanilla) to promote enteral intake, but are usually not well accepted by peds patients for oral use.
- Supplements may come in either ready-to-use (RTU) form or as powder formulas that needs reconstitution with water. RTU products are more expensive but decrease wastage as they have a long shelf-life when unopened. Powder formulas are only viable for 24 h after reconstitution and should preferably only be used when a dedicated tube feed room is available for the hygienic mixing of enteral products (Fig. 26.6).

> Keeping in mind the nutritional goals set out for this patient in the previous chapter, how would you calculate her requirements to be sure her dietary needs are met and malnutrition will be prevented?

Nutrition Support

There is no universal consensus with regard to the nutritional requirements, criteria for, timing of, and duration of nutritional interventions [2]. A patient identified with a high nutritional risk should be considered for early nutrition intervention to prevent further deterioration of the nutritional state [3].

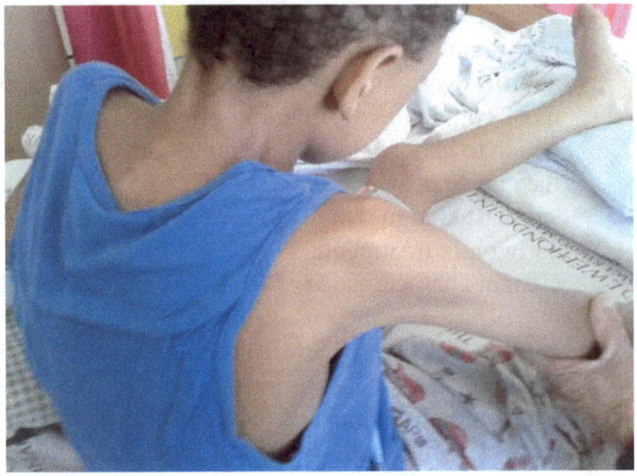

Fig. 26.6 Severe malnutrition

Nutritional Requirements

A variety of methods are available to estimate substrate needs. Indirect calorimetry is used as the gold standard to determine energy expenditure.

Energy [4]

The minimum amount of energy required by the human body to maintain all essential bodily functions is known as the basal metabolic rate (BMR).

A study done by Den Broeder et al. in children with a solid tumor, showed an increase in BMR that could be explained by the fact that the tumor consisted of metabolically active tissue. BMR values returned to normal after chemotherapy courses were successfully administered. The increase in metabolic rate may differ between patients with different tumor types and the fact that individuals respond differently to therapy.

Sources suggest the BMR be adjusted by a selection of stress factors or combined stress and activity factors to counter the effect of the solid tumor and still allow for optimal growth and activity.

The Schofield weight and height equation is recommended to calculate the estimated energy requirements for children >1 year old. The result should be adjusted by using a combined stress and activity factor of 1.5–1.8 on diagnosis and tapered during maintenance therapy or after the tumor was surgically removed.

For Severe Acute Malnutrition (SAM) the WHO's ten steps may be followed to prevent refeeding.

Table 26.6 The RDA for age should be used for those patients who have a normal weight-for-height ratio (>90 %)

RDA for proteins [10]	Age (years)	Proteins (g/kg)
Infants	0–0.5	2.2
	0.5–1	1.6
Children	1–3	1.2
	4–6	1.1
	7–10	1.0
Males	11–14	1.0
	15–18	0.9
Females	11–14	1.0
	15–18	0.8

Proteins [4]

For patients with greater requirements (refer to high-risk patients identified in Factors that Influence Nutritional Status [4]), adjust protein to 1.5–2.0 times the RDA. Should ideally not exceed 4 g/kg/day [4] (Table 26.6).

Fats [4]

During infancy about 40–50 % of consumed energy is provided by fats. For healthy children >2 years old, the recommendation is much less at <30 % of total energy derived from fats. Hepatic dysfunction may decrease lipid clearance and fats may have to be restricted. A recommendation of <2 g/kg fat per day is recommended in neutropenic children. Adequate fat intake is also an important source for fat-soluble vitamins A, D, E, and K.

Carbohydrates [5]

Adjust carbohydrate intake based on in-hospital glycemic control.

Fluid [4]

Normal fluid requirements for age should be followed except if the patient is fluid restricted because of medical reasons (i.e., during renal or cardiac failure) (Tables 26.7 and 26.8).

Micronutrients and Minerals

The supplementation of vitamins is controversial at best. Some studies show supplementation with anti-oxidants during chemotherapy may interfere with drug efficacy and is therefore not recommended [3, 4].

Table 26.7 Fluid requirements for age [11]

Age	mL/kg
0–3 months	150
4–6 months	130
7–9 months	120
10–12 months	110
1–3 years	95
4–6 years	85
7–10 years	75
11–14 years	55
15–18 years	50

Table 26.8 Another commonly used method of calculating fluid requirements is the Holliday-Segar equation [12]

First 10 kg	100 mL/kg/day
Second 10 kg	50 mL/kg/day
Every kg after this	20 mL/kg/day

The pediatric oncology dieticians interest group (PODIG) suggest that vitamin supplementation is not indicated in patients with good intake of a variety of foods, those receiving full enteral feeds, and those complying to oral supplementation drinks regimens [3]. Patients receiving blood transfusions may not need further iron supplementation [3]. They also discourage the use of mega dose single or combination vitamins, and rather suggest intake of age-appropriate multivitamins that do not exceed the recommended daily amount (RDA) [3]. More evidence is needed to support recommendations for use (Fig. 26.7).

Once the dietary requirements are calculated how would you successfully administer the nutrients?

Types of Nutritional Intervention

There are three categories for nutrition intervention to help ensure nutritional goals are met. The level of intervention will vary depending on several factors discussed in Factors that Influence Nutritional Status [4] and this decision should be discussed with the dietician, family, and multidisciplinary team. Psychological and socioeconomic factors should also be taken into account [2].

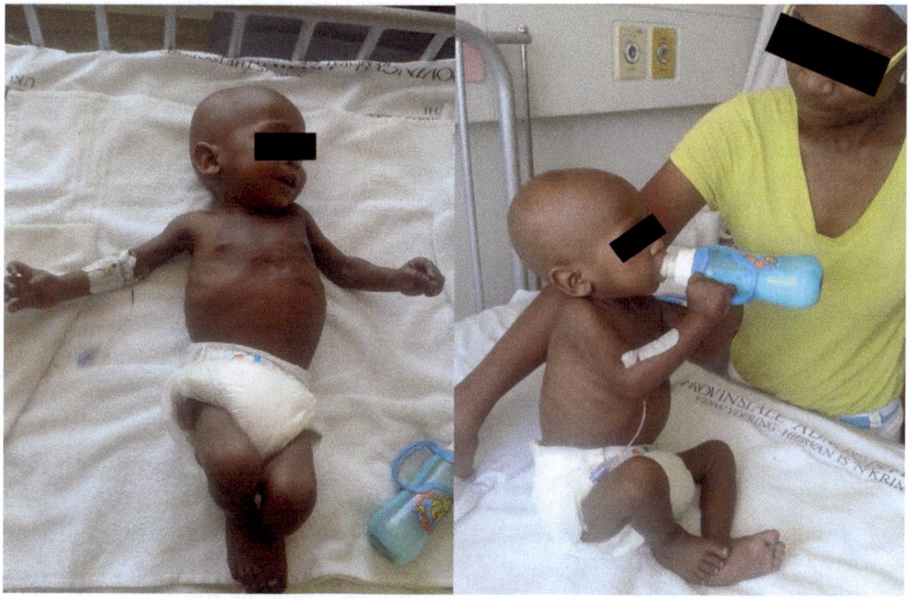

Fig. 26.7 A malnourished patient who refuses to eat solids and drinks liquids only

Supplementation

Most patients show better compliance to prescribed diets when nutrition education about the importance of optimal intake is done early on during the initial steps of treatment planning. The combination of education with supplementation was found to effectively prevent development of malnutrition in well-nourished children with less advanced disease, and those who are in remission or on maintenance therapy [4].

Supplementation to the ward diet should be considered if a reduced intake of the ward diet is noted but there is no change in nutritional status [3]. The effect of supplementation and intake of nutrient-dense meals were found to be more pronounced once patients were discharged, as there were fewer interruptions to meal times for various reasons like blood tests, etc. [4]. Strategies to supplement oral intake include:

- Education on how to increase energy and protein intakes or which are the food stuffs that are more energy dense [3].
- Dietary supplements should preferably be age-appropriate [3]. This may depend on stock available at one's institution or the affordability of products once a patient is discharged. Practical information can be provided at discharge on using fortified household products.
- Ward diet changes can be implemented to accommodate taste fatigue or treatment-related side-effects.

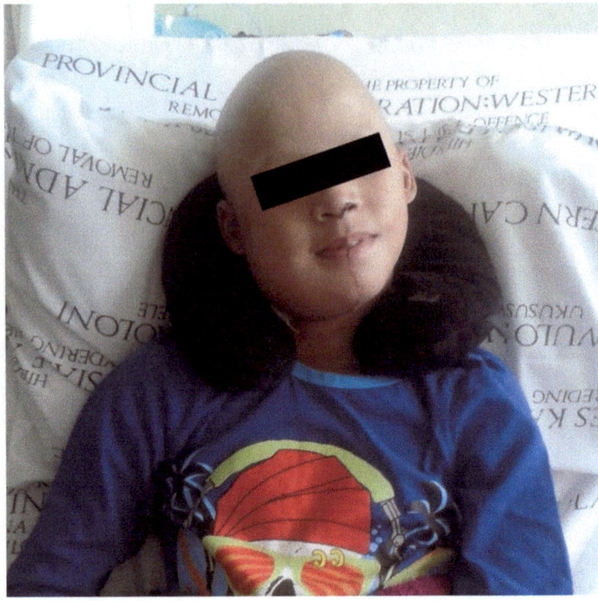

Fig. 26.8 A patient post-segmental right mandibulectomy, free fibula flap and selective neck resection, in need of supplementation as even the soft ward diet is difficult for him to take in

- Continued monitoring of weight changes and intake is advised. Cut-off values for progression to enteral feeds should be drawn up and implemented if changes in nutritional intake occur [3] (Fig. 26.8).

> Our 2-year 4-month-old patient is currently receiving her third cycle of chemotherapy. She is miserable and despondent. For the past 3 days she refuses to open her mouth or even take her beloved milk feeds; further investigation reveals she suffers from severe mucositis and has also developed a bout of acute diarrhea. Her weight has dropped to 11.5 kg (11.5 % weight loss since diagnosis), her weight-for-height ratio is on the 0 z-score and her MUAC is now 11.5 cm.

Enteral Nutrition

Enteral nutrition (EN) is the preferred and safest way to provide feeds to a patient who has proper gut function [2, 4]. Not only does it benefit the patient by preventing intestinal atrophy and bacterial translocation, toxicity, and complications of intravenous infusions [1, 2, 5] but is considered a more acceptable feeding route for children, and proves more physiological and cost-effective [4]. A positive correlation between the duration of provision of enteral feeds and increases in weight and MUAC were also found [4].

Early enteral interventions should be considered prophylactically in high-risk patients, specifically for those malnourished at diagnosis [3]. Recommendations for nasogastric feeds include using a soft bore polyutherane NGT (French 8 or 10). Patients with low platelet counts may also need additional platelet cover [4]. Nightly feeds may be considered as a practical way to encourage oral intake during the daytime and progression onto full oral intakes [4].

Entry Criteria for the Provision of EN [2–4]

- Total weight loss of >5 % since diagnosis.
- Weight-for-height ratio <90 % OR W/H < −2 *Z*-score.
- A decrease of two percentiles in current percentile for weight or height.
- Adipose energy reserves determined by triceps skinfold thickness <5th percentile for age and gender.
- Voluntary food intake <70 % of estimated requirements for 3–5 days with no improvement with prescription of supplementary drinks.
- Anticipated gut dysfunction for >5 days as a result of treatment in well-nourished patients.
- High nutritional risk based on tumor type and oncology treatment regimen.
- Bone marrow transplant as a treatment for any tumor.
- Severe mucositis <3 days.

Administration of EN is usually done via a nasogastric tube, but gastrostomies or jejunostomies may be considered in patients [3] (Figs. 26.9 and 26.10):

- Receiving an intensive treatment protocol and who are prone to developing mucositis.
- Receiving head or neck therapy.
- Who require long-term nutrition support for >2 months.
- Who do not accept/tolerate NGTs.
- Who are older and prefer this route.
- With severe vomiting for 3–5 days [2].

Choosing the Type of Feed [4]

Two standard, polymeric feeds with concentration ranging from 1 to 1.5 kcal/mL were both found to be tolerated well. In one study the use of the more concentrated formula did not increase GIT side-effects and seemed to significantly improve arm anthropometry and weight-for-height ratios. Indication for the use of semi-elemental formulas includes compromised gut function, malabsorption, diarrhea, and prolonged poor oral intake (>5 days). Polymeric and semi-elemental formulas exist for both infants <12 months and children >1 year (Table 26.9).

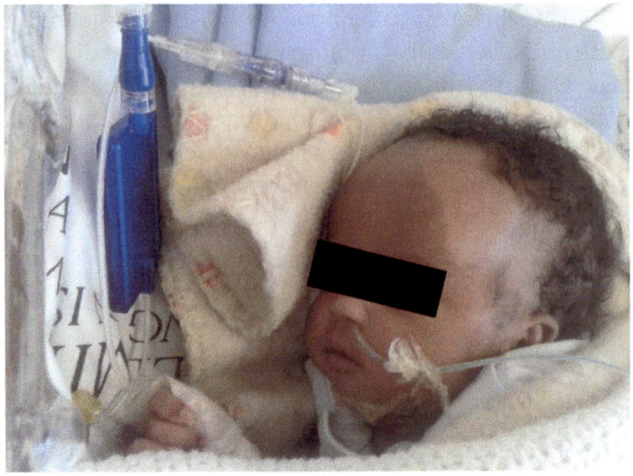

Fig. 26.9 A baby with nasogastric tube in situ

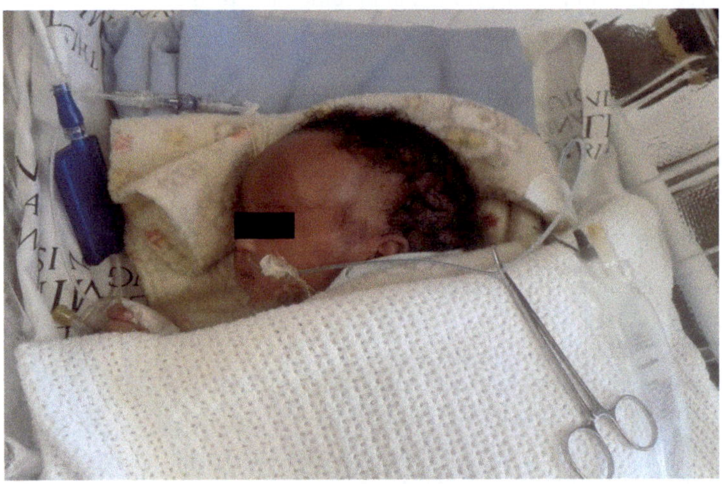

Fig. 26.10 The NGT is clamped in between feeds. Also note blue filter for TPN administration. This patient is receiving both TPN and trophic feeds via NGT

New onset abdominal distention causes the patient discomfort. She only tolerates a quarter of the prescribed enteral feeds, her weight now at 9.8 kg. To meet requirements and prevent further weight loss the feed is increased slowly, but this only results in vomits and further electrolyte derangements. She is very weak and lethargic.

Table 26.9 One can also use the following flow chart to decide which type of feed to use

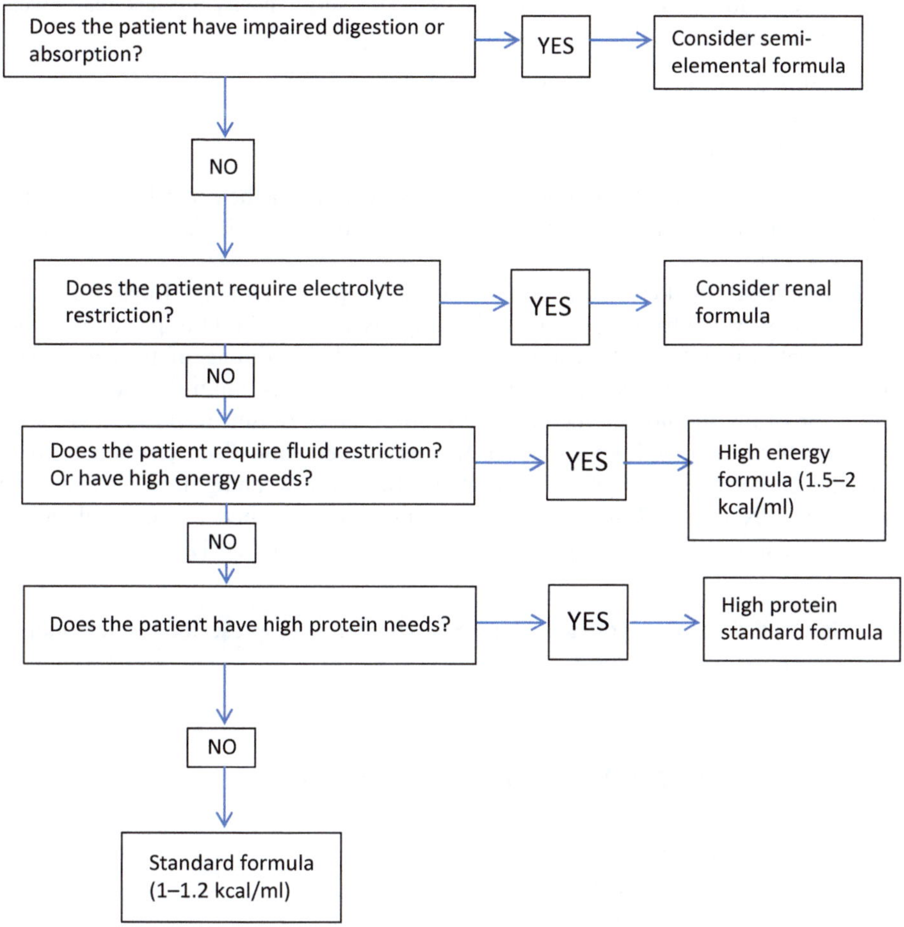

Parenteral Nutrition

Parenteral nutrition (PN) may be used as a sole provider of nutrients (TPN) or in combination with EN interventions. This will ensure requirements are better met while still stimulating the gut and preserving intestinal integrity [3].

Criteria for Administration of PN [2–4]

- Anticipated gut dysfunction that may last for >5 days

  - most commonly found in severe mucositis and enteritis, typhlitis, neutropenic enterocolitis, ileus, bowel obstruction, postsurgical chylous ascites, severe graft versus host disease (GVHD) involving the GIT

- Inability to meet requirements via EN alone
- Severe vomiting or diarrhea
- Severe pancreatitis

The administration of PN should preferably be done via the central venous route, with strict adherence to the aseptic technique and the institution's own TPN protocol [3, 4, 13].

Biochemical markers may be monitored as per Screening Tools for Early Detection of Malnutrition [8] or the institutions existing in TPN protocol. Daily assessments of GIT function are warranted to indicate timing of trophic enteral feeds. Enteral feeds should be built up slowly while TPN is diminished accordingly. Provision of PN should only be limited to short periods of time as potentially harmful side-effects include higher risk for infections, metabolic disorders, hepatotoxicity, and cholestatic liver injury [13]. Guidelines for weaning from PN suggest stopping TPN once >70–75 % of the requirements are met via the oral/enteral route—consult your in-house protocol [13] (Figs. 26.11 and 26.12).

What criteria would you use to assess whether your prescribed nutritional intervention was effective?

Suggested Goals for Nutritional Repletion [4]

- Weight for age or weight for height >90 %.
- Arm fat area >5th percentile.
- Subscapular skinfold >10th centile.
- MUAC > 14.5 cm/norm for age group (Fig. 26.13).

Management of Side-Effects [4]

Table 26.10

The patient was successfully weaned onto oral feeds and regained most of her appetite. Although she has not reached her admission weight yet, she is a much happier child and is also ambulant. The mother wants to know what the future holds for them, including nutritional support at home.

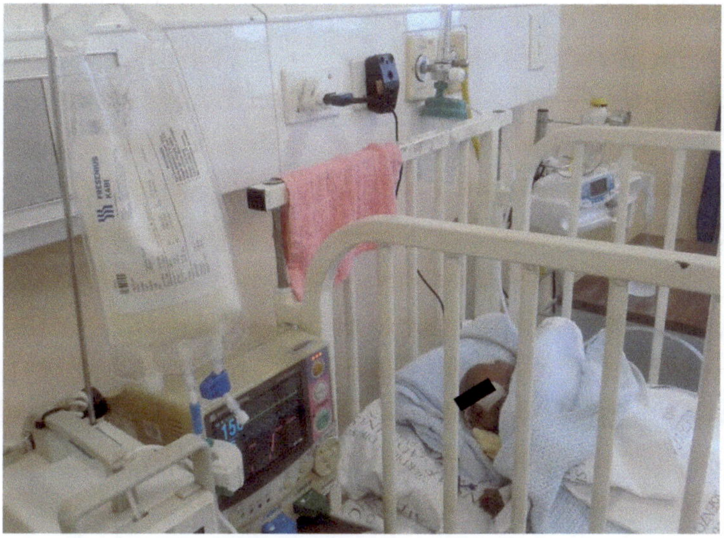

Fig. 26.11 A patient receiving TPN via CVP (all in one bag)

Fig. 26.12 A TPN bag

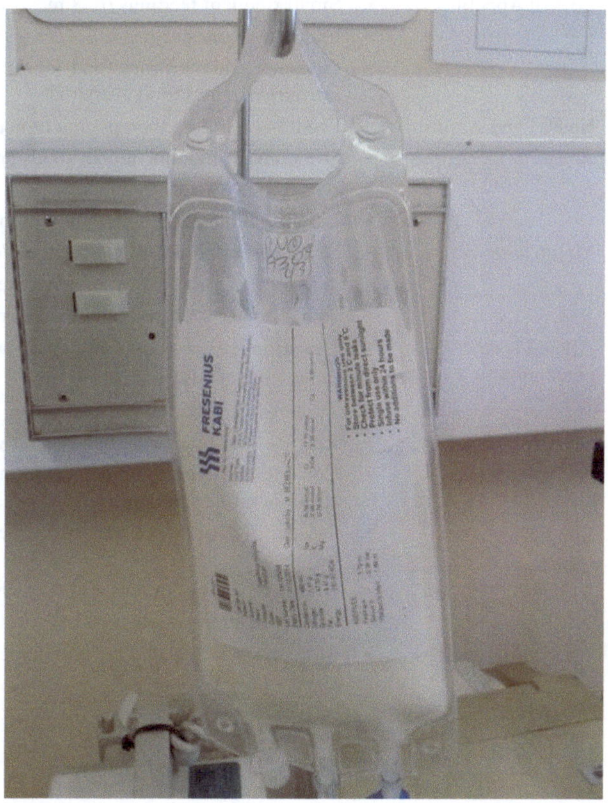

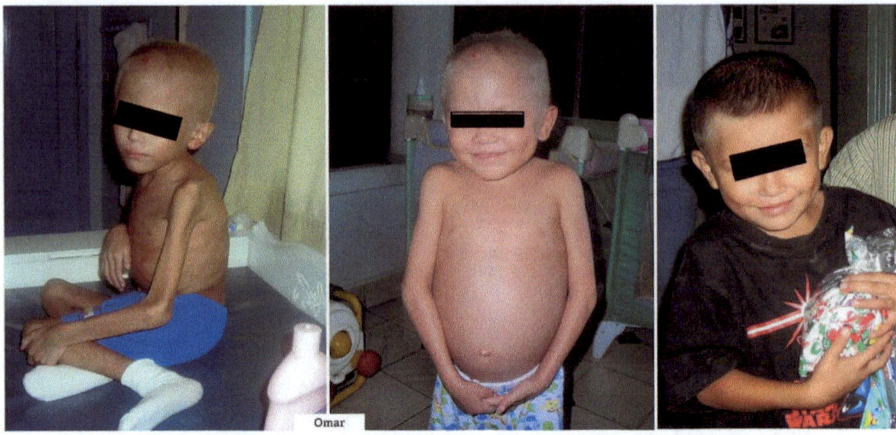

Fig. 26.13 Effective refeeding of a severely malnourished patient (*Source*: fmscblog.com)

Table 26.10 Strategies to improve oral intake during cancer treatment

Loss of Appetite	• Small frequent feedings (6–8 meals and snacks per day)
	• Encourage nutrient-dense beverages between meals
	• Offer favorite nutritious foods during treatment-free periods to prevent acquired food aversions
Nausea and vomiting	• Feed 3–4 h before therapy that typically causes nausea and vomiting
	• Offer small amounts of cool foods and encourage slow eating
	• Avoid foods with strong odors
	• Offer liquids between and not with meals
Mouth sores	• Serve soft or pureed bland food and/or liquids
	• Add butter, gravy, sauce, or salad dressing to moisten foods
	• Avoid highly seasoned, and hard or rough foods
Altered taste perception	• Use stronger seasonings and avoid excessively sweet foods
	• Offer salty foods
	• Try new flavored foods
Mucositis	• Risk factors: Intensive chemotherapy or upper GIT radiotherapy
	• Consider glutamine supplementation 0.3–0.5 g/kg/day from admission through duration of course
	• Powder glutamine is cost-effective, easy to use, well tolerated, and tasteless
	• Add to beverages or soft, moist foods
	• Not for use in patients with hepatic and/or renal failure
	• More evidence needed for glutamine use

Long-Term Planning

The literature suggests that survivors of pediatric cancers (especially ALL and AML) are at high risk for developing obesity and related endocrine problems later in life. This may be attributed to steroid use or treatments that influence a patient's height and ultimately weight-for-height ratio, potential body composition changes, and reductions in physical activity [4]. Effort should be made to prevent this occurrence with the main focus of "treatment" being nutrition education and motivation for sufficient physical activity [4, 5].

Advice Upon Discharge

- Patients should ideally be accompanied with a referral letter for continuing nutritional support once transferred to a referral hospital or special-care facility.
- Government nutrition supplementation schemes may exist that will provide the patient with free specialized products to supplement the home diet. The dietician should place qualifying patients on these schemes at discharge.
  - Guidance may be given to parents who can afford commercially available nutritional supplements as used in hospital.
  - Practical guidelines for increasing energy and protein density of affordable, home diet ingredients can be relayed if poor socioeconomic status is present.
- Emphasis must be placed on weight maintenance by recommending a healthy, varied diet at home. Additional advice may be given on food safety guidelines for neutropenic patients [4].

Follow-Up

Accurate record keeping of trends in ABCD (anthropometry, biochemistry, clinical, and diet history), regular evaluation of the patient's clinical condition is essential to ensure early detection of malnutrition and will provide grounds to timeously produce tailor-made nutritional plans.

Monitoring of anthropometrical and biochemical measures should occur at every outpatient visit, ideally on a monthly basis, and record kept of positive or negative trends. Caregivers with appropriate tools at home (such as scales, measuring tape) may be able to track weight and MUAC trends weekly at home offering additional insight, especially when assessing high-risk patients. Nutritional interventions should be adapted according to patient outcomes and ideally be done in consultation with the family to ensure compliance with the prescribed plan.

References

1. Sala A et al (2004) Children, cancer, and nutrition—a dynamic triangle in review. Cancer 100:677–687
2. Bauer J, Jurgens H, Fruwhald MC (2011) Important aspects of nutrition in children with cancer. Adv Nutr 2:67–77
3. Selwood K et al (2010) Nutrition in children and young people with cancer. Royal College of Nursing Working Group
4. Cape Town Metrolpole Pediatric Interest Group. Nutrition in the pediatric oncology patient. Completed 2007, Reviewed 2009
5. Mozby T, Challinor J (2012) Overview of nutrition in pediatric oncology. Oncopedia
6. WHO Growth Charts with Z-scores. Accessed http://www.who.int/childgrowth/standards/chart_catalogue/en/
7. WHO growth charts. Arm circumference-for-age standards. Accessed http://www.www.who.int/childrowth/standards/en/
8. The Stamp screening tool. http://www.stampscreeningtool.org
9. Garofolo A, Lopwez FA, Petrilli AS (2005) High prevalence of malnutrition among patients with solid non-hematological tumours as found by using skinfold and circumference measurements. Sao Paulo Med J 123(6):277–281
10. RDA for proteins. In: McCallum PD, Polisena CG (eds) (2000) The clinical guide to oncology nutrition. American Dietetic Association
11. Shaw V, Lawson M (2001) Clinical paediatrics dietetics, 2nd edn. Blackwell Science, Oxford
12. Meyers RS (2009) Pediatric fluid and electrolyte therapy. J Pediatr Pharmacol Ther 14:204–211
13. Department of Health, Directorate: Nutrition (2014) Draft National Parenteral Nutrition Practice Guidelines for Pediatrics

Chapter 27
Pain in Pediatric Oncology

Case Presentation

A 2-year-old boy is admitted for suspicion of neuroblastoma after complaining of a vague pain in his limbs for 15 days. His mother reports that he no longer plays and that it is difficult to bathe him. The child also changes his position frequently. Examination is difficult because the child is not allowing this. Abdominal palpation found an abdominal mass.

- How will you assess the pain in this child?
- What treatment do you suggest?
- What information would you give to the parents regarding the use of the proposed treatment?
- A bone marrow aspiration is planned. What do you recommend to prevent procedural pain?

Pain is one of the main symptoms in pediatric oncology. It is an unpleasant sensory and emotional experience caused by physical or perceived injury. The development of neoplastic diseases is revealed or complicated by pain, and may be related to the underlying disease, but more often linked to diagnostic or therapeutic procedures. In Africa, because of late-stage diagnosis of the disease, pain control is one of the priorities of caregivers. This is important, as it contributes significantly to humanizing care, improving the quality of life, and improving adherence to the treatment program by patients and their families.

Mechanisms of Pain

There are two main mechanisms of pain that can sometimes be identified.

D.C. Stefan, M. Harif, *Pediatric Cancer in Africa*,
DOI 10.1007/978-3-319-17936-0_27

Nociceptive pain is related to tissue damage causing excess painful stimulation. In this type of pain neurological pathways are intact. These pains are most frequently encountered and correspond to those observed in trauma, burns, or compression. The intensity is usually proportional to etiological factors.

Neurogenic or neuropathic pain is related to peripheral or central nervous system damage. The neoplastic (or other) lesion causes inhibition of sensory neurological stimuli. In this situation, slight stimulation (hyperpathia) or non-painful stimulation (allodynia) give rise to intense pain. The patient may also describe abnormal sensations of tingling or prickling (paresthesias), sometimes an unpleasant sensation (dysesthesia), or shooting pains. Examination may reveal hypoesthesia (a reduced sense of touch) or anesthesia (no sensation of touch or pain).

Clinical Expression of Pain in Children

Pain signs and symptoms vary according to the age of the child, the sociocultural context, the mechanism of pain and whether it is acute or chronic in character. Therapeutic tests may sometimes be necessary for the diagnosis of an unusual painful condition.

An infant experiences pain as anxiety or agitation. This may be interpreted as an aggression or punishment and is expressed as anger by the small child. Teenagers are more discreet, and the pain may even be denied, especially when it comes to a boy. Previous painful experiences can also have an impact on the mode of expression, as well as the sociocultural and family context, which may be encouraging or suppressing the complaint.

Acute pain is easy to diagnose, particularly when related to a diagnostic or invasive treatment. The child thus expresses pain through agitation, shouting, or by inconsolable crying. The child may also exhibit an antalgic gait, protect the painful area or be able to point to the location of pain.

Chronic pain has a more discreet expression, and is often linked to underlying cancer. The child unexpectedly becomes quiet, and sometimes confined to bed. He/she may also be sad and apathetic and can develop psychomotor inertia. The pain is sometimes denied by the child and/or the parents.

Nociceptive pain is easier to diagnose, while neuropathic pain sometimes requires careful investigation.

Assessment of Pain

The assessment of pain is an important step in order to provide adequate treatment and to monitor its effectiveness. The assessment must take into account the opinions of the parents regarding possible changes in behavior and the quality of sleep, especially in infants and small children. The caregiver should explain to the child, according to his/her ability of understanding, the principles of the assessment and its objectives.

Pain should be self-assessed by the patient and should also be assessed by a health care worker.

Self-Assessment

Self-assessment can only be performed when the child has reached a certain level of maturation to do so, and in practice this will not be possible in a child younger than 5 or 6 years old. There are multiple ways of evaluation, but the principle is not to simply ask the child whether there is pain or not, but obtain information about the intensity of the pain.

The simplest way is *the simple verbal scale* which is to ask the child if the pain is mild, moderate, or severe, but this is still a very rough estimate.

The Visual analogue scale (VAS) is the most commonly used tool for self-assessment (Fig. 27.1). The side with a triangle of which the base is the maximum pain (10) and the summit is the absence of pain (0) is shown to the patient. The child has to move the cursor at the level of the triangle corresponding to the intensity of the pain. The scale is placed vertically, with the base of the triangle positioned at the top. On the other side is a scale ranging from 0 to 10 corresponding to pain intensity.

The faces scale is also used in the self-assessment of pain (Fig. 27.2). A series of faces expressing increasing degrees of pain are shown to the child. Each face corresponds to a score of 0, 2, 4, 6, 8, or 10. This method presents the risk of confusion by the child between his/her emotional state and pain.

Other questionnaires, and more or less playful tools can also be used to reach the best way of quantifying pain.

Heteroassessment

Heteroevaluation is pain assessment performed by the caregiver. Because of their inability to use self-assessment tools, this assessment is required in small children and infants. In older children with mental retardation or difficulties of expression, this method is also preferred. Good communication with parents is a valuable aid in this assessment. The evaluation takes into account behavioral changes, verbal and body expression and changes of some physiological constants. Evaluation methods vary according to the acute or chronic characteristics of pain. Various scales are used.

The evaluation of *acute pain* in the newborn and infant may be made depending on facial expressions according to the Neonatal Facial Coding System (Table 27.1). The objective scale of pain (OPS) (Table 27.2) may be used in older children.

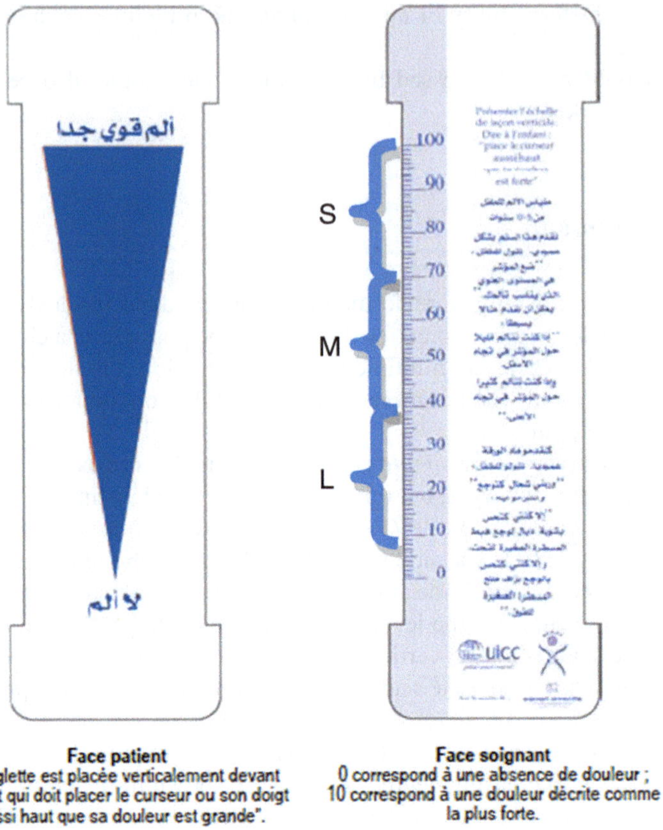

Fig. 27.1 Visual analogue scale for self-evaluation of pain. *S* severe pain; *M* moderate pain; *L* mild pain

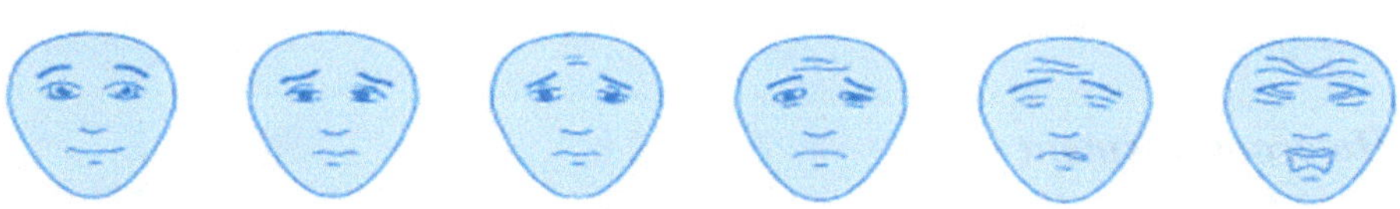

Fig. 27.2 The faces scale for the self-assessment of pain

Prolonged pain can also be assessed according to several rating systems. The Gustave Roussy Child Pain Scale includes ten items on a 0–4 intensity scale, where 0 is the absence of signs, 1 the doubtful presence of a sign, 2 the discreet presence of the sign, 3 is a clear sign and 4 the expression of severe pain. This scale evaluates the voluntary expression of pain, its direct signs, and possible psychomotor atony (Table 27.3). However, this requires an availability of the care team to be able to evaluate all items. Even if it is not used, it is interesting to read it carefully

Table 27.1 Neonatal facial coding system (NFCS) for the heteroevaluation of acute pain of the newborn and infant

Criterion	Score: absent 0/present 1
Eyebrow bulging	
Eyelids squeezed tight	
Nasolabial furrow accentuated	
Mouth open	

Table 27.2 Objective pain scale (OPS) for the heteroevaluation of acute pain in infant and small child

Score	0	1	2
Crying	Absent	Present and responds to nurturing	Present but does not respond to nurturing
Movements	None or relaxed	Restless, changes position constantly	Disorderly and intense unrest with a risk of trauma
Agitation	Child asleep or calm	Gentle/mild, can be comforted to lessen agitation	Hysterical, cannot be comforted
Verbal expression (not possible in very young child)	Child asleep or states no pain	Complains of mild pain, cannot localize pain, overall discomfort	Moderate, verbally or points to designated localized pain. Legs drawn up to trunk, fists clenched. The child touches the painful area or tries to protect it
Variations in blood pressure	Less than 10 % increase	Increase 10–20 %	More than 20 % increase

to understand various ways of expression of pain in this setting. A simpler version is preferred by most teams (Table 27.4).

At the end of these different assessments the pain is considered mild when the score is less than 4, moderate if the score is between 4 and 7 and severe beyond 7.

Drug Treatments of Pain

The treatment of pain must be a function of the type of pain and its intensity. This must be regularly adapted according to repeated evaluation. The treatment must be systematic and not on demand. In addition, side effects must be prevented as far as possible.

The World Health Organization proposed three levels for the classification of analgesic drugs according to their power:

Level 1: non-opioid analgesics (paracetamol and nonsteroidal anti-inflammatory drugs) proposed for mild pain.

Table 27.3 Gustave Roussy Child pain scale for the heteroevaluation of chronic infant and child pain

Item	0	1	2	3	4
1: Positioning for pain at rest	Absence of particular antalgic position/can adopt any preferred position	Seems to avoid certain positions	Avoids certain positions but does not appear uncomfortable	Chooses an obvious antalgic position which gives some relief	Unsuccessful to adopt an antalgic position and fails to get comfortable
2: Lack of expressiveness	Alert and lively, with animated expression	Appears a bit dull and impassive	Lack of facial expression, inexpressive eyes, muttering/ monotonous voice, slow verbal flow	Many of the previous signs are marked	Face rigid. Blank stare. Speaks with effort
3: Spontaneous protection of painful areas	No attempt to protect	Avoids violent contact	Protects the body, avoiding and moving away from any touch	Is visibly concerned to restrict any bodily touch	All the child's attention is focused on protecting the affected area
4: Expressing complaints	No complaints	"Neutral" complaints no emotional expression, and without any effort to say if there is pain	At least one of the following signs:	In additional previous signs, the child:	The child is groaning, sobbing, or pleading when complaining of pain
	The child does not mention that there is pain		– A raised concern about possible pain	– Attracts attention to clearly state the pain	
			– Uses whining voice to say there is pain	– Requests medication	
			– Expressive face accompanying the complaint		
5: Pain avoidance when moving	No discomfort. Movements are flexible and with ease	Some movements cause discomfort	Takes precautions when making certain movements	Clearly avoids certain movements and generally moves with caution	Avoids too painful movements, will need help to move

Item	0	1	2	3	4
6: Lack of interest in surroundings	Full of energy, interested in the environment, able to concentrate and amuse himself	Is interested in his environment, but without any enthusiasm	Gets bored easily, but can be stimulated	Unable to play. He watches passively	Apathetic and indifferent to everything
7: Reaction when being moved	Can be moved without paying attention	Pays attention when being moved	In addition to previous score, shows person to take care when being moved	In addition to previous score (2) holds back caregiver's hand or guides the movements	Opposed to any initiative of the caregiver or ensures that no move is made without his permission
8: Indicates painful areas	No indication of any pain at any time	Verbal indication only, of painful sensation somewhere, without giving details	In addition to previous score, the child uses a vague gesture to indicate painful area	Points to a specific painful area	In addition to previous score (3), the child describes confidently and precisely where the pain is
9: Reactions to examination of painful areas	No reaction triggered by the examination	Is reticent while being examined but not otherwise	During the examination, there is at least one of these signs: stiffness of the examined area, tension of the face, sudden crying, holding his breath	In addition to previous score (2), the child changes color, sweats, moans, or tries to stop the examination	The child's reactions make it almost impossible to examine the painful area
10: Slowness and infrequency of movements	Child's movements are expansive, lively, quick, varied, and he takes some pleasure in them	The child is a little slow, and moves without any vivacity	One of the following signs:	Many of the previous signs are marked	The child appears to be stuck on the spot, although nothing seems preventing him from moving

(continued)

Table 27.3 (continued)

Item	0	1	2	3	4
			– Delayed movements		
			– Restrained movements		
			– Slow gestures		
			– Starts motor activity infrequently		

Table 27.4 Heteroevaluation scale of prolonged pain

Signs of pain	0	1	2
Somatic complaints	None	Complaints about having pain	Complaints with groaning sobbing, crying, or pleading
Interest in surroundings	The child is interested in his environment	Loss of enthusiasm, interest in activity only when encouraged	Complete inhibition, apathy, indifference, and lack of any interest in environment
Antalgic position	The child can take up any position without any complaints	The child has chosen an obvious antalgic position	Unsuccessful to find an antalgic position
Slowness and infrequency of movement	Extensive, intense, quick, and diverse movements	Slow gestures, restricted movements, and rare initiatives	Child is motionless in his bed, though nothing seems preventing him from moving
Reaction on examination when being moved	Examination and movement without any problem	Asks the examiner to "be careful," protects the painful area, detains or guides the caregiver's hand	Impossible to access the painful area or opposition to any initiative of the caregiver on movement

Level 2: proposed painkillers are weak opioids such as codeine for moderate pain.
Level 3: use of strong opioids, particularly morphine for severe pain.

Treatment of pain, and particularly morphine, is not easily available in many parts of Africa. However, appropriate treatment is affordable in most cases.

Treatment of Nociceptive Pain

Mild pain can be controlled with paracetamol. Given at the correct dose and on a regular basis this may be sufficient. The recommended oral dosage is 15 mg/kg every 6 hours. For medication administered per rectum, the dosage must be increased to 30 mg/kg, followed by 20 mg/kg every 6 hours. The injectable form of paracetamol can be used at a dose of 60 mg/kg/day in a 15-minute intravenous infusion. Intravenous paracetamol is not more efficacious than the oral form, and should only be used when oral intake is difficult or not possible. The injectable form is however more expensive. Nonsteroidal anti-inflammatory drugs (ibuprofen, niflumic acid, diclofenac, etc.) may also be used. Corticosteroids may be recommended if there are contraindications to the use of nonsteroidal anti-inflammatory drugs. In visceral spastic pain the use of antispasmodic medication is necessary.

In moderate pain the painkillers of choice are level 2. The main molecule in this category is codeine. The dosage is 0.5–1 mg/kg every 6 hours. Side effects are vomiting, nausea, sedation, and constipation. This may be administered in combination with paracetamol. Tramadol, nalbufine, and buprenorphine are also part of this class of painkillers.

Severe pain requires the use of strong opioids, and particularly morphine. Immediate-release oral morphine is used at a dose of 0.2 mg/kg every 4 hour (or 1.2 mg/kg/day). Pain relief is usually noticed after 20–30 minutes. An increase of 50 % may be necessary to control the pain. It is then recommended every 8 hours until adequate analgesia is obtained. In chronic pain the use of slow-release oral morphine is recommended. The initial dosage is 1 mg/kg/day given in two doses. Intravenous morphine is administered preferably via continuous infusion, either through a patient-controlled analgesia (PCA) pump or electric syringe pump. It is advisable to do a titration by injecting a dose of 0.1 mg/kg followed every 5 minutes by doses of 0.025 mg/kg, until a satisfactory level analgesia has been obtained. The injected total dose corresponds to the dose required for 4 hours and can then be administered in repeated short perfusions, or ideally, continuous infusion. The side effects of morphine are respiratory depression, sedation, nausea, constipation, urinary retention, pruritus, and hallucinations. Fentanyl is also used in this type of pain as an alternative to intravenous morphine possibly using PCA pumps. The transdermal (patch) is also available. This is administered every 72 hours.

Treatment of Neuropathic Pain

The nociceptive pain analgesics are inefficient in this type of pain. *Tricyclic antidepressants* are efficient in controlling prolonged pain, dysesthesia, and allodynia. Amitryptyline is started at the initial dose of 0.3 mg/kg and gradually increased to achieve a dose of 1 mg/kg/day. Their action is noticeable only after a week. *Antiepileptic drugs* are used for paroxysmal pain especially in shooting pains.

Preventative Treatment of Pain Related to Invasive Procedures

In the practice of pediatric oncology, procedural pain is quite common. This contributes significantly to the deterioration of the quality of life and the negative feelings towards procedures in caregivers as well as in children and their parents.

Various approaches can be used to prevent this kind of pain. The main tools are EMLA (Euretic Mixture of Local Anesthetics) cream and MEOPA (nitrogen monoxide-oxygen mixture) inhalation.

EMLA cream consists of two local anesthetics, lidocaine and prilocaine. This is a transcutaneous anesthesia of 3 mm in depth 1 hour after application and 5 mm after 2 hours. The main indication is venipuncture, but can also be used when performing an arterial puncture, when accessing a portocath, before a lumbar puncture, and when placing catheters.

The MEOPA is composed of an equimolar mixture of 50 % oxygen and 50 % of nitrogen monoxide. Efficiency is obtained after 3 minutes of a continuous inhalation. The MEOPA may be used to prevent pain during painful procedures of short duration, such as lumbar punctures, bone marrow aspiration, dressings, and in some cases of venipuncture or other painful interventions.

Alternative Treatment of Pain

These methods can be very effective when used alone or in combination with medication. The main tools are physical methods and cognitive-behavioral techniques. In Africa, traditional medicine can be helpful. This should be used with or without conventional medication.

Physical methods include exercise, physical therapy, and massage. They can significantly reduce the stress. Neurostimulation and other local treatments, including hot or cold treatment can be efficient for inflammatory pain.

Cognitive-behavioral methods include relaxation, distraction or hypnosis, which may also be contributory to the reduction of pain. They are most often recommended in iatrogenic pain.

Key Points

- Pain in Pediatric Oncology is more frequently related to invasive procedures and treatment than the underlying disease.
- Nociceptive pain is related to tissue damage.
- Neuropathic pain is related to neurological injury, and gives rise to paresthesia, hyperpathia, and allodynia.
- Evaluation of pain is important for appropriate diagnostic and treatment:
  - In older children and adolescents, self-assessment by the visual analogue scale or the scale of the faces provides an insight of the intensity of the pain.
  - In small children, infants, and the newborn, heteroevaluation is the only method to evaluate pain using adapted scales.
- Treatment is adapted to pain intensity. The recommendations are:
  - In mild pain, non-opioid analgesics (paracetamol and nonsteroidal anti-inflammatory).
  - In intermediate pain, weak opioids such as codeine.
  - In intense pain, opioid analgesics are required, particularly morphine.
  - Tricyclic antidepressants and antiepileptic drugs should be used in neuropathic pain.

Suggested Reading

Hockenberry MJ, McCarthy K, Taylor O et al (2011) Managing painful procedures in children with cancer. J Pediatr Hematol Oncol 33:119–127

Schmitt C, Theobald S, Fabre N et al (2006) Standards, options and recommendations for the management of procedure-related pain (lumbar puncture, bone marrow aspiration or biopsy, blood sampling) in children with cancer. Bull Cancer 29:73–83

Schmitt C, Theobald S, Fabre N, Kasparian C, Séblain C, Boutard P et al (2006b) Standards, options and recommendations for the management of procedure-related pain (lumbar puncture, bone marrow aspiration or biopsy, blood sampling) in children patients with cancer (summary report). Bull Cancer 93:805–811

World Health Organization (1998) Cancer pain relief and palliative care in children (therapeutic strategies). World Health Organization, Geneva, p 14

Yao A, Coze C, Traoré F et al (2013) Prise en charge de la douleur de l'enfant attaint de cancer en Afrique: Etat des lieux au sein du groupe franco-africain d'oncologie pédiatrique. Arch Pédiatrie 20:257–263

Chapter 28
Nursing Care Principles in Pediatric Oncology

Nurses play a major role in care of children with cancer and they contribute significantly to the successes of curing the patients in pediatric oncology (Fig. 28.1). In many high income countries, pediatric/hematology oncology nursing is recognized as a subspecialty in the nursing educational system.

In Africa, nursing care is one of the weakest components(links) in the care for children with cancer. Nursing shortage, a lack of and constant rotation to other pediatric or adult wards are all handicaps and their constant mobility and transfer to other children or adults wards is a handicap for appropriate development of care in this setting. In most parts of Africa there are no dedicated education programs in nurses' schools in hematology and oncology.

The Nurse Educator

Having dedicated nurses for educating children with cancer and their families and training new nurses is one of the strategies that proved to be very efficient in developing countries.

The nurse educator should be an experienced nurse in the pediatric oncology team and who leads the training program. He or she should be in charge of educational program to ensure compliance with all developing compliance with all developing nursing staff's clinical skills and knowledge.

The nurse educator in high income countries has been a long established advance nursing role.

However despite major progress in the field of nursing and acceptance of the importance of such a nurse educator, most Sub-Saharan countries do not benefit from this form of nursing intervention.

D.C. Stefan, M. Harif, *Pediatric Cancer in Africa*,
DOI 10.1007/978-3-319-17936-0_28

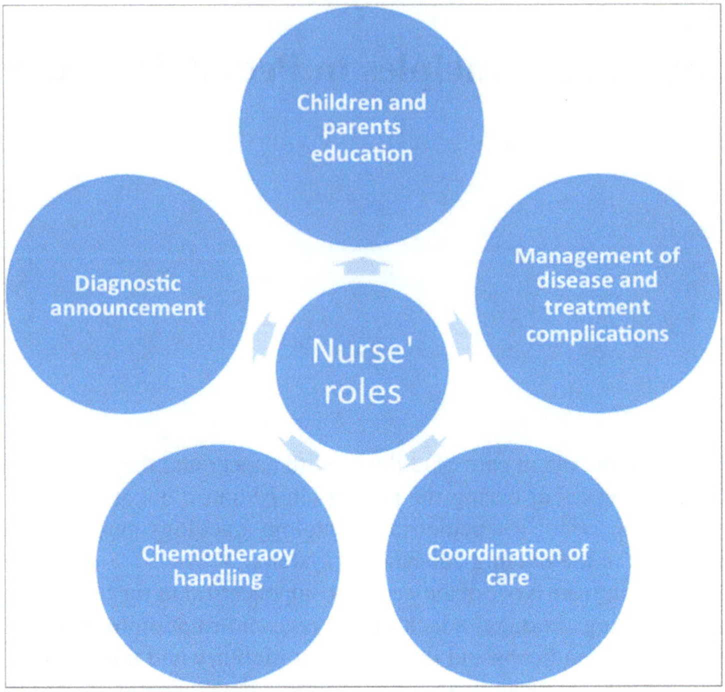

Fig. 28.1 Roles of pediatric oncology nurses

Diagnosis and Treatment Plan

Establishing a good communication with the family and child with cancer is crucial for appropriate care. The objective of the education process is to give the families and children appropriate information in order to ensure that they are well informed about the diagnosis, treatment, and prognostics and achieve their full support and understanding. In many low income settings, where parents and families may not have more than a primary education and little exposure to biomedical health care(as opposed to tradional healing) explaining a childhood cancer diagnosis and treatment can be challenging.

The initial information regarding the diagnosis and the treatment options is the responsibility of the attending physician. However, the nurse should participate in this session by providing more practical details and supplemental information based on their expertise. Also the nurse is part of the team and offers emotional and moral support to the entire family. In Africa, treatment abandonment remains a significant problem as many parents and caregivers do not return with the child for the completion of cancer therapy once the child is diagnosed or the therapy has started.. A good relationship from the beginning between the medical staff and the family is essential in order to establish and inspire the confidence of the family and the child (if old enough) to continue and complete the treatment.

Children and adolescents should be involved in this process according to their maturity. The parents can decide if other family members should be included.

Parent/Patient Education

Patient and parent education is an important component of the medical care. In Africa, it is also a powerful tool to address the abandonment of treatment. Poverty and illiteracy are of great impact in the adherence to treatment. The nurses are usually more efficient in establishing close relationships with the parents. This is because they spend more time together with the patient and the family and may have a good understanding of the familiy's community.

Patients and families should be informed about the diagnosis of the child, treatment, and follow-up plans.

Role of the Nurse in Organization of Care

Care of children with cancer is complex and requires intervention of various teams and sometimes from professionals in different hospitals. Organizing the care of patient is crucial in order to have good communication between the teams and appropriate planning of care. Nurses play an important role in coordinating multiple professional teams. It is important to ensure appropriate contact with parents and caregivers throughout the duration of child'scare and follow-up.

Preparation and Administration of Chemotherapy

Preparation and administration of chemotherapy is the responsibility of the nurse in most hospitals in Africa however that is changing in many hospitals including Sub-Saharan Africa too.

In some hospitals or units, the preparation of chemotherapy and administration might be allocated to the doctors as well. Chemotherapy has a narrow therapeutic index with high risk of toxicity. Protocols can also be very complex. If the nurses are responsible for preparation and administration of the chemotherapy, a pharmacist and/or a physician should offer support and supervision. In most parts of Africa, nurses are preparing chemotherapy. For preparation safety, personal protective equipment (gloves, gowns and masks with face shield or googles) and an appropriate biohazard cabinet are critical (Fig. 28.2). This is important to protect the nurse-froms any chemotherapy contamination. A system for double checking the chemotherapy order before mixing chemotherapy and before administering the che-

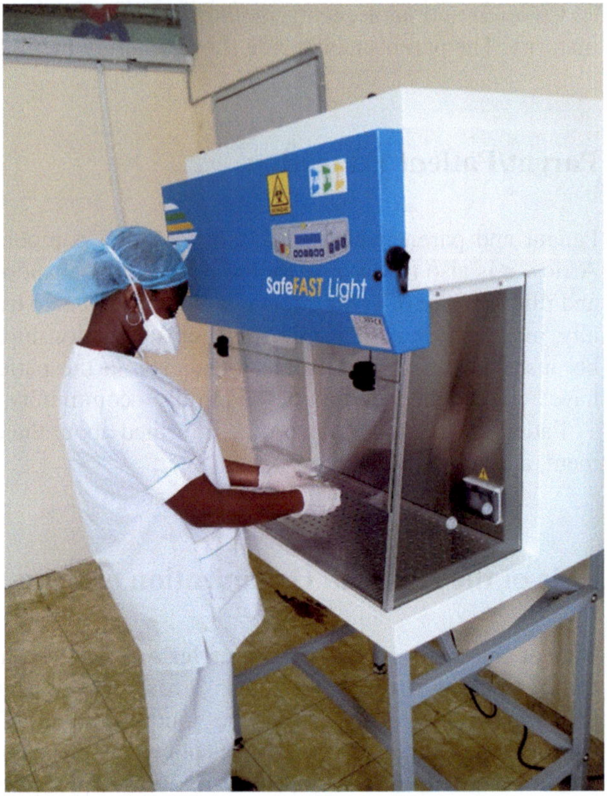

Fig. 28.2 Preparation of chemotherapy in Abidjan

motherapy to the child is essential to reduce the risk of errors in chemotherapy including preparation and administration. The nurse must respect the 5 rights of medication administration, which includes right patient, right drug, right dose, right route and right time. Accurate weights and heights measurements are the responsability of the nurses to verify when the chemotherapy dosing is calculated. Daily careful documentation of all chemotherapy given and that which is held is important for maintaining an accurate record of the child's progress in the treatment protocol. This is an essential nursing responsability.

During chemotherapy administration close monitoring of the patient is required. Special attention should be given to possible extravasation of chemotherapeutic agent and allergic reactions. It is important that all pediatric oncology units have a clear procedure(posted) and all nurses are well trained in extravasation and allergic reactions and have the medication required to treat these events.

Nurses should explain to the patient possible side effect of the treatment and if the treatment can be given at home all information should be given regarding the doses, the time and safe handling and also when to report side effect and whom to report to with a telephone number.

Infection/Hygiene

In Africa, hygiene remains a real problem in pediatric oncology units where children re compromised. Nurses should explain to the patient and the caregivers the special risk of infection in children with cancer and immunocompromised settings.

The most efficient preventive measure of infection remains proper hand washing before and after any contact with the patient. Hospital staff should be good role models and insist that parents, caregivers, visitors also wash their hands frequently with water and soap or hand/rub sanitizer. Nurse educator should insist that the hospital provides hand/rub sanitizer which is an efficient and cheap preventive measure along with hand washing in settings where clean water or sinks, soap and paper towels are limited. Communal towel cloths harbour germs and should not be used at sinks with water.

Fever in neutropenic patient is a real emergency situation. Once a neutropenic child (immunocompromised due to cancer treatment) has fever there is an 8 hour timeframe interval before they will be in septic shock. Early intervention is the key of infection control. Therefore the nurses are responsible to inform the physicians and to obtain blood cultures and evaluation of any suspected areas which should be done promptly. Broad spectrum antibiotic should be started afterward as soon as possible.

When the patient is discharged, the nurse should inform the family of the importance of coming or contacting as soon as possible to the hospital in case of fever. Patients should avoid the crowded areas, public transportation and any contact with other person having a fever or any suspected infection. The child should also avoid exposure to mold and animals and wear if necessary a surgical facial mask.

Vomiting

Nausea and vomiting are significant side effects of chemotherapy. Nausea and vomiting can induce nutritional and metabolic disturbances. Nurses should be able to evaluate the risk of vomiting according to the chemotherapy and radiation therapy regimen. Treatment is usually adapted to the risk and also to the individual child's previous experience.

There are several medications that may mitigate nausea and vomiting and these should be explored with the physician. In addition there are some distraction strategies which can be used by nurses in order to help the child to cope with the side effects.

Mucositis

Oral mucositis is a frequent complication of chemotherapy and radiotherapy. This side effect can be very painful and compromise nutrition. Good oral hygiene should be insured before and during treatment using frequent rinsing with saline solution and soft toothbrush. Oral cold substance seems to prevent induced mucositis lesions if given during administration of chemotherapy. Adequate pain treatment should be insured when needed so the child does not suffer and will continue to eat and drink if possible.

Pain Management

Pain is a very frequent complaint of children with cancer and contribute significantly in quality-of-life degradation. Pain can be related to cancer but is also frequently related to invasive diagnostic procedures and treatment. Inadequate pain prevention and control can be the cause of treatment abandonment.

Nurses have an important role in pain evaluation and control. The nurse should be taught to use appropriately the tools of pain evaluation in each nursing shift and ideally a pain scale is posted in the unit. In case of invasive procedure the child should be informed and adapted analgesia should be implemented. Local anesthetic cream when available should be used in less invasive procedure including venipuncture and lumbar puncture.

Psychological Support

A child receiving cancer therapy causes disruptions in the family routines, finances, emotional and spiritual balance. The nurse can be a key figure to help families to adjust and cope with all changes a family experiences. Listening to parents, caregivers and the patients to hear what are the most distressing issues and then strategizing with the family on how to access available resources and/or to accomodate the changes is a fundamental nursing task. The nurse educator can be instrumental in providing the staff nurses with training and resources in this important supportive care.

Practical Recommendation in Limited Resource Settings

- Nurse's knowledge and skills in pediatric hematology/oncology are essential in educating the patients and families, on chemotherapy handling, in management of disease and treatment complications, and in coordination of care.
- The team should identify a nurse as educator for nurses and parents;
- Nurses should

- Participate in diagnostic announcements
- Actively participate in patient education
- Organize and coordinate care for the patient
- Manage chemotherapy preparation and administration
- Participate in prevention, evaluation, and care of infection, vomiting, mucositis, and pain. Provide patient and families with psychological support

Suggested Reading

Al-Qudimat MR, Day S, Almomani T, Odeh D, Qaddoumi I (2009) Clinical nurse coordinators: a new generation of highly specialized oncology nursing in Jordan. J Pediatr Hematol Oncol 31:38–41

Day SW, Segovia L, Viveros P, Banfi A, Rivera GK, Ribeiro RC (2011) Development of the Latin American Center for Pediatric Oncology Nursing Education. Pediatr Blood Cancer 56:5–6

Day SW, Garcia J, Antillon F, Wilimas JA, McKeon LM, Carty RM, Alarcon P, Pui C-H, Ribeiro RC, Howard SC (2012) A sustainable model for pediatric oncology nursing education in low-income countries. Pediatr Blood Cancer 58:163–166

Monnet S, Thinlot C, Douçot M-S, Hamdoud Z, Patte C (2015) Formation d'infirmiers éducateurs africains dans le cadre du GFAOP (Groupe franco-africain d'oncologie pédiatrique). Rev Oncol Hématol Pédiatr 3:101–103

Day S, Challinor J, Hollis R et al (2015) Pediatric Oncology nursing care in low-middle income countries: A need for baseline standards cancer control 111

Chapter 29
Chemotherapy Induced Nausea and Vomiting

Case Presentation

A 14-year-old girl presented with a swollen, painful right knee, and a biopsy of the mass confirmed osteogenic sarcoma. Chemotherapy (cisplatinum and adriamycin) was initiated as soon as the staging process had been completed. One hour after the first cisplatinum infusion was commenced, the girl complained of severe nausea and then vomited profusely for the rest of the day. She received appropriate antiemetic treatment and improved, although she was still nauseous and vomited occasionally during the 3 days of chemotherapy.

When the patient had to be admitted for the second cycle of chemotherapy 3 weeks later, she started feeling nauseous on the way to hospital and vomited as soon as she entered the hospital ward.

Discuss the Following Definitions Regarding Chemotherapy-Induced Nausea and Vomiting (CINV): Acute vs. Delayed Vomiting and Anticipatory Vomiting (Table 29.1)

What Are the Risk Factors for the Development of CINV in Children?

1. Children older than 6 years, especially adolescents.
2. Female gender.
3. High expectation of nausea and vomiting, even before starting treatment.
4. Moderate to high emetogenic risk of the chemotherapeutic agent.

D.C. Stefan, M. Harif, *Pediatric Cancer in Africa*,
DOI 10.1007/978-3-319-17936-0_29

Table 29.1 Definitions

Acute vomiting	Expulsion of stomach contents within 24 hours after administration of chemotherapy
Delayed vomiting	Expulsion of stomach contents 2–5 days after administration of chemotherapy. Classically associated with cisplatinum as well as with cyclophosphamide, doxorubicin, and ifosfamide
Anticipatory vomiting	A learnt response of vomiting, which occurs prior to the administration of chemotherapy. This is more common in children with a history of motion sickness or a previous negative post-chemotherapy nausea and vomiting experience

5. Chemotherapy dose.
6. Concurrent radiotherapy to the abdomen

Discuss the Differential Diagnosis of Nausea and Vomiting in a Cancer Patient

1. Direct intra-abdominal effects of the tumor, e.g. stretching of the intra-abdominal organs or gastrointestinal tract obstruction.
2. Raised intracranial pressure.
3. Complications of recent abdominal surgery.
4. Other drug-induced vomiting, e.g. opioids, antibiotics, sedation agents, antiepileptics, etc.
5. Infection, e.g. gastroenteritis, urinary tract infection, septicemia, etc.
6. Organ dysfunction, e.g. abnormal liver function, renal dysfunction.
7. Acute pancreatitis.
8. Metabolic causes, e.g. hypokalemia (ileus), hyperglycemia, hypercalcemia, etc.
9. Peptic ulcer disease, i.e. esophagitis, gastritis, peptic ulcer.
10. Psychiatric cause, e.g. anxiety.

Tabulate the Emetogenic Risk of Chemotherapeutic Agents (Table 29.2)

Discuss the Characteristics and Use of Antiemetic Agents Available for Use in Children

Since it is extremely important to prevent nausea and vomiting, rather than treat it once it occurs, the antiemetic agent(s) should be administered 30 minutes prior to chemotherapy. This should be given on a strict schedule and not as needed while chemotherapy is still being administered.

Table 29.2 Emetogenic risk of chemotherapeutic agents and prevention/treatment

Level of emetogenic risk	Percentage of patients who experience nausea and vomiting	Drugs	Antiemetic treatment
Level 4 (high)	>90	Cisplatin, Cyclophosphamide (>1.5 mg/m^2), Dacarbazine, Dactinomycin, Cytarabine (intravenous dose ≥1 g/m^2)	5-HT3 antagonist PLUS Dexamethasone (plus Aprepitant in adults; clinical trials ongoing in pediatric patients)
Level 3 (moderate)	30–90	Carboplatin, Cyclophosphamide (≤1.5 g/m^2), Daunorubicin, Doxorubicin, Idarubicin, Ifosfamide, Cytarabine (Intravenous dose <1 g/m^2 or intrathecal dose), Epirubicin, Irinotecan, Methotrexate >1 g/m^2, Carmustine, Lomustine	5-HT3 antagonist PLUS Dexamethasone
Level 2 (low)	10–30	Cytarabine (≤100 mg/m^2), Etoposide, Gemcitabine, Methotrexate, Mitoxantrone, Fluorouracil, Paclitaxel, Topotecan, Procarbazine	5-HT3 antagonist or single dose dexamethasone or dopaminergic antagonist
Level 1 (minimal)	<10	Vinblastine, Vincristine, Vinorelbine, Fludarabine, Bleomycin, Busulfan, Cladribine, Rituximab, L'asparaginase, 6 Mercaptopurine, Thioguanine, oral Methotrexate	No need for routine antiemetic therapy

Antiemetic therapy may be needed for several days after the administration of chemotherapy, depending on the individual patient, the diagnosis, possible complications, as well as the chemotherapy regimen.

The Complete Drug Information Pamphlet Should Be Studied for Each Drug Mentioned Below

5-HT3 Antagonists

5-HT3 antagonists revolutionized the prevention and treatment of CINV in the early 1990s. Serotonin receptors are situated on the vagal nerve ends, enteric neurons in the gastrointestinal tract as well as in the chemoreceptor trigger zone in the brain. In response to chemotherapy, the enterochromaffin cells in the mucosa of the small bowel releases serotonin, while stimulating the 5-HT3 receptors, leading to a vagal afferent stimulus which causes nausea and vomiting. 5-HT3 receptors are indicated for use when chemotherapeutic agents of moderate to high emetogenic risk are administered, to prevent nausea and vomiting associated with radiotherapy and for postoperative prevention. Granisetron and ondansetron, the first two 5-HT3 antagonists, are more effective for the management of acute nausea and vomiting than for delayed vomiting. Oral and intravenous preparations are available and are equally effective. There are few side effects associated with these drugs. A promising new agent, palonosetron, appears to be more effective than granisetron and ondansetron, and has been approved for use in children from age 1 month old. Unfortunately, this is not yet widely available.

Kytril (Granisetron) is eliminated by the liver, but dose adjustments are not required in patients with liver failure, nor with renal failure. Its safety has not been established in children younger than age 2 years. In children aged 2–16 years, a dose of 10–40 mcg/kg IV (maximum 1 mg per dose) can be used 12 hourly. Studies in adult patients have shown that a daily dose of 2 mg is just as effective as a 12 hourly dose of 1 mg. Side effects are usually mild and include headache, constipation, asthenia, diarrhea, abdominal pain, and dyspepsia. QT prolongation is another possible adverse effect, thus care needs to be taken if prescribing granisetron concurrently with other drugs known to cause QT prolongation. Serotonin syndrome may occur when granisetron is used together with serotonergic drugs, such as some antidepressants, fentanyl, and tramadol. The clinical symptoms and signs of this syndrome include an altered mental state, autonomic instability, neuromuscular symptoms, seizures, and gastrointestinal symptoms.

Zofran (Ondansetron) is extensively metabolized and 5 % is recovered in urine. No dose adjustment is needed. The side-effect profile is similar to that of granisetron. The concurrent administration of apomorphine is contraindicated, since severe hypotension may occur. The pediatric (6 months to 18 years) intravenous dose is 0.15 mg/kg/dose (maximum 16 mg per dose) with the first dose given 30 minutes before chemotherapy, the second dose 4 hours after the chemotherapy has been given/started and the third dose 8 hours after the first dose. The oral dose for patients 4–11 years is 4 mg three times per day in the same schedule as the intravenous dose.

Dexamethasone

Dexamethasone is a glucocorticosteroid with multiple indications for use, but has not been approved as an antiemetic. However, its use in the prevention of acute and delayed CINV has been well established. It is most effective when used in conjunction with other antiemetic agents. The mechanism of action is still unclear, although it is known that it has a central action in the brain. The pediatric dose is 0.25–0.5 mg/kg once or 6 hourly and it can be given for up to 5 days, especially when delayed vomiting is expected. This is especially useful to reduce cerebral edema as a cause for nausea and vomiting. However, it should not be used in a patient with a systemic fungal infection. Multiple side effects are possible, and careful monitoring of patients is important. Hypertension, glucose intolerance, Cushing syndrome as well as peptic ulcer disease is frequently seen.

Benzodiazepines

Lorazepam (Ativan) is useful in the prevention of anticipatory vomiting at an oral dose of 0.02–0.06 mg/kg/dose 8–24 hourly, to be taken the evening prior to chemotherapy, as well as the morning of treatment. Alprazolam (0.005–0.02 mg/kg/dose 6–8 hourly) may also be used. Behavioral therapy should also be utilized in the management of anticipatory vomiting.

Other Agents

Metoclopramide (Maxalon, Reglan, etc.) is a dopamine receptor antagonist that has a lower efficacy in preventing CINV, and side-effects occur more frequently, especially unpleasant extrapyramidal effects. When given intravenously and at high doses it is most effective. The recommended intravenous dose is 1–3 mg/kg 30 minutes before chemotherapy and then 2–4 hourly for up to five doses.

Prochlorperazine (Compazine, Stemetil, etc.) is a phenothiazine, which has an effect on the central and peripheral dopaminergic receptors. This can be given via any administration route, but is not indicated for use in children younger than age 2 years. Prochlorperazine is effective in preventing CINV associated with low to moderate emetogenic risk chemotherapy as well as preventing nausea associated with radiotherapy. It may be of value in preventing and treating delayed vomiting. There is a significant potential for side effects including extrapyramidal effects and hypotension.

A neurokinin-1-receptor antagonist (aprepitant) is the newest antiemetic agent, and Fosaprepitant is available in an oral and an intravenous preparation. If used together with dexamethasone, the dose of dexamethasone has to be reduced by 50 %. Clinical trials are currently being conducted in the pediatric population.

Other agents that have been studied, but are not in clinical use, include cannabis and ginger.

What Is the Most Appropriate Preventative Treatment for Each of the Levels of Emetogenic Risk of Chemotherapeutic Agents? (Table 29.3)

Non-pharmaceutical interventions may also provide relief of symptoms to patients. The following dietary modifications may be of benefit to some patients: eat dry foods, such as toast or biscuits, sit up for at least 1 hour after a meal, eat bland, soft

Table 29.3 Advised antiemetic agents for chemotherapy agents with different emetogenic risk levels

Level of emetogenic risk	Antiemetic treatment
Level 4 (high)	5-HT3 antagonist plus dexamethasone (plus aprepitant in adults; clinical trials ongoing in pediatric patients)
Level 3 (moderate)	5-HT3 antagonist plus dexamethasone
Level 2 (low)	5-HT3 antagonist or single dose dexamethasone or dopaminergic antagonist
Level 1 (minimal)	No need for routine antiemetic therapy

foods, eat meals in a well-ventilated room, rinse the mouth before and after a meal, and try sucking hard candies (peppermints). Hypnosis, relaxation exercises, behavioral therapy, and acupuncture may be tried in older children.

Suggested Reading

1. www.cancer.gov/cancertopics/pdq/supportivecare/nausea/healthProfessional. Accessed 24 Feb 2015
2. Gopal RS, Gopaul S, Gibson F, Houghton E, Craig JV, Light K, Pizer B (2010) Antiemetic medication for prevention and treatment of chemotherapy induced nausea and vomiting in childhood (Review). The Cochrane Collaboration. The Cochrane Library 2010, Issue 9
3. Hesketh PJ (2008) Chemotherapy-induced nausea and vomiting. N Engl J Med 358(23):2482–2494
4. Jordan K (2007) Guidelines for the anti-emetic treatment of chemotherapy-induced nausea and vomiting: past, present and future recommendations. Oncologist 12(9):1143–1150

Chapter 30
Patient Support Groups

Childhood cancer can affect any child anywhere regardless of culture, financial well-being, education or the country where the child lives. Parents should not feel that they are to blame for their child contracting cancer. For this reason, having a child diagnosed with cancer, is one of the most life-changing challenges a family will ever have to face. The childhood cancer journey is often a very lengthy one, with initial treatment taking from a couple of months to a couple of years, with long-term after effects having to be negotiated for many years thereafter. Therefore, parent support groups and foundations have been, and need to be, formed throughout the world to help families cope with this journey.

There is a great disparity between high-income and middle–low-income countries in the quality of services and treatment available to patients and their families. Childhood cancer parent support groups and foundations often form a therapeutic alliance with the healthcare providers at treatment centers to overcome the challenges that are faced jointly by all stakeholders.

Overview

Growth of Parent Support Groups

The first known childhood cancer support group was started in 1968 by two fathers in Japan. They recognized the need to provide psychosocial support for each other and other families in the ward; understanding that as parents of children with cancer, they better understood the cancer journey that parents of newly diagnosed children will need to undertake.

The idea was noticed by some Americans visiting Japan, and in 1970 a Childhood Cancer Support Group called Candle Lighters was started in the USA. Their focus

D.C. Stefan, M. Harif, *Pediatric Cancer in Africa*,
DOI 10.1007/978-3-319-17936-0_30

was mainly to assist bereaved parents. In the 1970s and 1980s more countries followed suite, and many more parent support groups were founded.

In Hanover, Germany in 1992, members of parent support groups were invited by the German parent support group, Deutsche Leukämie-Forschungshilfe (DLFH), to attend a meeting at the SIOP conference. This was the first time that a parent, Ulrike Baum, was invited to address the conference at the opening ceremony of SIOP and made the voice of parents of children with cancer heard by the healthcare professionals present.

In 1993, parent support groups from 16 countries from Europe and the USA met in Valencia, Spain, to draft the constitution for an international body to represent parent support groups globally. The International Confederation of Childhood Cancer Parent Organizations (ICCCPO) was signed in 1994 in Valencia, with the mission "To share information and experience in order to improve access to the best possible care for children with cancer everywhere in the world".

The ICCCPO grew steadily over the years, from the 11 original members in 1994 to 171 members from 88 countries in 2014. In 2014, the name ICCCPO was changed to Childhood Cancer International (CCI) which currently has 181 members from 90 countries.

Definition

A Childhood Cancer Parent Support Group consists of a group of individuals with the common purpose of addressing matters of concern involving children with cancer, their families and the treatment they receive. From here forward the term "Childhood Cancer Foundation" (CCF) will be used to describe all groups involved with children with cancer. These groups may consist only of parents of children who have been diagnosed with cancer, of groups that have no parents involved, or a combination of both. They could be formally registered (which is recommended) or informal, which would depend largely on the aims of the CCF and the level of enthusiasm and expertise of the members of the group.

Other commonly used terms are:

Parent: meaning parents of children diagnosed with childhood cancer.
Non-parents: those who share the same concerns as parents, but who have not had a child diagnosed with cancer.
NPO: non-profit organization.

Situation in Africa

Most children, who get childhood cancer (80 %), live in developing countries such as Africa [1] where the survival rate is much lower than those in developed countries. The incidence of childhood cancer from birth to age 19 years in a developed country such as the USA, is 1 in 285 children and adolescents [2]. In Africa, the incidence of childhood cancer is estimated at 94 cases per million [3]. However, as there are so few accurate, reliable childhood cancer registries on the African continent, this number may not reflect the true picture. Although there are some cancers that are thought to be caused by familial or genetic factors, and even less caused by environmental factors, in most cases (probably around 90 %) the cause is still unknown.

In Africa in 1997, there were only three known CCFs (Egypt, Morocco and South Africa). Since 2008, this position has changed dramatically with CCI having 25 members from 16 countries in 2015. There may be more CCFs that support children with cancer in Africa who are not members of CCI.

Typical Areas of Involvement

In Africa, childhood cancer affects not just the child and the family, but often the whole community. For the parents, this can mean major changes, such as having to leave their job or their farm. Siblings may feel abandoned by their parents, with all the focus now being centered on the ill child. Grandparents have a double burden, as they try to finds ways to help not only their child, but also their grandchild. For the community, among other things, it can be the need to run the farm or taking care of the family left behind at their home.

CCFs, especially in Africa, step in where the government or health services do not provide adequate care for the child with cancer. There are even rare examples where CCFs have built dedicated childhood cancer hospitals in their country.

Parent and Child Support

Parent-to-Parent

Helping new parents understand the diagnosis and the need to complete treatment protocols is a very important part of such support. Other activities could include: where new parents are welcomed into the ward and made to feel part of the cancer family by other parents who have been there for a while; basic coping skills for ward-life; one-on-one chats; explanations why it is necessary to complete treatment; preparing both patients and parents psychologically for medical procedures; discussion groups; information on the hospital layout; and where to shop.

Practical Support

Support is provided for needs such as: funding for transport to-and-from the treatment centers; food parcels for families left behind at home; extra food in the wards; clothing; wigs for the children; wheelchairs; medical devices to be used at home and prostheses. One of the most important services, is providing "parent homes." These facilities house the parents and the patient while being treated, since their own homes are often a long distance from the treatment centers. Some CCFs are also able to arrange that children with cancer and their families have a brief holiday to get away from ward-life and have a few days or normal family life for a while. Others even supplement the loss of income of the caregiver or parent who needs to give up their job to look after their child who is ill.

Adolescents and Young Adults

Recent research suggests that adolescents and young adults (AYA) with cancer (age 15–20 years) should form a group separate to that of young children (age 0–14 years) as their medical and psychological needs differ. In most countries in Africa, AYAs are treated in adult oncology wards on adult protocols, despite recent research indicating that AYA cancers following a pediatric protocol have better outcomes. Internationally, websites and chat rooms have been established so that AYAs can support one another. There are wards, in Africa, especially for AYAs where their unique needs are better addressed, however, at the time of writing there were few. CCFs actively assist with establishing such wards where they are allowed by health departments and hospital administrators. Literature specifically for this group is also available from many CCFs globally through CCI.

Ward Volunteers

Volunteers help entertaining the children by reading or playing with them. These volunteers could also help with translation in general, but especially when health-care professionals communicate the disease. They can also help with many others aspects of ward-life such as: personnal hygeine practices, answering telephones, filing, arranging transport, organizing information packs, completing forms for illiterate parents or caregivers, cleaning, cooking, distributing gifts and clothing and accompanying patients to other areas of the hospital.

Play and Music Therapy

CCFs organize volunteers and professionals to offer support through play therapy to address issues such as, accepting their diagnosis; how to cope with life in a hospital ward; hygiene; addressing their angers; overcoming fears of medical procedures; understanding of death; and alleviation of pain by listening to music.

Recreation

Patients and their families are offered a break from ward-life by organizing birthday parties, outings to places of interest, as well as attending special camps for children with cancer and possibly also their siblings in some countries.

Survivor Groups

Survivors form groups to offer support to one another on how to meet the challenges of long-term survival. They also advocate for change by governments and other institutions to address issues, such as discrimination when applying for work, health insurance being loaded, etc. There is a group called, Childhood Cancer International Survivors Network, run by survivors that can be contacted through www.iccpo.org.

Palliative Care

Some CCFs provide a palliative care service where treatment centers are understaffed or staff are overworked and unable to take adequate care of those for whom cure is no longer an option.

Bereavement Support

Families are assisted with the cost of funerals and the transport of the deceased child back home. Forming special bereavement support groups to assist in long-term support of the family. Arranging annual bereavement services, regular meetings for bereaved parents where they are addressed by experts in the field. Appointing bereavement counsellors specially trained to assist parents, siblings and relatives.

International and Regional Conferences

CCFs help organize an annual international conference for all stakeholders in childhood cancer matters, but with an emphasis on issues affecting the activities of CCFs. This usually takes place at the same venue where SIOP has their annual Conference. Regional conferences are also organized in the following regions: Africa, Asia, Europe, Latin America, North America and Oceania.

Treatment Center Support

Ward Improvements

CCFs make provision for the following needs at the treatment center:

- Furnishings, such as bedding, window coverings, painting of the walls, floor covering.
- TV sets, video games, radios, games for the children. Specially equipped playrooms where this is possible.
- Renovate rooms as lounges for parents, provide recliners next to beds where possible.

- Fridges for parents' use and medical supplies.
- Fully stocked kitchens where parents can prepare food, or where volunteers can prepare food for the parents and children.
- Washing machines and driers only for use in the cancer wards for bedding and clothing of patients and their caregivers. This reduces "shrinkage" of, particularly, special bedding that is sent to the hospital's central laundry for cleaning.
- Some CCFs renovate entire facilities to make them suitable for the care of children with cancer.
- There are some cases in Africa and globally, where CCFs have been responsible for building an entire childhood cancer children's hospital.

Medical and Hospital Equipment

To a larger or lesser extent, some governments do not provide suitable or sufficient medical equipment for the effective care of children with cancer. CCFs provide support in the following ways: organize safety cabinets for mixing drugs, or supply, maintain and repair medical equipment, such as bedside monitors, syringes and needles, drugs, beds, infusion pumps, ultrasound equipment, etc.

Healthcare Professionals Support

Volunteers

CCFs train and manage volunteers, who help with ward admin, such a filing, supervise the playroom or toy bank, washing bedding, etc.

Extra Personnel

CCFs pay the entire salary or supplement the salary of extra staff in the ward, such as nurses, doctors, pathologists, psychologists, palliative care specialists, social workers, data-capturers for the childhood cancer registry, clerks, researchers, and personal assistants.

Scholarships and Stipends

CCFs provide funds for healthcare professionals, who do not have sufficient (or any) funding to attend conferences and special courses that will improve their knowledge. This could also mean paying for the subscription to specialist medical journals and the purchase of books.

Advocacy and Awareness

One of the key roles of a CCF is to advocate for the improvement of care that children with cancer receive. CCFs often team up with other key role-players in childhood cancer, such as The World Health Organization (WHO), Union for International Cancer Control (UICC), UNICEF, and SIOP when advocating on an international stage. Areas that CCFs cover among other things are:

Advocacy

- For governments to include a comprehensive cancer control programme for children with cancer as well as childhood cancer treatment guidelines.
- For affordable, accessible, sufficient and effective childhood cancer drugs.
- For free cancer treatment for children with cancer.
- For comprehensive healthcare insurance for children, especially those with cancer.
- For laws that ensure employment is not terminated for parents who need to accompany their child for treatment.
- For the provision of sufficient and well-trained healthcare professionals at treatment centers.
- For lobbying the education of the child while in hospital, and for the full integration of the child back into the education system without discrimination once treatment has been completed.
- For dedicated, well-equipped childhood cancer wards.
- For adequate facilities and supply of soap for washing of hands by healthcare professionals and visitors to the pediatric oncology wards.
- For the age of children admitted to pediatric oncology wards in Africa to be raised to 19-years old.
- For adolescents and young adults (age 15–25 years) to be recognized as a separate group than adults, and to be treated on appropriate protocols.
- For adequate training of students at tertiary medical training centers about the early warning signs of childhood cancer.
- To support a programme that trains primary healthcare workers, family doctors, doctors at secondary hospitals and traditional healers on the early detection of childhood cancers, and the correct referral procedures.
- For the distribution of early Warning Sign's Posters at all primary healthcare facilities.
- To parents of newly diagnosed children about the importance of completing treatment.

Awareness

- About childhood cancer that it is not contagious and is curable.
- Of the early warning signs of childhood cancer.

- That childhood cancer is different from adult cancers.
- That as other communicable diseases are controlled, childhood cancer will become one of the leading causes of premature death among children.
- That childhood cancer is already the second highest cause of premature death among children in many countries.
- Of safe use of drugs when at home.
- Of the importance of general hygiene for a cancer patient when at home.

Information and Education

Evidence-based information has been published which is written at an appropriate level so that it is easy for patients and their families to comprehend. Such material is available in a number of languages and is culturally sensitive. Many CCFs also have special websites where information is available. Information covers aspects such as:

- The type of childhood cancers in non-medical adult language.
- Booklets written for children to help them understand their cancer and their own cancer journey.
- Coping mechanisms for parents, siblings and grandparents.
- Safe use of drugs at home.
- Information for school teachers and students who have a child with cancer in their classroom.
- The importance of basic hygiene.
- Nutrition.
- Immediate and long-term effects of cancer drugs.

How to Form a Support Group

Where to Start

We strongly recommend that you read this in combination with the booklet "Your Group is not Alone" produced by Childhood Cancer International (see "Suggested Reading"). Examples of material mentioned below are also available from CCI through their head office.

Step 1: Someone needs to volunteer to start the process of forming a CCF. Often it happens that the need for support is recognized by one of the ward's medical staff, who would then identify a parent or caregiver and approach them about the possibility of starting a CCF to support the children and their families, as well as the ward staff.

Step 2: This person (or persons) will need to identify others, with potential, to assist with the process. This is often the defining moment in the development of a group and usually the most difficult. If individuals with the necessary skills to run an organization successfully are not identified from the pool of parents and caregivers available, then non-parent volunteers or professionals will need to be identified. The importance of identifying individuals who are joining for the correct reasons and not to fulfil personal, self-centered agendas need to be emphasized. This group will need to decide on the following:

- The name of the organization
- The objectives of the group
- Whether it be run and managed by parents only, or non-parents, or a combination of both. Here it is strongly suggested that the group be parent-run, meaning parents are in control of the organization
- Whether it be a formal group or informal group
  - An informal group will be a loosely structured group fulfilling a common purpose who could work under the umbrella of another NPO.
  - A formal group will have a constitution, bank account, elected committee or board, will be registered as an NPO or charity with the relevant government authority and will have its own logo.
  - Will the group be entirely run by volunteers or will salaried staff be employed to run the daily operational side of things. This will depend on the funding available to the CCF.
- Will the CCF serve only the local treatment center or will it have a national footprint with branches. CCFs can evolve from being local to serving multiple treatment centers as they grow and evolve. Those with a national footprint can also be a body that unites a number of local organizations with a common objective under one national umbrella organization.

Step 3: Appoint an interim committee who will need to oversee the further development of the group.

Step 4: A formal group should have someone to assist with drawing up the CCFs constitution, which among other things addresses the following matters: name; vision and mission; objectives and aims; membership matters; finance and governance matters; ethos of the group; structure of the group and roles and responsibilities; committee positions with their roles and responsibilities; meetings and annual general assembly; staffing; changes to the constitution; and winding up.

Step 5: Decide on a logo and if needed a tagline too.

Step 6: Have the CCF registered at the relevant government authority responsible for NPOs or charities. However, it may be possible to start with operating services ahead of formal registration.

Step 7: Open a bank account, with a minimum of three signatories, which we highly recommend in case one is out of town. Always have any two to sign off any payments.

Step 8: Appoint an auditor or audit firm to prepare the annual financials.

Step 9: Do a baseline survey of what the conditions are in the ward so that any improvements can be measured after the group starts with the support. If the treatment center or country does not have a childhood cancer registry, it is important to request statistics on the incidence of childhood cancer, in the areas where your CCF will be active, from the head of the unit.

Step 10: Develop a business plan for the group which should include: deciding on the activities that the CCF will best be able to cope with within the first year of existence; how and who will do these; what resources will be required, and how these will be secured; completion dates; and what are the desired measurable outcomes.

Step 11: If you are going to have ward volunteers, who will be working with the children and their families as well as the healthcare staff, decide on the recruitment criteria and assessment of ward volunteers, how they will be trained and supported, their roles and responsibilities, who they will be, and who will manage them.

Step 12: A Memorandum of Understanding should be signed with the head of the unit and hospital administration. This should happen as soon as possible, so that all parties are clear about their roles, responsibilities, limitations and assistance that will be offered from both sides.

Step 13: Decide on the CCFs communication policy and procedure. This could include who will address the media and who will check the accuracy of any material that the CCF releases to the public.

Challenges

CCFs, especially parents, and healthcare teams should work together to overcome the typical challenges faced in Africa. All of these can be addressed and managed with information that is available through organizations like Childhood Cancer International (previously named ICCCPO (www.icccpo.org). Some of the major challenges include:

Late Presentation

Children are diagnosed late, which results in their chances of survival being compromised.

Malnutrition

In these children, malnutrition is often caused by their inability to absorb the nutrients required because of the cancer they have, and the side-effects of the treatment they are receiving. In Africa, many newly diagnosed patients sometimes arrive in the ward severely malnourished because of other economic or climatic factors.

Abandonment

Patients interrupt treatment or discontinue treatment for a variety of reasons.

Diagnostic Delays

There is a lack of suitably equipped laboratories that are able to diagnose patients in their own countries.

Improving Supportive Care

Less intense supportive care leads to treatment-related mortality and needs to improve from diagnosis to end-of-life care.

Poor Communication

This would include such issues as: little or no communication about the disease to the parents; illiterate parents, lack of translators; little contact with parents once they return home, often because of no street addresses; lack of understanding different customs and traditions; and parent groups not welcomed by heads of the ward.

CCF Members

Where issues exist, such as volunteers who are not trained in hospital protocol; over-eager volunteers; healthcare professionals who view parents as "interfering and inferior"; and inconsistent delivery of undertakings, CCF members can intervene.

Continued Education

Children who need to stay in hospital for any length of time and are away from their regular school, need to be educated while in hospital.

Ethics

There are many ethical dilemmas faced by healthcare professionals such as: clinical trials; who makes the decisions affecting the child and his/her treatment; and data management.

Lack of Reliable Childhood Cancer Registries

The true childhood cancer burden in a country is unknown, since data on the incidence of childhood cancer is incomplete or non-existent.

Access to Safe Affordable Drugs

In some African countries, access to drugs is often limited by the high costs, and at times where parents are expected to source and fund the drugs needed to treat their child. These drugs are often bought on the black market with no guarantee that these are not counterfeit drugs; no or limited health insurance; shortages, unavailability of required drugs.

Funding

This could include matters such as: raising funds in low-income countries; volunteers vs. salaried staff; differences in spending priorities between healthcare professionals and CCF members; accounting for funds raised.

Hygiene

There may be no facilities for basic hygiene, such as ablutions, soap for washing hands, understanding among parents and families of basic hygiene.

Theft

Sometimes it happens that donations of food, ward furnishings, medical equipment and drugs are stolen by visitors, volunteers, parents, ward staff or the healthcare personnel.

A Cancer Child Is Replaceable

The belief that parents should have another baby and let the ill child die.

Hospital Detention

The practice in some countries where patients and their parents are detained by the hospital authorities until outstanding bills have been settled.

Groups in Africa

Below is a list of CCFs in Africa, however, there may be others unknown to the author.

Egypt: Alexandria Group of Childhood Cancer Care (AGCCC)
Ethiopia: Mathiwos Wondu - YeEthiopia Cancer Society (MWECS). www.mathy-cancersoc.org
Tesfa Addis Parents Childhood Cancer Organization TAPCCO
Cameroon: North West Childhood Cancer Parent Organization in Cameroon (NWCCPOC)
Ghana: Ghana Parents Association for Childhood Cancers (GHAPACC) www.gha-pacc.org
Kenya: Childhood Cancer Initiative
Hope for Cancer Kids
Malawi: Children's Cancer Club. www.childrenscancermalawi.org
Cancer Survivors Quest. www.csq.rossal.net
Morocco: AMAL (Association des maladies atteints de leucémies)
L'Association L'Avenir. www.lavenir.ma
Noujoum. www.noujoum.org
Namibia: Namibia Childhood Cancer Parents Support Organization (NaCCapso)
Nigeria: Children Living with Cancer Foundation (CLCWF). www.clwcf.org
Simara Children Cancer Foundation. www.simaraccf.com
Senegal: ASEAC
Sierra Leone: Rowaca Cancer Group - Sierra Leone (RCG-SL). rowacacancersl.webs.com/
South Africa: CHOC Childhood Cancer Foundation South Africa. www.choc.org.za
Little Fighters Cancer Trust. www.littlefighters.org.za
Tanzania: Tumaini la maisha Tanzania. www.tumainilamaisha.org
Uganda: Bless a Child Foundation. www.blessachildfoundation.org
Zambia: Kayula Childhood Cancer Foundation (KCCF). www.kayulachildhood-cancer.org
Zambian Childhood Cancer Foundation (ZACCAF). www.zaccaf.org
Zimbabwe: Children's Cancer Relief. www.kidzcanzimbabwe.org
Zimbabwe Parents of Children with Cancer Association

Where to Get Further Information

CCI

Childhood Cancer International formerly known as The International Confederation of Childhood Cancer Parent Organizations. An International organization with around 181 CCF members from 90 countries. This website is currently, but will be changed. (www.icccpo.org)

SIOP

The International Society for Pediatric Oncology. SIOP has a division called the PODC: Pediatric Oncology in Developing Countries that focuses on issues in developing countries. (www.siop.nl)

UICC

Union for International Cancer Control. An international group focusing on cancer control and the reduction in the inequity and burden of cancer globally. (www.uicc.org)

St Jude Children's Research Hospital

The leading research hospital in the world on childhood cancer. They also have a website (www.cure4kids.org) that provides support and advice for doctors in other countries. (www.stjude.org)

IARC

The International Association of Cancer Registries. An organization that is part of the WHO responsible for the publication of global cancer statistics. Very useful for those wishing to start a childhood cancer registry, as they offer training and software. (www.iarc.fr).

Concluding Remarks

African culture traditionally has a strong sense of the community and its needs. This willingness to help one's fellow man, despite one's own situation, will result in countries, communities and individuals working together to find unique solutions to the challenges in Africa regarding childhood cancer. In doing so, every child with cancer should get the chance of survival that they so richly deserve.

References

1. American Cancer Society (2007) Global cancer facts and figures 2007. American Cancer Society, Atlanta
2. Ward E, Desantis C et al (2014) Childhood and adolescent cancer statistics, 2014. CA Cancer J Clin 64:83–103
3. Ferlay J, Shin HR, Bray F et al (2010) GLOBOCAN 2008 v2.0, Cancer Incidence and Mortality Worldwide: IARC CancerBase no 10 [Internet]. International Agency for Research on Cancer, Lyon
4. The Executive Committee of ICCCPO (The International Confederation of Childhood Cancer Parent Organizations) (2008) Your Group is not Alone. [Internet]. http://cms.onlinebase.nl/userfiles/c1icccpo/file/Handbook_FINAL.pdf

Suggested Reading

African Guide to Communicating the Diagnosis of Pediatric Cancer. Débora Lolonga (available in French and English)

What do parent groups/organizations do…and how do they do it? Mark Chesler (Vice President, ICCCPO). Extract from the ICCCPO Newsletter, V8, N2—Spring 2001). Available CCI website

Volunteer Development Programme. Barb Smeltzer—Kids Cancer Care Foundation of Alberta, Canada [Notes from the presentation given at the ICCCPO Workshops, Vancouver, Sept 2005]. Available CCI website

Your Group is Not Alone available and produced by Childhood Cancer International (formerly known as ICCCPO—The International Confederation of Childhood Cancer Parent Organizations). Available from CCI website

Chapter 31
Research and Ethics in Pediatric Oncology

Case Presentation

An 11-year-old girl presents with a distal metaphyseal osteosarcoma of the left femur, and lung metastases. Chemotherapy allowed a complete response of lung metastases and a slight volume reduction of the tumor of the thigh. The surgeon proposed an amputation, which was denied by the teenager and her parents. After 3 months of treatment abandonment, she returned to the hospital because of pain. Chest X-rays showed lung metastases. Treatment with second-line chemotherapy and radiotherapy is proposed on an experimental basis.

1. Would it would be ethical to proceed with this program?
2. Should it be discussed with the parents, who are illiterate?
3. Should the patient be informed?

Research on diagnostic and therapeutic approaches has been the main tool to improve the quality of care of childhood cancer in developed countries. Besides diagnostic and therapeutic approaches, the research may also involve epidemiology, organization, funding, and organization of care or the sociocultural aspects of pediatric oncology. Even though this group of diseases is rarely encountered compared to adult cancer, appropriately organized international teams made a great impact. This is now considered as a model in medical practice. In well-organized pediatric oncology units, up to 70 % of patients are included in prospective research programs. Patients enrolled in international network programs have also show to have a better outcome. Hence, among the competences that a team should have to support children with cancer, the ability to conduct research and participate with other teams in national and international programs, is of great added value.

However, research must respect the principles of ethics. The team should respect the basic principles of human rights, and pay attention to possible exploitation of

D.C. Stefan, M. Harif, *Pediatric Cancer in Africa*,
DOI 10.1007/978-3-319-17936-0_31

vulnerable patients and families for commercial purposes. In most countries, regulation to protect patients is implemented. One of the most effective ways of protection of persons is the use of a review by independent ethics committees.

Furthermore, the authors and editors of scientific publications have ethical obligations. For the publication of study results, investigators have to ensure the accuracy of their results. Negative as well as positive results should be published or made available. Funding, and any potential conflicts of interest must be clearly outlined in the publications.

In developing countries, searching for the best diagnostic and therapeutic approaches adapted to local settings is one of the best research fields. The rights of the child and their parents to get best possible care must always be respected.

Informed Consent

This is one of the fundamental ethical principles. Indeed, respect for the dignity and autonomy of subjects are at the basis of ethics. Children, their parents or their legal representatives must give their informed consent without any constraint or influence. Consent must be voluntary and reversible.

The information given to parents must enable them to understand the rationale for the study, the type of investigations, the expected results and potential risks (Table 31.1). They should also be informed of available alternatives and about the measures taken to protect confidentiality of their personal information. The process of consent must take into account the sociocultural context.

Information of Children and Relationship with Parents

The treatment of cancer in children requires a genuine alliance between the healthcare team and parents, and the relation should be established on the basis of mutual trust. The interests of the child must prevail in all cases. Parents must be convinced of the relevance of therapeutic choices. The use of traditional or alternative

Table 31.1 Rules of informed consent

• The information must be given in an understandable manner
• Explanations of the benefits and potential risks should be included
• The consent must be given prior to inclusion in the study
• The consent must be collected without any constraint or influence
• The consent must be well documented

Table 31.2 Ethical principles for conducting research in humans

• Protection of life, health, dignity, and privacy of the person
• This must be based on updated scientific literature and other relevant sources of information as well as appropriate experimentation carried out in laboratory and, where appropriate, on the animal
• Research topics should be aimed at improving the health, well-being, or human knowledge
• Research must be done by qualified persons and under the supervision of competent doctors
• The methodological choice must be adapted to the objective of the research and should answer the questions raised by the research
• The criteria for selection of the target population should be based on a scientific validity and not on economic vulnerability
• The risk must be reduced to the minimum, and in all cases be justified by a potential benefit to the patient or the community
• An assessment by a third party not involved in the study and in particular an Ethics Committee is recommended to avoid potential exploitation
• Duly obtained consent should be obtained after giving information to parents and possibly to the child
• Throughout the research, the investigator must ensure well-being of persons subjected to the research work, protect their personal data, give them an update of the study as needed and allow them to withdraw from the research if necessary

medicine can be a handicap to the treatment, but should not be systematically denied to the extent that there is no risk to the child.

Establishing a relationship of trust with the child is recommended. To do this, caregivers should avoid giving false information and take into account the cultural environment, the child's age and maturity for sensitive information.

In the relatively mature child and adolescent, his or her opinion should be taken into consideration. The help of a psychologist may be necessary.

The Fundamental Principles to Govern Medical Research

The Helsinki declaration, adopted by the World Medical Association in 1964, summarizes the basic principles to govern research involving human beings (Table 31.2).

The Ethics Committee

The Ethics Committee must be independent of the sponsor, investigator or any other form of undue influence. Membership must provide scientific resources, but also civil society, scholars, and theologians. This must ensure respect for the laws and regulations in place in the country, and should have the right to monitor the progress of ongoing studies. The investigator has the obligation to provide the Committee with information on the progress of the study and on the occurrence of significant adverse events. The investigator should also communicate to the Committee information on financing potential conflicts of interest as well as the procedures of inclusion of participating patients in the research program.

Adapted Diagnostic and Therapeutic Approach

The issue of use of developed country's diagnostic and treatment approaches in settings where resources are very limited is frequently raised. The capacity of the family and the healthcare system should be properly evaluated before applying those approaches. Adaptation of these approaches should be carefully studied and may need approval of the Ethics Committee. These approaches should nevertheless be evaluated regularly.

Ethics and End-of-Life

The management of the end-of-life period is difficult and sometimes raises ethical issues. Therefore, it is important that clarity on the objectives of care is observed between the patient, the parents, and the medical team. Progress in medical resuscitation techniques to artificially maintain life sometimes poses an ethical problem regarding the suspension of these therapies when there is no more hope of cure. In developing countries, the problem is frequent, given the difficulties of access to care and cultural considerations. Many families prefer that patients die at home. In all cases, good palliative care and, particularly, pain should be provided.

In the event of conflict between the healthcare team and family concerning the continuation of care, the opinion of the Ethics Committee is required. "Futile" treatment may indeed be challenged according to the sociocultural context (Table 31.3).

Table 31.3 Practical recommendations

• Clinical research must be justified by the benefit for the patient or for new scientific knowledge
• An independent Ethics Committee must validate the relevance and the methodology of the research
• Informed consent is a major component in clinical research
• Adaptation of diagnostic and treatment approaches in resource-limited countries should also be closely monitored as clinical research projects
• End-of-life care can pose an ethical problem when they mobilize significant resources without anticipated benefit

Suggested Reading

Committee on Bioethics of the American Academy of Pediatrics (1995) Informed consent, parental permission, and assent in pediatric practice. Pediatrics 95:314–317

Emanuel EJ, Wendler D, Grady C (2000) What makes clinical research ethical? JAMA 283:2701–2711

Devine S, Dagher RN, Weiss KD, Santana VM (2008) Good clinical practice and the conduct of clinical studies in pediatric oncology. Pediatr Clin North Am 55:187–209

Joffe S, Fernández CV, Pentz RD et al (2006) Involving children with cancer in decision-making about research participation. J Pediatr 149:862–868

Varelas PN, Abdelhak T, Hacein-Bey L (2008) Withdrawal of life-sustaining therapies and brain death in the intensive care unit. Semin Neurol 28:726–735

Burns JP, Truog RD (2007) Futility: a concept in evolution. Chest 132:1987–1993

Chapter 32
Health Economics

Case Scenario

A 3-year-old child who lives in Johannesburg (South Africa) is diagnosed with nephroblastoma. The parents brought him to the hospital very late as the child lives with his grandmother in a rural area and visits the parents only twice a year. The grandmother did not observe the swelling of his abdomen. His disease is advanced with multiple lung metastasis (stage IV).

What is the cost of his treatment and is it cost-effective to treat him? Is it cost-effective to treat childhood cancer in your country?

What is the information required in order to be able to calculate the costs?

If the same child would have presented much earlier with a stage 1, what would have been the cost of treatment?

Introduction

South Africa is an upper-mid income country with a population of around 51 million people.

Children represent 31 % of the total population. Applying the described incidence of 110–140 new cases per million, it is expected to report an annual new number between 1600 and 2000 children diagnosed with cancer in South Africa. However the total number reported annually does not exceed 700 new cases (the overall age-standardized average annual incidence rate is 45/million).

The per capita GDP of the country is US$5916.46 and the medical treatment (including oncology) in the government institutions is free for all children below the age of 6 years, while modest income-based contributions are required for older children.

D.C. Stefan, M. Harif, *Pediatric Cancer in Africa*,
DOI 10.1007/978-3-319-17936-0_32

Guidelines to determine the cost and evaluate the cost-effectiveness of treatment are stipulated in the WHO's "Guide to cost-effectiveness analysis" and "Burden of Disease" reports. They suggest the detailed calculation of all expenses related to treatment and to measure these costs against Years of Life Lost (YLL), Disability-Adjusted Life Years (DALYs) and the per capita Gross Domestic Product (GDP) of the country help guide important decisions regarding the optimal application of resources.

The Global Burden of Disease working group has set the different Disability Weights for different diseases.

So, What Is Health Economics?

Health Economics is one of the many branches in economics, an applied field in medicine that allows for the systematic and rigorous examination of the problems faced in promoting health for all.

It has been also defined as "a branch of economics concerned with issues related to efficiency, effectiveness, value, and behavior in the production and consumption of health and healthcare". In broad terms, health economists study the functioning of healthcare systems and health-affecting behaviors (such as smoking).

The concept of health economics can be explained in layman language as the study of economical functioning of healthcare system in an economy. It involves matters affecting the health of individuals in a society. An example of application of the health economics is the study of cigarette smoking and its effects on the economy from the health expenses perspective. Economics bills have been introduced to curb smoking-related expenditures and healthcare.

Why Is it Important to Understand the Health Economics of Childhood Cancer in Africa?

On a continent which is affected by major other causes of diseases, childhood cancer and the treatment of childhood cancer may not appear as a priority or cost-effective intervention. In most high-income countries, cancer represents the leading cause of non-accidental death in children older than 1 year. While infection accounted for 64 % of global deaths in the first 5 years of life in 2010, major shifts in both the magnitude and causes of childhood mortality have occurred in many developing countries. Worldwide, an increased number of countries dealt with an impressive decline in childhood mortality from 1990 to 2011 following a better and more efficient infectious disease control program.

The essential understanding of health economics in Africa (as anywhere else in the world) is based on the high rate of achievability of cure. In high-income countries, at present more than 80 % of children with cancer are cured. Although cure rates in low-mid-income countries are much lower, there are many examples of successful treatment with adapted regimens, with innovative ways of collaborating with developed centers amongst which twinning is one of them.

In societies in which cancer may be seen as a death sentence, the treatment of childhood cancer may offer the opportunity to demonstrate high cure rates in a manageable number of patients especially if the diagnosis is made early enough and basic infrastructure is present.

What Is a Direct Cost?

The direct cost is the total expenses directly related to the treatment of a patient and can be divided into direct medical and direct non-medical costs. Direct medical costs, includes all charges attributed to investigations, medication, staffing, cost of hospital admissions, etc.

Direct non-medical costs include personal expenses incurred by the patient and family including travel cost and additional paid caregiver time.

What is an indirect cost? This is the financial input to establish and manage treatment programmes. Cost of central administration of intervention and cost of developing interventions and skills required to deliver care.

What Is Cost-Effectiveness?

Cost-effective healthcare aims to gain the maximum benefit from the financial input required to obtain treatment goals.

Guidelines to determine the cost and evaluate the cost-effectiveness of treatment is stipulated in the WHO's "Guide to cost-effectiveness analysis" and "Burden of Disease" reports. They suggested the detailed calculation of all expenses related to treatment and to measure these costs against Years of Life Lost (YLL), Disability-Adjusted Life Years (DALYs) and the per capita Gross Domestic Product (GDP) of the country help guide important decisions regarding the optimal application of resources. The Global Burden of Disease working group has set the Disability Weight for all major diseases (e.g., non-Hodgkin lymphoma at 0.09).

Cost-effectiveness is defined as the ratio of monetary expense required to avert 1 Disability-Adjusted Life Year (DALY) to the annual gross domestic product (GDP) per capita in a country.

A ratio of 3:1 is considered cost-effective and a ratio of 1:1 is considered very cost-effective.

Health Outcomes

If information from the literature regarding disability weight and average duration of disability of a type of cancer (in this case nephroblastoma) specific to a country (e.g.: South Africa) is available, the total number of disability-adjusted life years (DALYs) due to the disease can be calculated. Using standard methods from the WHO Global Burden of Disease working group, the total number of DALYs due to the disease are calculated by adding the years of life lost (YLL) due to ill health, disability or early death, with the years lived with disability (YLD). Years of life lost (YLL) without treatment is calculated by subtracting the estimated age at death without treatment from the standard life expectancy in the specific country, multiplied by the absolute annual number of cases of the disease. Years lived with disability (YLD) is calculated by multiplying the estimated duration of illness with and without treatment by the disability weight for disease (as set by the Global burden of Disease working group) and the incident number of cases.

Another Example: Cost of Burkitt Lymphoma in South Africa

Using the WHO-CHOICE framework for generalized cost-effectiveness to estimate the cost-effectiveness of treating Burkitt lymphoma in South Africa. Cost-effectiveness is defined as the ratio of the monetary expense required to avert 1 DALY to the annual gross domestic product (GDP) per capita of South Africa. Thus, using 2010 GDP per capita data, if the cost to avert 1 Daly is equal or less than $34800 it is cost-effective to treat Burkitt Lymphoma and if it is $11600 or less it is regarded as very cost-effective.

Future Directions

Part of future direction is the inclusion of health economics in the curriculum of all medical schools in order to understand the value of costs and cost-effectiveness of the therapeutic interventions.

The knowledge could serve as a platform for informing governments and health officials in developing further policies and regulations in a country.

Further research is needed into finding the most effective way of treating various different childhood malignancies in the setting of different resource constraints. Studies identifying how to prevent common causes of treatment failure in low- to mid-income countries should also be conducted.

Take-Home Messages

- Financial objections are often raised to the treatment of childhood cancer in resource-constrained settings; policymakers and laypersons may assume that any such treatment is prohibitively expensive. This assumption is often unsupported.
- Knowing the cost of treatment of the most common childhood cancers in a country as well as calculating their cost-effectiveness is essential in formulating policies and supporting the advocacy for free treatment of all children affected by cancer.
- The cost of the most common cancers in children is not prohibitive and represents an investment of the government in the future of the country, especially in countries where the young population represents in some cases more than half of the population of that specific country.

Suggested Reading

Bhakta N, Martiniuk ALC, Gupta S, Howard SC (2013) The cost effectiveness of treating paediatric cancer in low-income and middle-income countries: a case-study approach using acute lymphocytic leukaemia in Brazil and Burkitt lymphoma in Malawi. Arch Dis Child 98:155–160

Hendrickson KC, Rimar J (2009) Patterns of hospital resource utilization of children with leukemia and CNS tumors : a comparison of children who survive and those who die within 3 years of diagnosis. Nurs Econ 27:35–44

Norum J, Angelsen V, Wist E, Olsen JA (1996) Treatment costs in Hodgkin's disease: a cost-utility analysis. Eur J Cancer 32:1510–1517

Russell HV, Panchal J, Vonville H, Franzini L, Swint JM (2013) Economic evaluation of pediatric cancer treatment: a systematic literature review. Pediatrics 131:e273–e287

Stefan DC, Stones D (2009) How much does it cost to treat children with Hodgkin lymphoma in Africa? Leuk Lymphoma 50:196–199

WHO (2008) The global burden of disease. http://www.who.int/healthinfo/global_burden_disease

Chapter 33
Developing Support Network in Africa

International support is vital in planning further activities in pediatric oncology in Africa.

As the main causes of morbidity and mortality of the Sub-Saharan continent remain related to infection and malnutrition, there is a transition and a focus on the improvement of preventive measures globally. The burden of cancer is slowly more recognized in the world and a range of interventions is planned for the future.

The lack of resources and lack of local childhood cancer awareness impact negatively on the population.

Cancer care is complex and might appear expensive and unaffordable as it needs constant expertise, organization, medication and supplies that are most of the time all interconnected to the social aspects and wealth of the country.

National cancer plans and implementation of the plans in the limit of a realistic budget is one of the first steps in moving forward.

International support and network contribute to the improvement of care of children with cancer through shared expertise and protocols, education and training, collaboration based on research, improvement of pathology services and radiology amongst many other components.

It is interesting to note that developing pediatric oncology activity in any hospital has a positive impact on general care in the hospital. Developing multidisciplinary approach, infection control, improvement in pathology diagnosis and radiology area activities with positive impact on many other disciples and care for patients.

There are many requirements for success of a collaboration and for establishing an efficient network. We are mentioning only a few in the following paragraphs.

- **Ethical aspects:** Ethics is an important component in developing any program. It is essential to ensure that all actions have benefits for patient. Collaboration based on research that would have no impact on care for children in Africa should not be considered.

D.C. Stefan, M. Harif, *Pediatric Cancer in Africa*,
DOI 10.1007/978-3-319-17936-0_33

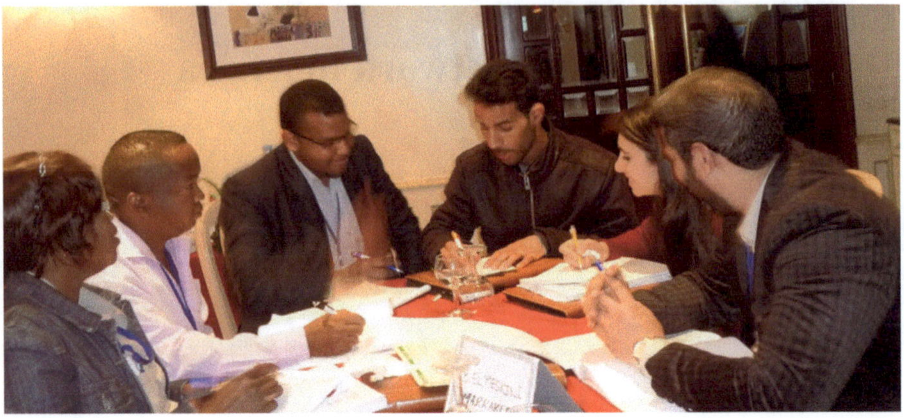

Fig. 33.1 Nurse pediatric oncology intensive course

- **Local leadership:** Local commitment is vital and each program should have a champion. The local caregivers need to be fully involved, understand the project and the benefits and have the capacity to mobilize stakeholders for the advocacy of the children.
- **Long-term commitment:** The program between two centers should be considered for several years. Only continuous support may have significant impact. In Africa, political instability has a major negative impact on sustainability. Any program should take this into account and also address the difficulty to maintain good experts in the program.
- **Comprehensive approach:** In order to be successful, any support program should include all caregivers who need to be regularly involved and evaluated.
  - **Education:** Education is the key tool to develop competences in various disciplines. Education is addressed to the physicians, but also nurses (Fig. 33.1), pathologists, surgeons and all other members of the team (dieticians, social workers, occupational therapists, pharmacists, etc) involved in the care of children with cancer. Education includes amongst others professional training and visit of experts.
  - **Evaluation:** The program should be evaluated on a regular basis. Specific indicators should be identified at the beginning of the activities and provide time allocated to address the challenges.
  - **Clinical research:** This is an important component of infrastructure of any pediatric oncology program. Any clinical research program should address local issues. Approaches addressing late presentation, malnutrition, abandonment of treatment programs, less intensive chemotherapy regimen are those of best impact. Sharing and reviewing data are very efficient in making progress in care.

- **Twinning:** The twinning concept (or paring/matching a pediatric oncology unit in developing country with a unit in a developed country) has proved to be very effective in several areas. Twinning can also include two units from Africa where the most developed unit offers support to another one (e.g. twinning between the pediatric oncology at Tygerberg Hospital in South Africa with the unit in Windhoek, Namibia)

Example of Successful Networks in Africa

Various initiatives are in place and more continue to develop continuously.

- **French African Pediatric Oncology Group (GFAOP)** is a French-speaking group founded in 2000 by Professor Jean Lemerle in Paris. The group has put in place pilot units in pediatric oncology in several sub-Saharan countries. The support included supply of medication, salaries for nurses and continuous education. The group started different programs for Burkitt lymphoma and Wilms tumor and then extended the program to acute lymphoblastic leukemia, Hodgkin disease and retinoblastoma. Recently, the GFAOP launched the African School of Pediatric Oncology with the support of Foundation Sanofi-Espoir with the involvement of the French and Moroccan universities. The African school offers a diploma in pediatric oncology. The Moroccan foundation Lalla Salma contributed to a program for housing parents of children with cancer during the duration of treatment (Fig. 33.2).

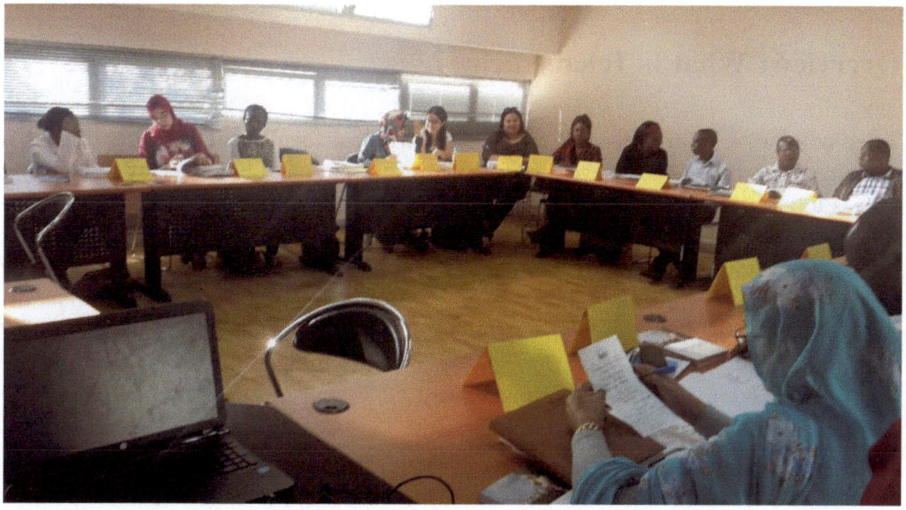

Fig. 33.2 Students at the African Diploma of Pediatric Oncology in Rabat

Information and Communication Technologies

Information and communication technologies (ICTs) have great potential to address some of the challenges faced by both developed and developing countries in providing accessible, cost-effective, high-quality healthcare services. Telemedicine uses ICTs to overcome geographical barriers, and increase access to healthcare services. This is particularly beneficial for rural and underserved communities in developing countries—groups that traditionally suffer from lack of access to health care.

Historically radiology and pathology were among the first high spread applications to be impacted by the use of ICTs, as the use of counselling between specialists is very important in these fields of medicine.

In many countries scientific institutions are involved with the development of telemedicine solutions in the absence of national telemedicine agencies or policies.

The importance of evaluation within the field of telemedicine cannot be overstated: the field is in its infancy and while its promise is great, evaluation can ensure maximization of benefits. ICTs can be costly, as well as the programmes using them to improve health outcomes. Indeed, the most frequently cited barrier to the implementation of telemedicine solutions globally is the perception that the cost of telemedicine is too high.

While developing countries are more likely to consider resource issues such as high costs, underdeveloped infrastructure, and lack of technical expertise to be barriers to telemedicine, developed countries are more likely to consider legal issues surrounding patient privacy and confidentiality, competing health system priorities, and a perceived lack of demand to be barriers to telemedicine implementation.

Actually, ICTs potentially are the most cost-effective set of solutions and tools to make possible the diffusion of practice in medicine.

Overview: What Is Telemedicine?

Telemedicine, a term coined in the 1970s, which **literally means "healing at a distance,"** signifies the use of ICT to improve patient outcomes by increasing access to care and medical information. **Recognizing that there is no one definitive definition of *telemedicine*—**the World Health Organization has adopted **the following broad description:** *"The delivery of healthcare services, where distance is a critical factor, by all healthcare professionals using information and communication technologies for the exchange of valid information for diagnosis, treatment and prevention of disease and injuries, research and evaluation, and for the continuing education of healthcare providers, all in the interests of advancing the health of individuals and their communities."*

Some distinguish telemedicine from telehealth with the former restricted to service delivery by physicians only, and the latter signifying services provided by health professionals in general, including nurses, pharmacists, and others. However, in many circumstances, telemedicine and telehealth are synonymous and used interchangeably.

Four elements are essential to telemedicine:

1. Its purpose is to provide clinical support.
2. It is intended to overcome geographical and social barriers, connecting users who are not in the same physical location and developing conditions.
3. It involves the use of various types of ICTs.
4. Its goal is to improve health outcomes.

Plenty of applications are included in telemedicine definition, both interactive and not. Some examples are telecounseling with Voice over IP and Web Conference tools, remote access to medical records software, digital imagins as teleradiology and telepathology, eOncology solutions, conferences and lessons broadcasting, eLearning facilities, remote surgery and robotic applications, home care solutions, eHospital and several others.

Barriers to Telemedicine Development

Telemedicine implementation largely remains a privilege of high-income countries, nevertheless it could be of great utility and efficacy in low-income countries lacking appropriate healthcare facilities by allowing for the performance of good level healthcare practices.

The most frequently reported barrier to the implementation of telemedicine solutions was the perception that telemedicine programmes were too expensive to implement. While this is true for some programmes, others, as discussed above, can be implemented using pre-existing infrastructure and low-cost technologies and are therefore relatively inexpensive. Many ICT solutions are consolidated into common use for decades and could be easily oriented to telemedicine.

For example, asynchronous data store-and-forward measures such as e-mail services have been found to be usable in areas with limited bandwidth to successfully deliver telemedicine across a variety of medical specialties and international environments.

Still, these findings emphasize the need to build on existing resources and infrastructure, and introduce other simple, already available low-cost telemedicine solutions within the context of the community to provide the basis for evaluation and further adoption. Start-up costs should be kept as low as possible to increase the likelihood of committed funding to support new innovations.

Another serious obstacle to the spread of telemedicine is the "Digital Divide" problem. Digital Divide is economic and social inequality of peoples in their access, use or knowledge of ICTs. It is strongly related to the development level of the countries, the rate of internal democracy and available economic resources.

Although ICTs have an agnostic character to anthropological factors and potentially they can support the same service levels everywhere, the implementation of basic networking infrastructures in developing countries follows a patchy trend. Often in developing countries the latest consumer technologies become available before the support of basic transmission network is fully established.

A good national planning strategy is essential to ensure the development of pervasive facilities such as telemedicine, in an economic sustainability vision.

Key Messages

International support can be efficient in supporting and developing pediatric oncology activity in Africa.

The keys of success are development of local leadership, long-term commitment, comprehensive approach including education program, medication and supplies, and regular evaluation.

Use of new technology of communication and information becomes more accessible and proves to be efficient.

The system of cooperation between different pediatric oncology units uses the concept of twinning or a network model.

Various successful examples are in place including French African Pediatric Oncology Group, The International Network for Cancer Treatment and different successful African twinning programs.

Suggested Reading

http://www.gfaop.fr/
http://www.inctr.org/
Oberlin O, Harif M, Perilongo G, Valteau-Couanet D, d'Angio GJ, Patte C (2014) In memoriam—Jean Lemerle (1930–2014). Pediatr Blood Cancer 61(12):2333–2334
White Y, Castle V-P, Haig A (2013) Pediatric oncology in developing countries: challenges and solutions. J Pediatr 162(6):1090–1092

Index

D.C. Stefan, M. Harif, *Pediatric Cancer in Africa*,
DOI 10.1007/978-3-319-17936-0

I

Q

MIX
Papier aus verantwortungsvollen Quellen
Paper from responsible sources
FSC® C105338

If you have any concerns about our products,
you can contact us on
ProductSafety@springernature.com

In case Publisher is established outside the EU,
the EU authorized representative is:
Springer Nature Customer Service Center GmbH
Europaplatz 3, 69115 Heidelberg, Germany

Printed by Libri Plureos GmbH
in Hamburg, Germany